Color
Atlas of
Human
Anatomy

Library of Congress Catalog Card Number: 76-023581
International Standard Book Number: 0-8151-5823-8

Printed by Smeets-Weert, Holland
Reprinted January 1978
Reprinted June 1978
Reprinted January 1980

Color Atlas of Human Anatomy

R.M.H. McMinn

Sir William Collins Professor of Anatomy
Institute of Basic Medical Sciences
Royal College of Surgeons of England

R.T. Hutchings

Chief Medical Laboratory Scientific Officer
Department of Anatomy
Royal College of Surgeons of England

Year Book
Medical Publishers, Inc.
35 E. Wacker Drive
Chicago

To
Margaret and Marion,
Anne, Sam and Isabel

Contents

Acknowledgements

We are indebted to all those who over the years have contributed specimens to the Anatomy Museum of the Royal College of Surgeons of England, and especially to Dr D. H. Tompsett who also prepared the corrosion casts. (Full details of the methods used can be found in his book 'Anatomical Techniques', 2nd edition, 1970, Livingstone.) We are also grateful to Dr J. L. Cordingley of King's College London, Professor T. W. Glenister of Charing Cross Hospital Medical School, and Professor F. R. Johnson of the London Hospital Medical College for the loan of osteological material; to Dr Oscar Craig of St Mary's Hospital and King's College London for some of the radiographs; to Mr V. H. Oswal, consultant ENT surgeon at the North Riding Infirmary, Middlesbrough, for the coloured dissections of the ear; to those who acted as models; and to Mrs Gina Howes for typing the manuscript. Dr D. H. Bosman of the Royal College of Surgeons, Dr B. A. Wood of the Middlesex Hospital Medical School, and Professor J. W. Rohen of the University of Erlangen, West Germany, helped to check the key numbers.

The illustrations of Museum specimens are reproduced by courtesy of the President and Council of the Royal College of Surgeons of England, to whom we express our thanks.

Preface

The object of this atlas is to assist undergraduates and postgraduates in the study of human anatomy. Of course, good textbooks and atlases already exist and by colouring arteries red and nerves yellow, for example, they are justly popular as aids to learning. But so often, and especially for newcomers to the subject, the interior of the body seems to look very different from the neat diagrams in the book, and we believe it is helpful to show body structures as they actually exist in suitably prepared specimens of the kind that students see in the dissecting room and meet in examinations. In this way we hope to bridge the gap between the description of the textbook and the reality of the body.

When a student is dissecting or being asked to identify a structure in an examination, when a physician is examining a patient, or when a surgeon is operating, they direct their gaze at any one time on to a fairly small area, and the size of the printed page has been carefully chosen so that the illustrations could be made approximately life-size. Obviously there are wide variations in body size and some illustrations may appear larger and others smaller than a student's own particular specimen. Occasionally the monocular vision of the camera lens may give rise to a minor degree of distortion compared with similar views in a drawing. It is all too easy to alter a drawing to include or exclude anything that is wanted or not wanted, but with actual specimens the camera has an all-embracing eye and the choice of a precise camera angle has been all-important in showing the proper relationships of structures to one another.

By displaying the parts of the body in their natural size we have been able to label structures by numbers overlying them and to avoid in most instances the use of unsightly leader lines, except for very small or crowded structures. For revision purposes students will be able to test their knowledge by covering up the numbered keys. Usually we have deliberately given different numbers to the same structure in similar dissections so that the student must exercise a judgement and cannot identify a structure simply by remembering a number from a previous picture (although in the case of bones a single key has been used for different views of the same bone in order to save space). In most illustrations numbering begins in the upper left part of the picture and proceeds in a clockwise direction, although it has not always been practical to adhere too rigidly to this scheme. Sometimes it has been considered helpful in large or complicated areas to label a structure more than once. An arrow instead of a leader line has been used to indicate that the structure referred to is under cover and out of sight just beyond the tip of the arrowhead. The short notes that accompany many of the keys either make a comment on the particular items in the specimen or draw attention to general points in the region concerned. They are not intended in any way to provide a comprehensive description of everything seen; our aim is to supplement existing texts, not to substitute for them.

In order to produce a volume of reasonable proportions both in size and in price we have had to be selective in choosing the illustrations from the material available to us. We have deliberately chosen a variety of cadaveric and museum specimens, since different methods of preparation and preservation give a range of appearances as far as colour is concerned, and the student must not imagine that all specimens will look the same no matter how they have been treated. It will always be impossible to please everyone all the time; for some there will be too much detail, for others not enough, but we believe that we have at least covered most of the items that are most important to most students. Although many of the minutiae of muscle attachments to bones are hardly necessary for most people, we have covered bones in some detail in view of the increasing difficulty of purchasing good specimens.

We would like to think that this book may be regarded as something more than just an aid to academic learning and the passing of examinations. The human body is indeed 'fearfully and wonderfully made', and we hope our attempt at exercising some degree of photographic artistry to display the interior of the body will lead to a wider appreciation of the fact that beauty of form is not limited to the exterior.

Head, Neck and Brain

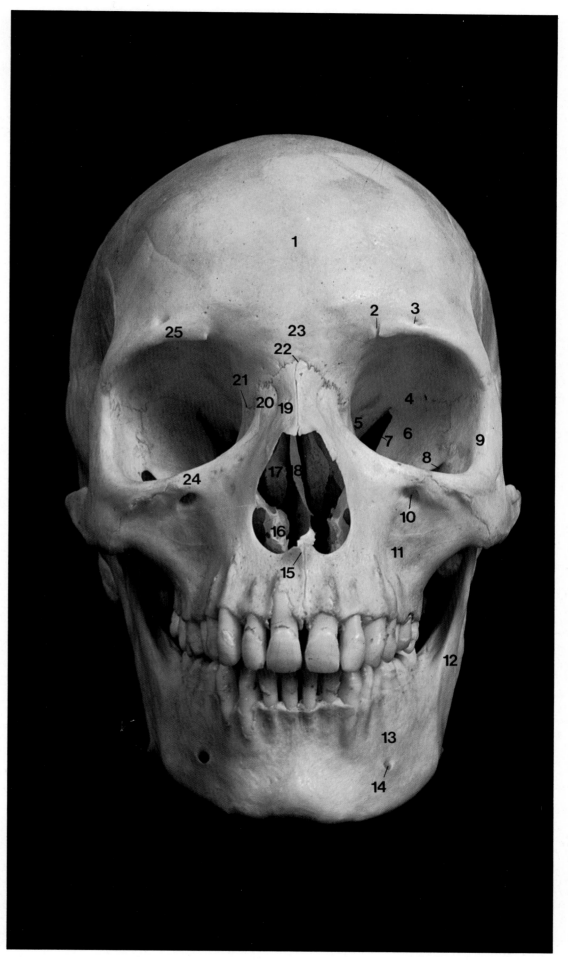

The skull, from the front
1 Frontal bone
2 Frontal notch
3 Supra-orbital foramen
4 Orbit (orbital cavity)
5 Lesser ⎫
6 Greater ⎭ wing of sphenoid
7 Superior ⎫
8 Inferior ⎭ orbital fissure
9 Zygomatic bone
10 Infra-orbital foramen
11 Maxilla
12 Ramus ⎫
13 Body ⎭ of mandible
14 Mental foramen
15 Anterior nasal spine
16 Inferior ⎫
17 Middle ⎭ concha
18 Nasal septum
19 Nasal bone
20 Frontal process of maxilla
21 Lacrimal bone
22 Nasion
23 Glabella
24 Infra-orbital margin
25 Supra-orbital margin

● Details of individual skull bones are given on pages 23–32, of the bones of the orbit and nose on page 18, and of the teeth on page 20.
● The supra-orbital, infra-orbital and mental foramina lie in approximately the same vertical plane.
● Strictly speaking the term skull includes the mandible, and the cranium refers to the skull without the mandible, but skull and cranium are often used interchangeably. The calvaria is the vault of the skull or skull-cap – the upper part of the cranium that encloses the brain.

The skull, from the front. Muscle attachments
1 Temporalis
2 Masseter
3 Orbicularis oculi
4 Procerus
5 Levator labii superioris alaeque nasi
6 Levator labii superioris
7 Zygomaticus minor
8 Zygomaticus major
9 Levator anguli oris
10 Nasalis
11 Buccinator
12 Depressor labii inferioris
13 Depressor anguli oris
14 Platysma
15 Mentalis

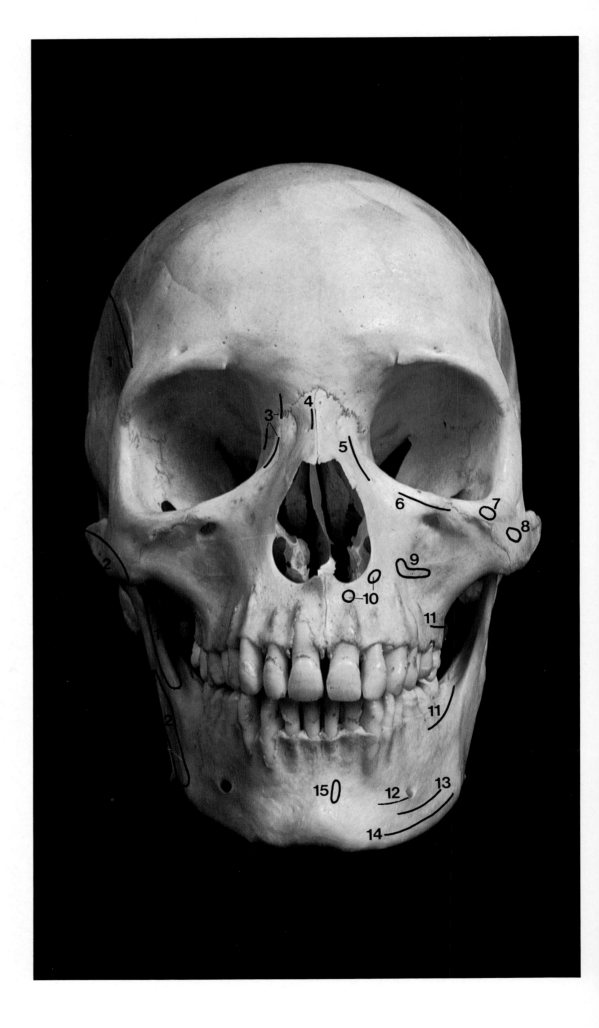

The skull, from the right
1 Parietal bone
2 Coronal suture
3 Frontal bone
4 Glabella
5 Nasion
6 Nasal bone
7 Frontal process of maxilla
8 Anterior lacrimal crest
9 Nasolacrimal groove
10 Posterior lacrimal crest
11 Lacrimal bone
12 Orbital part of ethmoid
13 Frontozygomatic suture
14 Zygomatic bone
15 Maxilla
16 Anterior nasal spine

17 Body ⎫
18 Ramus ⎪
19 Coronoid process ⎬ of mandible
20 Condyle ⎪
21 Mental protuberance ⎭
22 Mental foramen
23 Styloid process ⎫
24 Tympanic part ⎪
25 Mastoid process ⎪
26 External acoustic meatus ⎬ of temporal bone
27 Zygomatic process ⎪
28 Squamous part ⎭
29 Zygomatic arch
30 Greater wing of sphenoid
31 Pterion
32 Inferior ⎫
33 Superior ⎬ temporal line

34 Lambdoid suture
35 Occipital bone
36 External occipital protuberance (inion)

● Pterion is not a single point but an *area* where the frontal, parietal, squamous part of the temporal and greater wing of the sphenoid bone adjoin one another. It is an important landmark for the anterior branch of the middle meningeal artery which underlies this area on the inside of the skull.

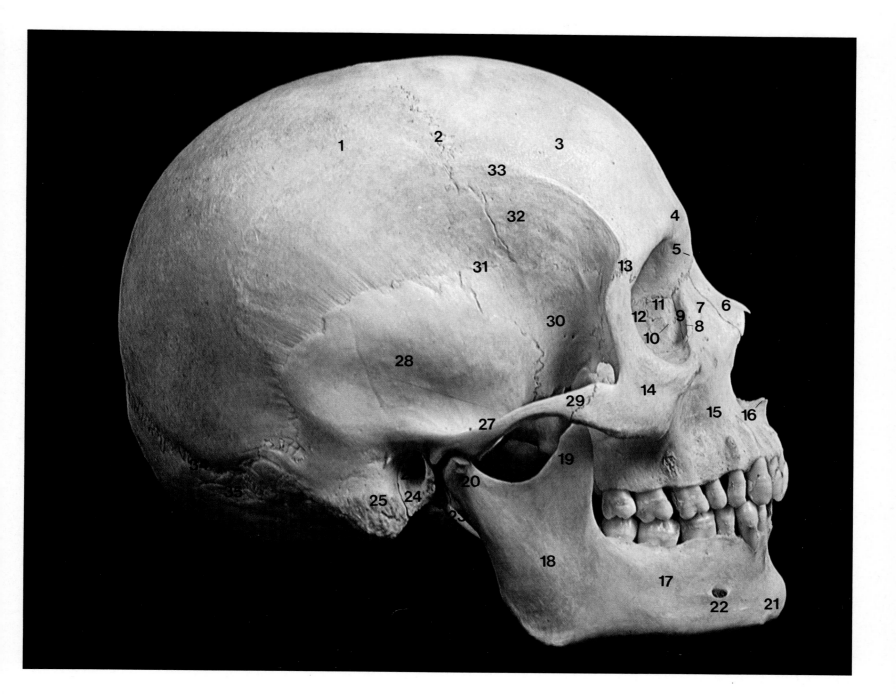

11

The skull, from the right. Muscle attachments
1 Occipital part of occipitofrontalis
2 Sternocleidomastoid
3 Temporalis
4 Masseter
5 Zygomaticus major
6 Zygomaticus minor
7 Orbicularis oculi
8 Procerus
9 Levator labii superioris alaeque nasi
10 Levator labii superioris
11 Nasalis
12 Levator anguli oris
13 Buccinator
14 Depressor labii inferioris
15 Depressor anguli oris
16 Platysma

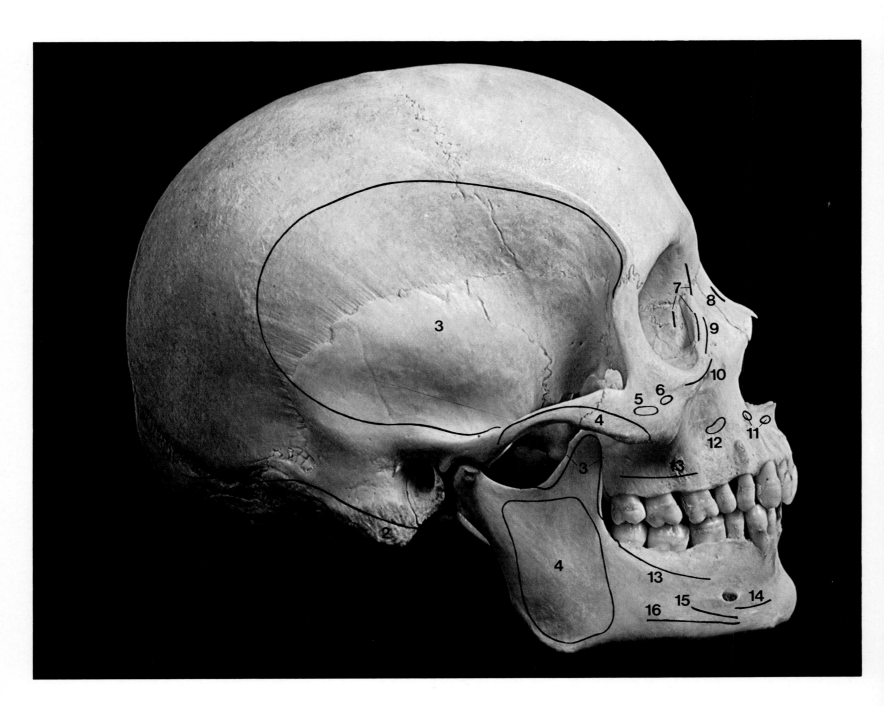

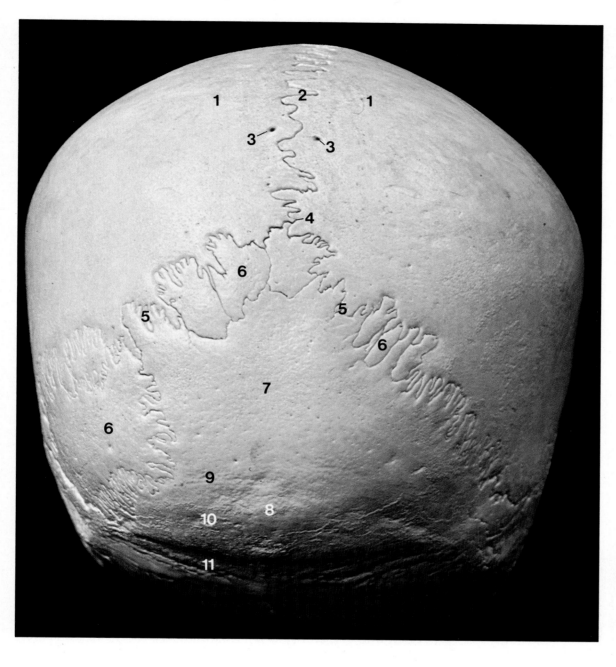

The skull, from behind

1 Parietal bone
2 Sagittal suture
3 Parietal foramen
4 Lambda
5 Lambdoid suture
6 Sutural bone
7 Occipital bone
8 External occipital protuberance (inion)
9 Highest ⎤
10 Superior ⎬ nuchal line
11 Inferior ⎦

● This cranium shows several sutural bones in the lambdoid suture, and one of them (on the left) is unusually large.

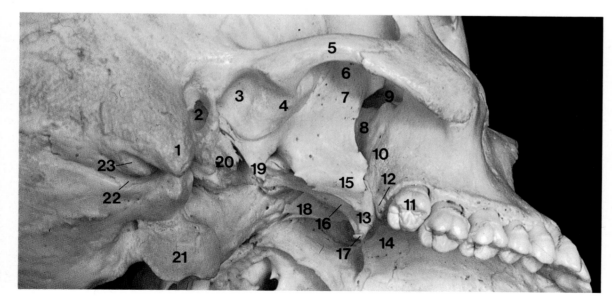

The skull. Right infratemporal region, obliquely from below and behind

1 Mastoid process
2 External acoustic meatus
3 Mandibular fossa
4 Articular tubercle
5 Zygomatic arch
6 Infratemporal crest
7 Infratemporal surface of greater wing of sphenoid bone
8 Pterygomaxillary fissure and pterygopalatine fossa
9 Inferior orbital fissure
10 Infratemporal (posterior) surface of maxilla
11 Third molar tooth
12 Tuberosity of maxilla
13 Pyramidal ⎤ process of
14 Horizontal ⎦ palatine bone
15 Lateral ⎤
16 Medial ⎦ pterygoid plate
17 Pterygoid hamulus
18 Vomer
19 Spine of sphenoid bone
20 Styloid process and sheath
21 Occipital condyle
22 Occipital groove
23 Mastoid notch

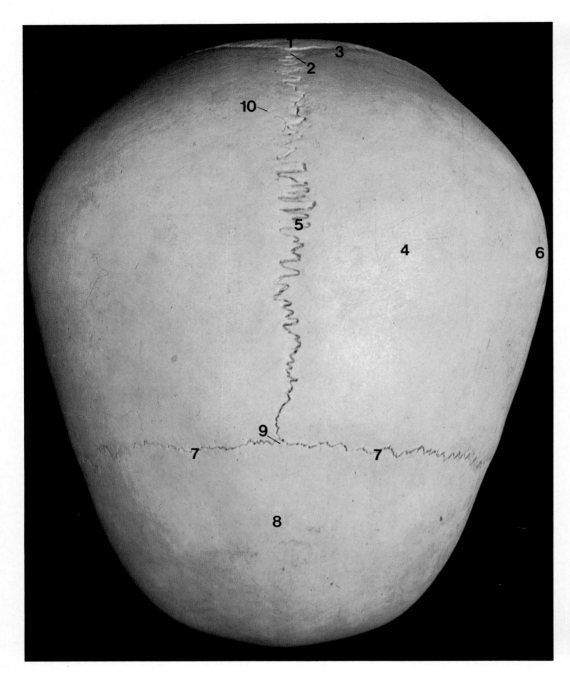

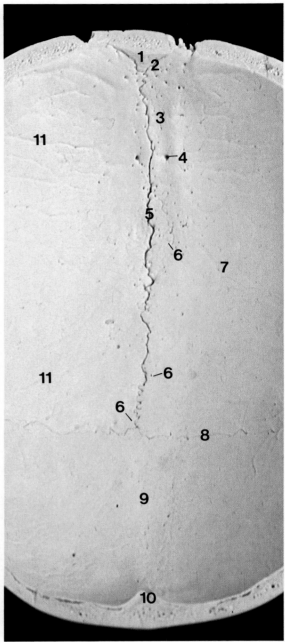

The skull, from above

1 Occipital bone
2 Lambda
3 Lambdoid suture
4 Parietal bone
5 Sagittal suture
6 Parietal eminence
7 Coronal suture
8 Frontal bone
9 Bregma
10 Parietal foramen

● In this skull the parietal eminences are prominent.

Internal surface of the cranial vault (midline region)

1 Occipital bone
2 Lambdoid suture
3 Groove for superior sagittal sinus
4 Parietal foramen
5 Sagittal suture
6 Depression for arachnoid granulations
7 Parietal bone
8 Coronal suture
9 Frontal bone
10 Frontal crest
11 Middle meningeal vessel markings

● The arachnoid granulations (through which cerebrospinal fluid drains into the superior sagittal sinus) cause irregular shallow depressions on the parts of the frontal and parietal bones that overlie the sinus.

**Inferior surface of the base of the skull
(from below and slightly behind)**

1 Incisive fossa
2 Palatine process of maxilla
3 Horizontal process of palatine
4 Greater palatine foramen
5 Lesser palatine foramina
6 Tuberosity of maxilla
7 Medial pterygoid plate
8 Pterygoid hamulus
9 Pyramidal process of palatine
10 Lateral pterygoid plate
11 Inferior orbital fissure
12 Infratemporal crest of greater wing of
   sphenoid
13 Zygomatic arch
14 Squamous part of temporal
15 Articular tubercle
16 Mandibular fossa
17 Petrosquamous fissure
18 Edge of tegmen tympani
19 Petrotympanic fissure
20 Squamotympanic fissure
21 Tympanic part of temporal
22 Styloid process
23 Stylomastoid foramen
24 External acoustic meatus
25 Mastoid process
26 Mastoid notch
27 Occipital groove
28 Mastoid foramen
29 Superior nuchal line
30 External occipital protuberance
31 Inferior nuchal line
32 External occipital crest
33 Foramen magnum
34 Condylar canal
35 Occipital condyle
36 Hypoglossal canal
37 Jugular foramen
38 Carotid canal
39 Spine of sphenoid
40 Foramen spinosum
41 Foramen ovale
42 Foramen lacerum
43 Pharyngeal tubercle
44 Scaphoid fossa
45 Palatinovaginal canal
46 Vomerovaginal canal
47 Posterior border of vomer
48 Posterior nasal spine

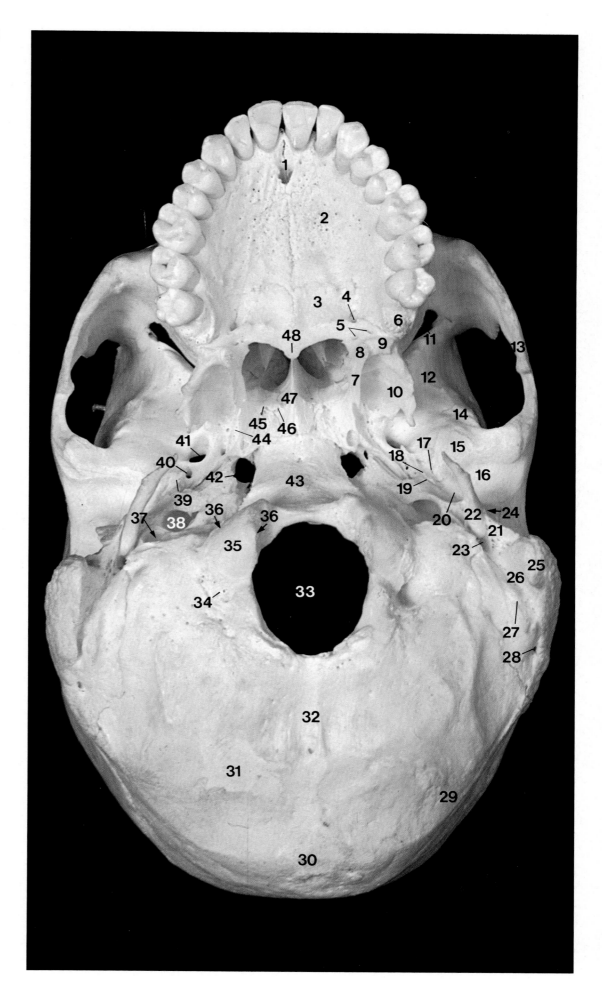

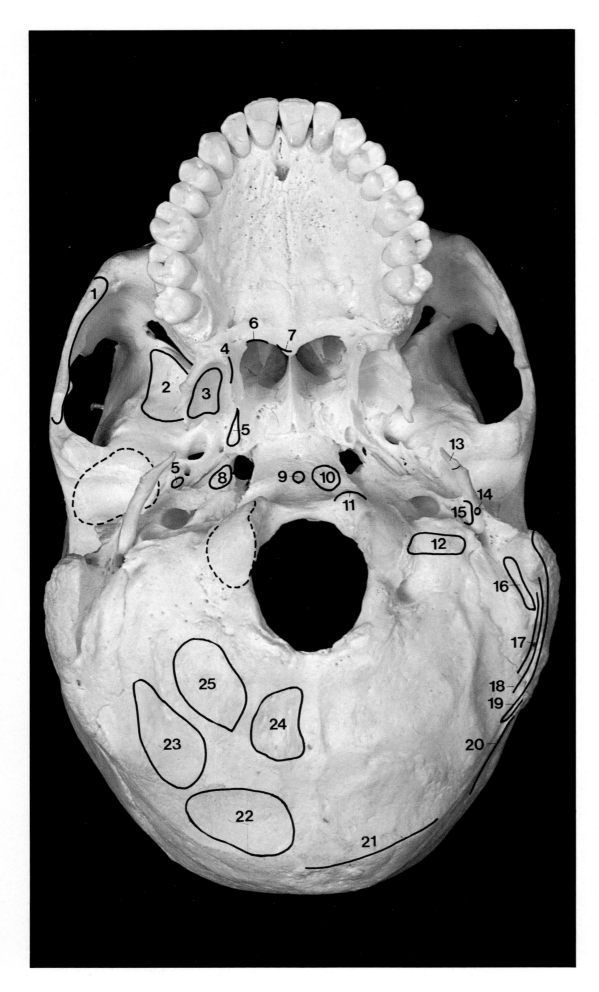

Inferior surface of the base of the skull.
Muscle attachments
(Capsule attachment, interrupted line)

1 Masseter
2 Upper head of lateral pterygoid
3 Deep head of medial pterygoid
4 Superior constrictor
5 Tensor veli palatini
6 Palatopharyngeus
7 Musculus uvulae
8 Levator veli palatini
9 Pharyngeal raphe
10 Longus capitis
11 Rectus capitis anterior
12 Rectus capitis lateralis
13 Styloglossus
14 Stylohyoid
15 Stylopharyngeus
16 Posterior belly of digastric
17 Longissimus capitis
18 Splenius capitis
19 Sternocleidomastoid
20 Occipital part of occipitofrontalis
21 Trapezius
22 Semispinalis capitis
23 Superior oblique
24 Rectus capitis posterior minor
25 Rectus capitis posterior major

Internal surface of the base of the skull (cranial fossae)

1 Diploë
2 Frontal sinus
3 Frontal crest
4 Foramen caecum
5 Crista galli
6 Cribriform plate of ethmoid
7 Groove for anterior ethmoidal nerve and vessels
8 Orbital part of frontal
9 Lesser wing of sphenoid
10 Jugum of sphenoid
11 Chiasmatic sulcus
12 Optic canal
13 Sella turcica (pituitary fossa)
14 Anterior clinoid process
15 Foramen rotundum
16 Greater wing of sphenoid
17 Foramen ovale
18 Foramen spinosum
19 Groove for middle meningeal vessels
20 Squamous part of temporal
21 Tegmen tympani
22 Petrous part of temporal
23 Groove for superior petrosal sinus
24 Arcuate eminence
25 Groove for sigmoid sinus
26 Groove for transverse sinus
27 Groove for superior sagittal sinus
28 Internal occipital protuberance
29 Parietal bone
30 Occipital bone
31 Foramen magnum
32 Hypoglossal canal
33 Jugular foramen
34 Groove for inferior petrosal sinus
35 Internal acoustic meatus
36 Clivus
37 Dorsum sellae
38 Posterior clinoid process
39 Carotid groove
40 Foramen lacerum
41 Trigeminal impression
42 Hiatus and groove for greater petrosal nerve
43 Hiatus and groove for lesser petrosal nerve

● The anterior cranial fossa is limited posteriorly on each side by the free margin of the lesser wing of the sphenoid.
● The groove for the superior petrosal sinus forms the boundary on each side between the middle and posterior cranial fossae.

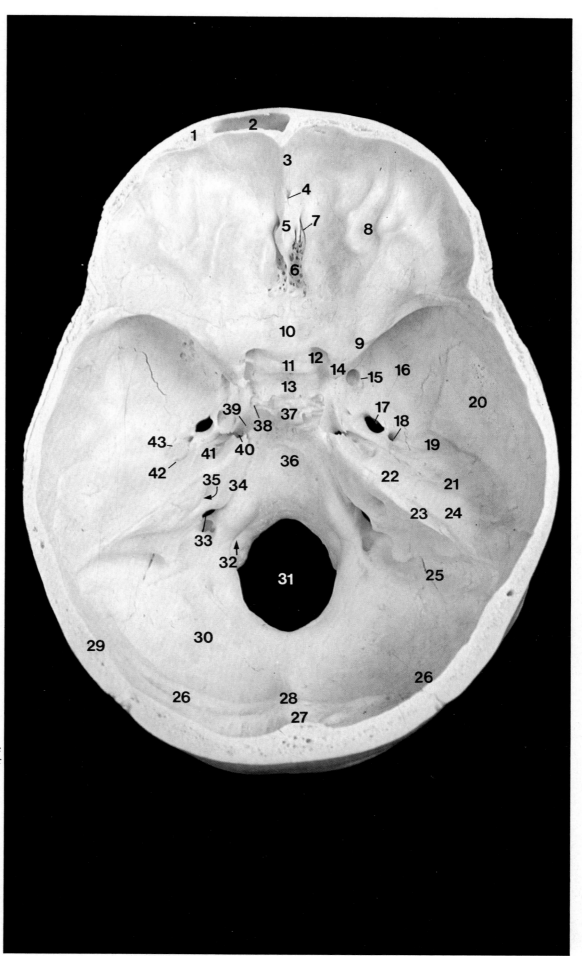

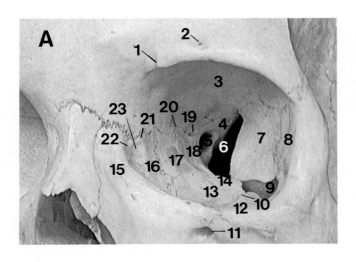

A Bones of the left orbit
1 Frontal notch
2 Supra-orbital foramen
3 Orbital part of frontal ⎤ forming
4 Lesser wing of sphenoid ⎦ roof
5 Optic canal
6 Superior orbital fissure
7 Greater wing of ⎤ forming
  sphenoid ⎥ lateral wall
8 Zygomatic ⎦
9 Inferior orbital fissure
10 Infra-orbital groove
11 Infra-orbital foramen

12 Zygomatic ⎤
13 Maxilla ⎥ forming
14 Orbital process of ⎥ floor
  palatine ⎦
15 Frontal process of ⎤
  maxilla ⎥ forming
16 Lacrimal ⎥ medial
17 Orbital plate of ethmoid ⎥ wall
18 Body of sphenoid ⎦
19 Posterior ⎤ ethmoidal foramen
20 Anterior ⎦
21 Posterior ⎤ lacrimal crest
22 Anterior ⎦
23 Nasolacrimal groove

B Lateral wall of the left nasal cavity, in a midline sagittal section of the skull
(The middle concha has been removed to show the ethmoidal bulla)
1 Occipital condyle
2 Hypoglossal canal
3 Groove for inferior petrosal sinus
4 Internal acoustic meatus
5 Clivus
6 Dorsum sellae
7 Sella turcica (pituitary fossa)
8 Sphenoidal sinus

9 Ethmoidal sinus
10 Superior concha
11 Ethmoidal bulla
12 Uncinate process
13 Frontal sinus
14 Inferior concha
15 Incisive canal
16 Hard palate
17 Maxillary sinus
18 Perpendicular plate of palatine
19 Sphenopalatine foramen
20 Medial pterygoid plate
21 Pterygoid hamulus

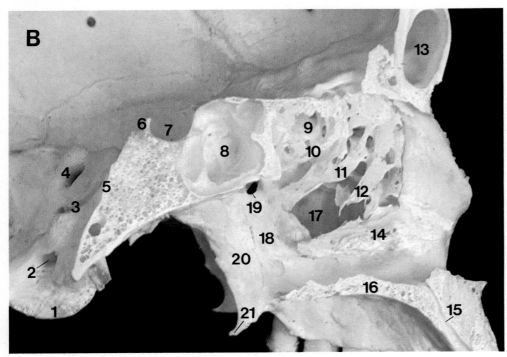

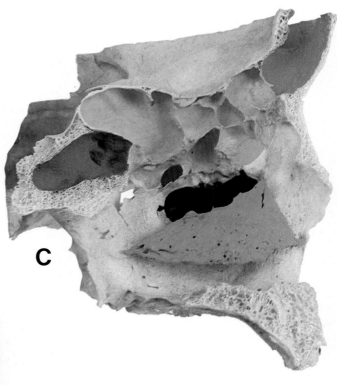

C The left paranasal sinuses, from a midline sagittal section of the skull
(The superior and middle conchae have been removed)
Dark blue, sphenoidal sinus
Yellow, ethmoidal sinus
Red, frontal sinus
Green, maxillary sinus
Light blue, inferior concha

● In the whole skull there are four pairs of paranasal sinuses – sphenoidal, ethmoidal, frontal and maxillary. Each ethmoidal sinus consists of a number of ethmoidal air cells.
● In this specimen the most posterior ethmoidal air cell is unusually large and extends backwards to overlap the sphenoidal sinus.

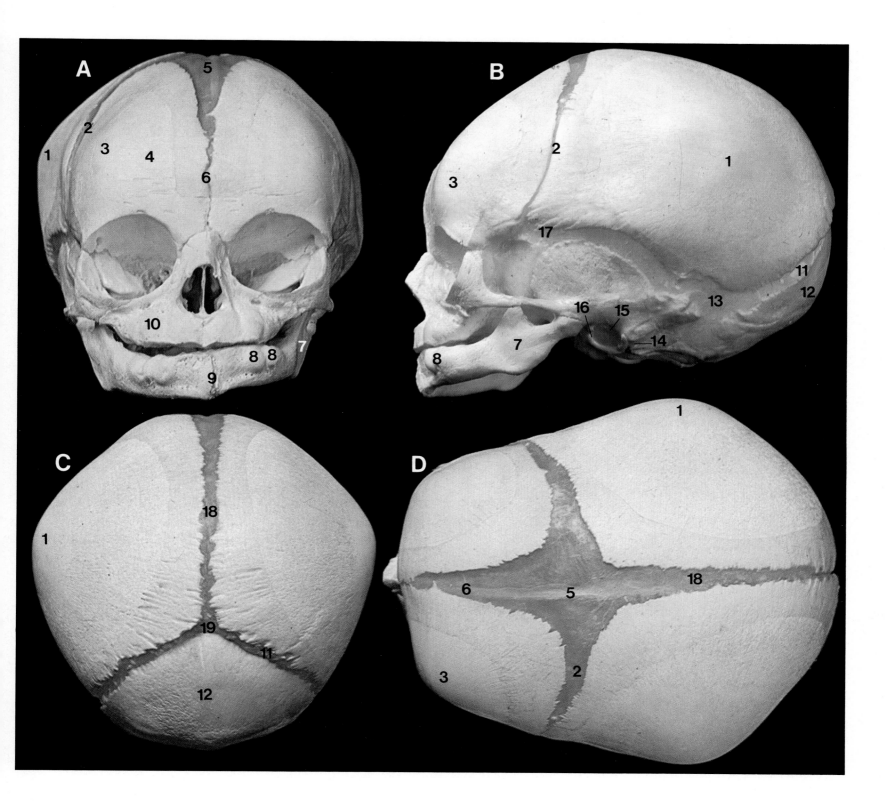

The skull of a full-term fetus, A from the front, B from the left and slightly below, C from behind, D from above

1 Parietal tuberosity
2 Coronal suture
3 Frontal tuberosity
4 Half of frontal bone
5 Anterior fontanelle
6 Frontal suture
7 Ramus of mandible
8 Elevations over deciduous teeth in body of mandible
9 Symphysis menti
10 Maxilla
11 Lambdoid suture
12 Occipital bone
13 Mastoid fontanelle
14 Stylomastoid foramen
15 External acoustic meatus
16 Tympanic ring
17 Sphenoidal fontanelle
18 Sagittal suture
19 Posterior fontanelle

● The face at birth forms a relatively smaller proportion of the cranium than in the adult (about one eighth compared with one half) due to the small size of the nasal cavity and maxillary sinuses and the lack of erupted teeth.
● The posterior fontanelle closes about two months after birth, the anterior fontanelle in the second year.
● Due to the lack of the mastoid process (which does not develop until the second year) the stylomastoid foramen and the emerging facial nerve are relatively near the surface and unprotected.

19

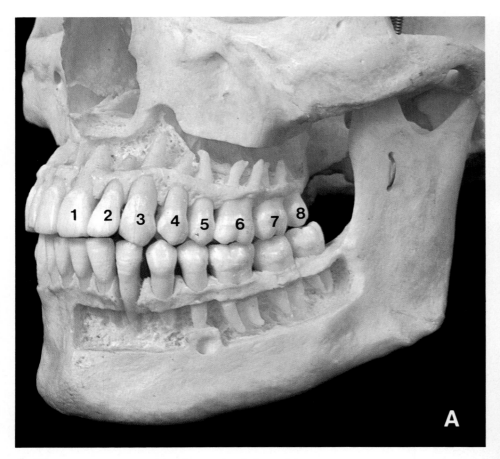

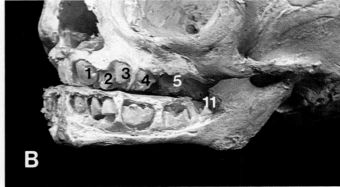

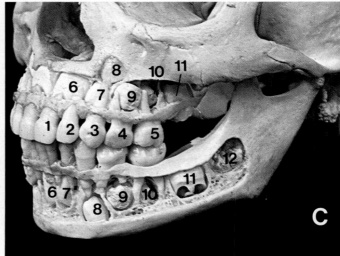

A The permanent teeth, from the left and in front

(With partial removal of alveolar bone to show the roots of the teeth, which are numbered and named on the left side)

1 Central ⎫
2 Lateral ⎬ incisor
3 Canine ⎭

6 First ⎫
7 Second ⎬ molar
8 Third ⎭

4 First ⎫
5 Second ⎬ premolar

● The corresponding teeth of the upper and lower jaws have similar names. In clinical dentistry the teeth are often identified by the numbers 1 to 8 (as listed here) rather than by name.

● The third molar tooth is sometimes called the wisdom tooth.

Upper and lower jaws from the left and in front, B in the newborn with unerupted deciduous teeth, C in a four-year-old child with erupted deciduous teeth and unerupted permanent teeth

1 Central incisor ⎫
2 Lateral incisor ⎪
3 Canine ⎬ of deciduous dentition
4 First molar ⎪
5 Second molar ⎭

6 Central incisor ⎫
7 Lateral incisor ⎪
8 Canine ⎪
9 First premolar ⎬ of permanent dentition
10 Second premolar ⎪
11 First molar ⎪
12 Second molar ⎭

● The deciduous molars occupy the positions of the premolars of the permanent dentition.

D The edentulous mandible in old age, from the left

● With the loss of teeth the alveolar bone becomes absorbed, so that the mental foramen and mandibular canal lie near the upper margin of the bone.

● The angle between the ramus and body becomes more obtuse, resembling the infantile angle.

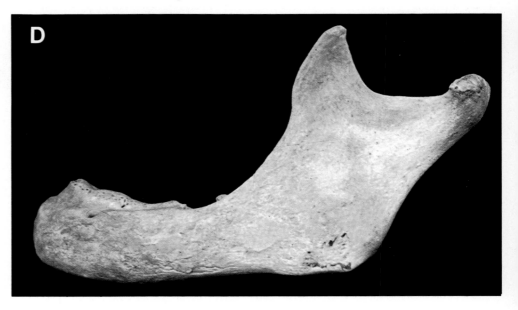

The skull, from the front. Cleared specimen
1 Frontal sinus
2 Frontal crest
3 Crista galli
4 Lesser wing of sphenoid
5 Optic canal
6 Superior orbital fissure
7 Greater wing of sphenoid
8 Maxillary sinus
9 Zygomatic arch
10 Mastoid process
11 Ramus ⎫
12 Body ⎭ of mandible
13 Nasal septum
14 Inferior concha
15 Infra-orbital margin
16 Supra-orbital margin

● Compare with the skull on page 9 and with the radiograph on page 73.

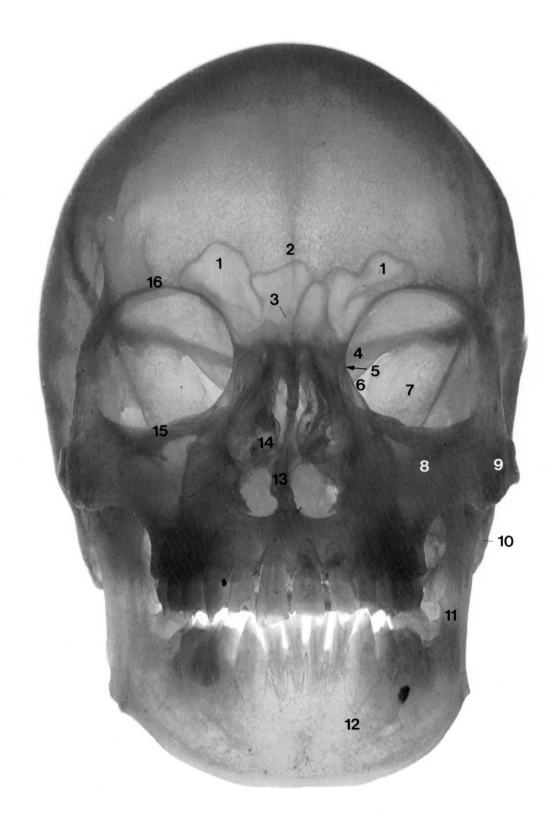

21

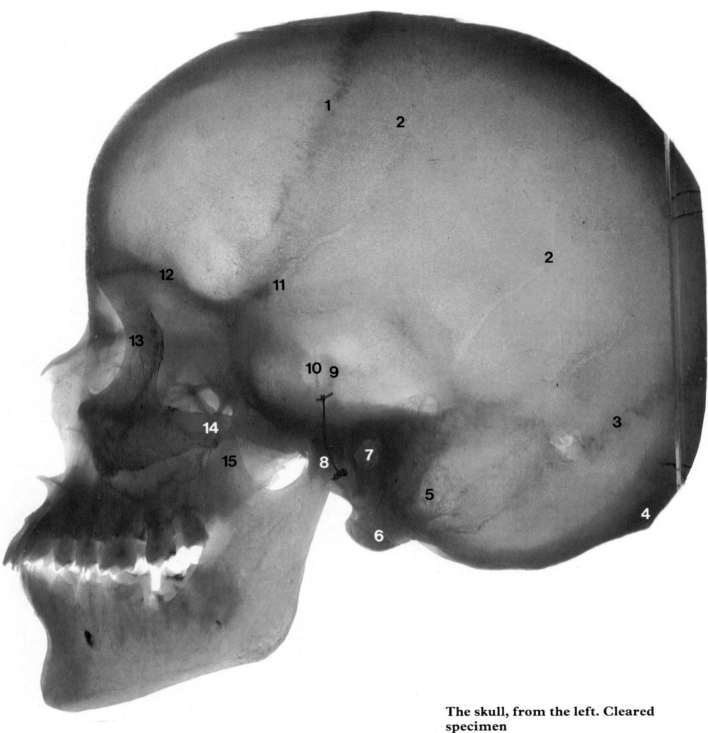

The skull, from the left. Cleared specimen
 1 Coronal suture
 2 Markings of middle meningeal vessels
 3 Lambdoid suture
 4 External occipital protuberance
 5 Mastoid air cells
 6 Mastoid process
 7 External acoustic meatus
 8 Condyle of mandible
 9 Dorsum sellae
10 Sella turcica (pituitary fossa)
11 Pterion
12 Roof of orbit
13 Orbital margin
14 Zygomatic arch
15 Coronoid process of mandible

**The mandible, A from the front, B
from behind and above, C from the
left and front**

1 Head
2 Neck
3 Pterygoid fovea
4 Coronoid process
5 Anterior border of ramus
6 Oblique line
7 Angle
8 Alveolar part
9 Body
10 Mental foramen
11 Mental tubercle
12 Mental protuberance
13 Base
14 Posterior border of ramus
15 Mandibular foramen
16 Mylohyoid groove
17 Lingula
18 Mylohyoid line
19 Submandibular fossa
20 Sublingual fossa
21 Superior and inferior mental spines
22 Mandibular notch
23 Digastric fossa
24 Ramus
25 Inferior border of ramus

● The head and the neck (including the
pterygoid fovea) constitute the condyle.
● The alveolar part contains the sockets for the
roots of the teeth.
● The base is the inferior border of the body, and
becomes continuous with the inferior border of the
ramus.
● In this mandible the third molar teeth are
unerupted.

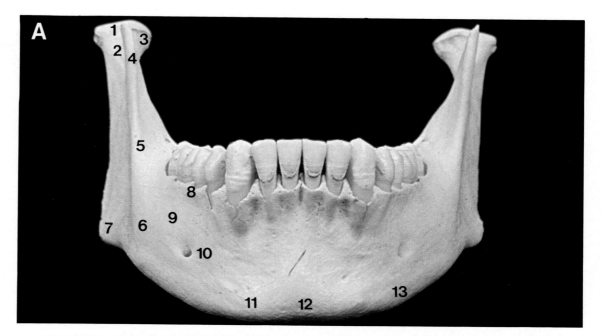

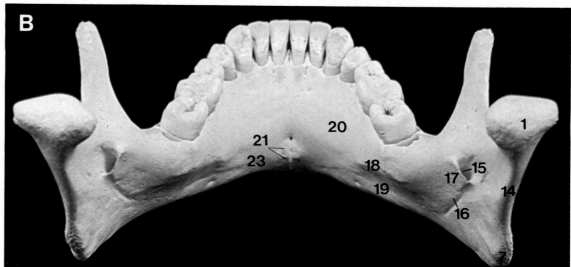

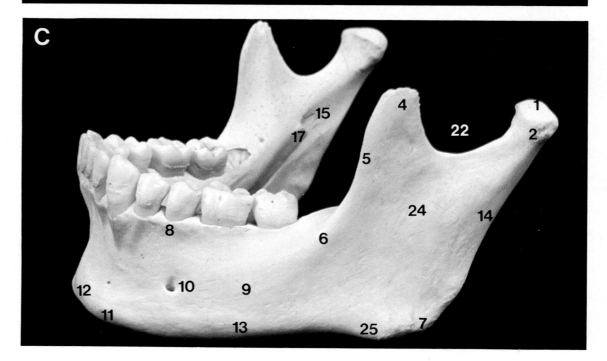

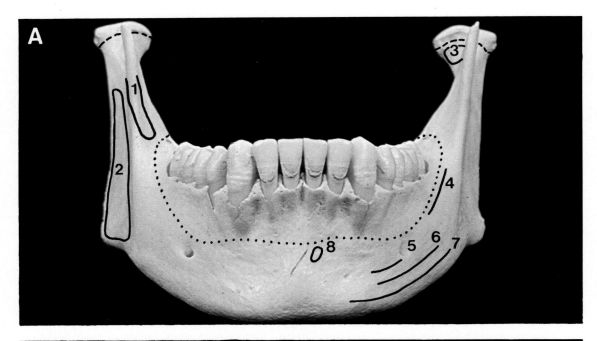

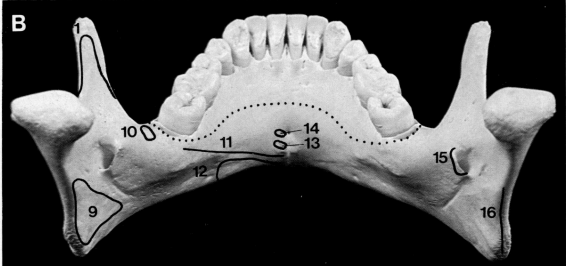

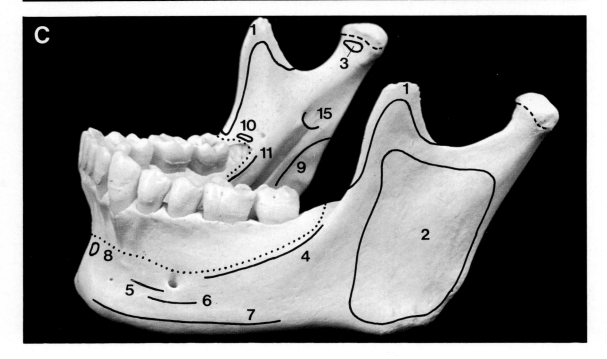

The mandible, A from the front, B from behind and above, C from the left and front. Muscle attachments

(Capsule attachment, interrupted line; the dotted line indicates the limit of attachment of the oral mucous membrane)

1 Temporalis
2 Masseter
3 Lateral pterygoid
4 Buccinator
5 Depressor labii inferioris
6 Depressor anguli oris
7 Platysma
8 Mentalis
9 Medial pterygoid
10 Pterygomandibular raphe and superior constrictor
11 Mylohyoid
12 Anterior belly of digastric
13 Geniohyoid
14 Genioglossus
15 Sphenomandibular ligament
16 Stylomandibular ligament

● The buccinator is attached to the alveolar processes of the maxilla and mandible opposite the three molar teeth. (Note that in this mandible the third molar has not yet erupted).

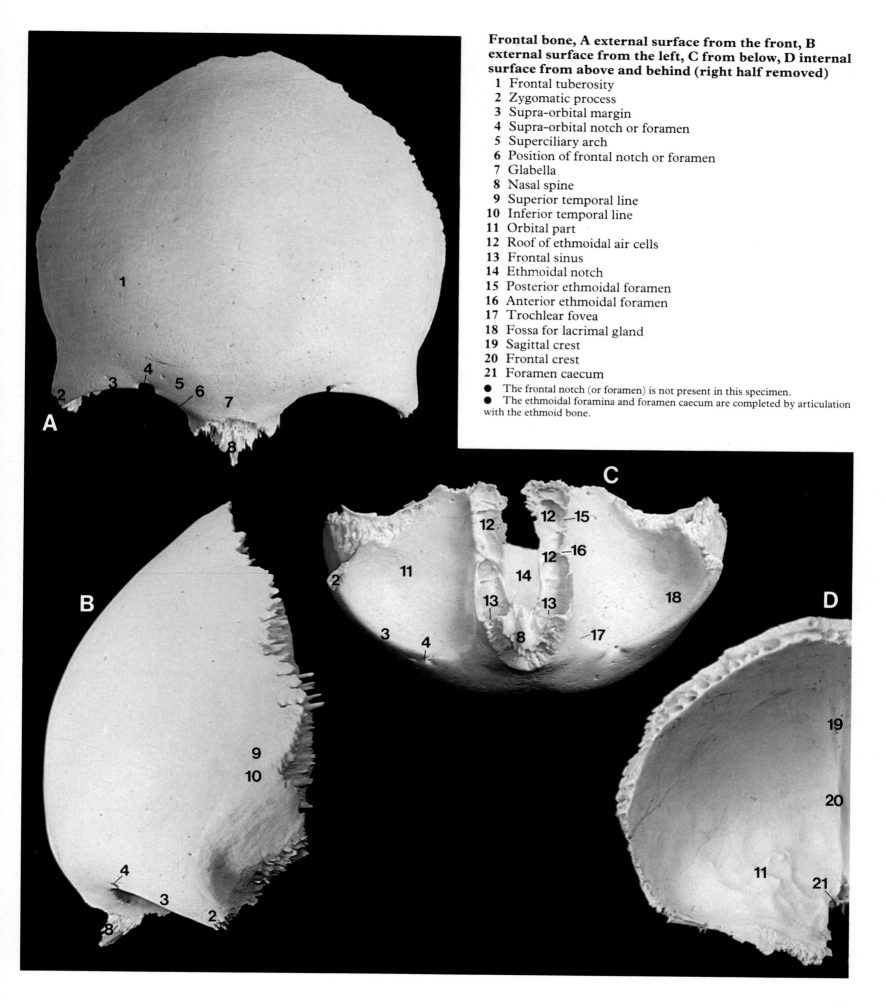

Frontal bone, A external surface from the front, B external surface from the left, C from below, D internal surface from above and behind (right half removed)

1 Frontal tuberosity
2 Zygomatic process
3 Supra-orbital margin
4 Supra-orbital notch or foramen
5 Superciliary arch
6 Position of frontal notch or foramen
7 Glabella
8 Nasal spine
9 Superior temporal line
10 Inferior temporal line
11 Orbital part
12 Roof of ethmoidal air cells
13 Frontal sinus
14 Ethmoidal notch
15 Posterior ethmoidal foramen
16 Anterior ethmoidal foramen
17 Trochlear fovea
18 Fossa for lacrimal gland
19 Sagittal crest
20 Frontal crest
21 Foramen caecum

● The frontal notch (or foramen) is not present in this specimen.
● The ethmoidal foramina and foramen caecum are completed by articulation with the ethmoid bone.

25

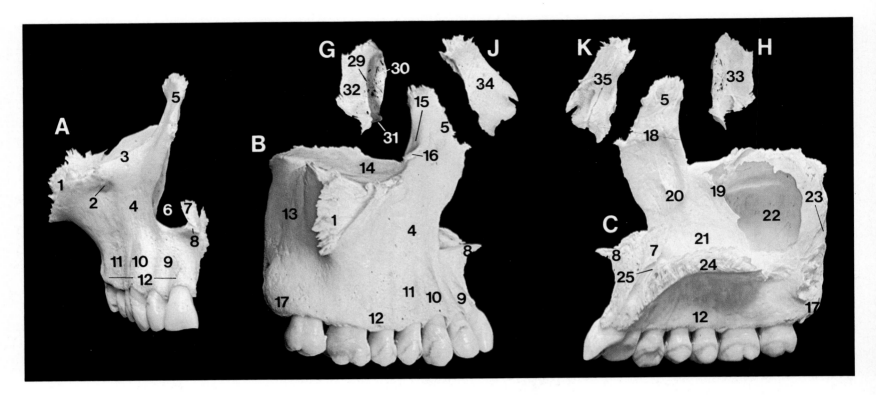

Right maxilla, A from the front, B from the lateral side, C from the medial side, D from below, E from above, F from behind

1 Zygomatic process
2 Infra-orbital foramen
3 Infra-orbital margin
4 Anterior surface
5 Frontal process
6 Nasal notch
7 Nasal crest
8 Anterior nasal spine
9 Incisive fossa
10 Canine eminence
11 Canine fossa
12 Alveolar process
13 Infratemporal surface
14 Orbital surface

15 Nasolacrimal groove
16 Anterior lacrimal crest
17 Tuberosity
18 Ethmoidal crest
19 Middle meatus
20 Conchal crest
21 Inferior meatus
22 Maxillary hiatus and sinus
23 Greater palatine canal
24 Palatine process
25 Incisive canal
26 Unerupted third molar tooth
27 Infra-orbital groove
28 Infra-orbital canal

Right lacrimal bone, G from the lateral side, H from the medial side

29 Posterior lacrimal crest
30 Groove for lacrimal sac
31 Lacrimal hamulus
32 Orbital surface
33 Nasal surface

Right nasal bone, J from the lateral side, K from the medial side

34 Lateral surface and vascular foramen
35 Internal surface and groove for anterior ethmoidal nerve

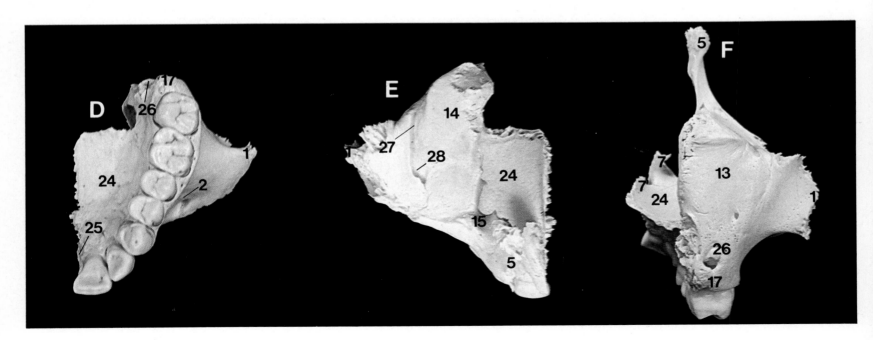

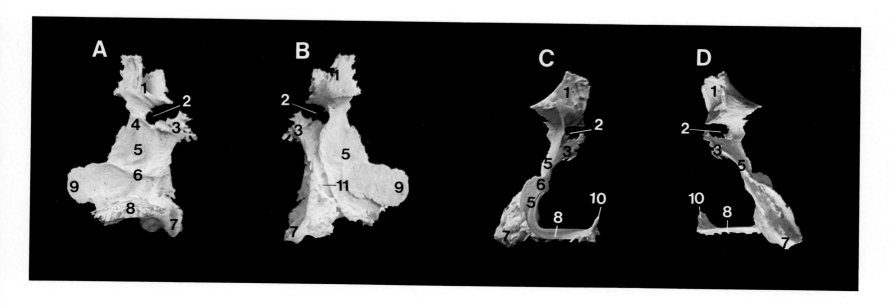

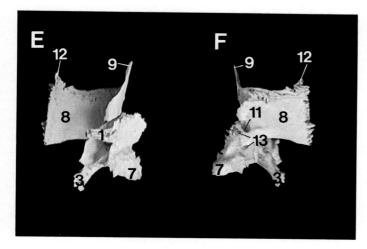

Right palatine bone, A from the medial side, B from the lateral side, C from the front, D from behind, E from above, F from below

1 Orbital process
2 Sphenopalatine notch
3 Sphenoidal process
4 Ethmoidal crest
5 Perpendicular plate
6 Conchal crest
7 Pyramidal process
8 Horizontal plate
9 Maxillary process
10 Nasal crest
11 Greater palatine groove
12 Posterior nasal spine
13 Lesser palatine canals

G Articulation of the right maxilla and the palatine bone, from the medial side

1 Palatine process of maxilla
2 Horizontal process ⎫
3 Maxillary process ⎬ of palatine
                     ⎭

● Compare with fig. C, opposite.

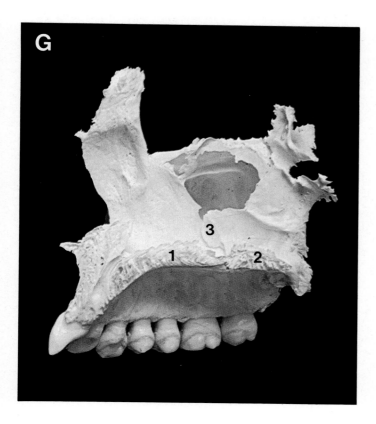

27

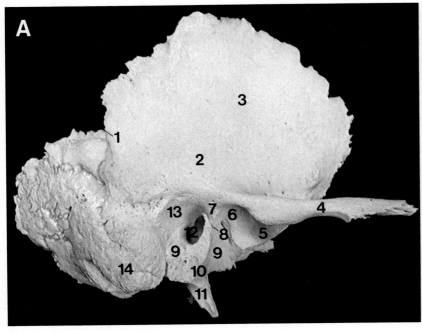

A

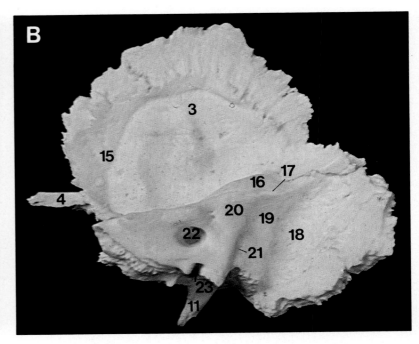

B

Right temporal bone, A external aspect, B internal aspect, C from above, D from below, E from the front

1 Parietal notch
2 Groove for middle temporal artery
3 Squamous part
4 Zygomatic process
5 Articular tubercle
6 Mandibular fossa
7 Postglenoid tubercle
8 Squamotympanic fissure
9 Tympanic part
10 Sheath of styloid process
11 Styloid process
12 External acoustic meatus
13 Suprameatal triangle
14 Mastoid process
15 Grooves for branches of middle meningeal vessels
16 Arcuate eminence
17 Groove for superior petrosal sinus
18 Groove for sigmoid sinus
19 Subarcuate fossa
20 Petrous part
21 Aqueduct of vestibule
22 Internal acoustic meatus
23 Cochlear canaliculus
24 Petrosquamous fissure (from above)
25 Tegmen tympani
26 Hiatus and groove for lesser petrosal nerve
27 Hiatus and groove for greater petrosal nerve
28 Trigeminal impression on apex of petrous part
29 Occipital groove
30 Mastoid notch
31 Stylomastoid foramen
32 Petrotympanic fissure
33 Edge of tegmen tympani
34 Petrosquamous fissure (from below)
35 Carotid canal
36 Canaliculus for tympanic branch of glossopharyngeal nerve
37 Jugular fossa
38 Mastoid canaliculus for auricular branch of vagus nerve
39 Jugular surface
40 Canal for tensor tympani
41 Auditory tube

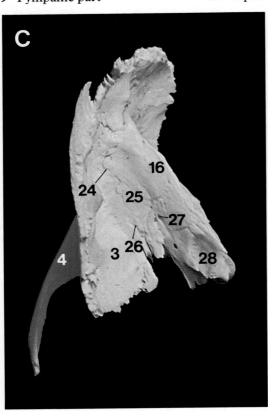

C

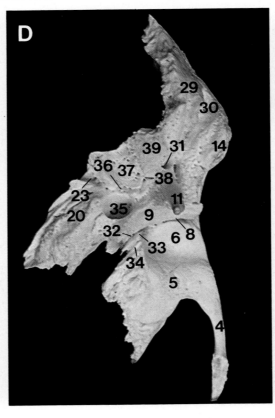

D

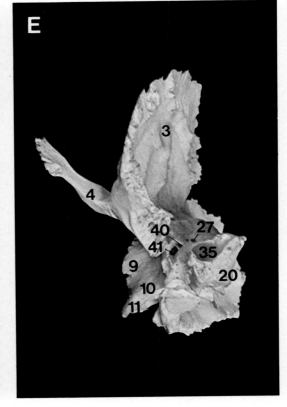

E

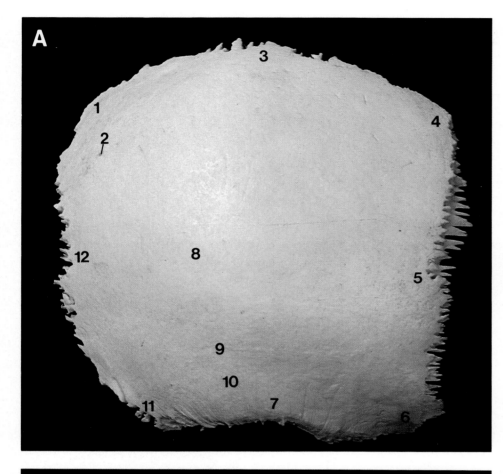

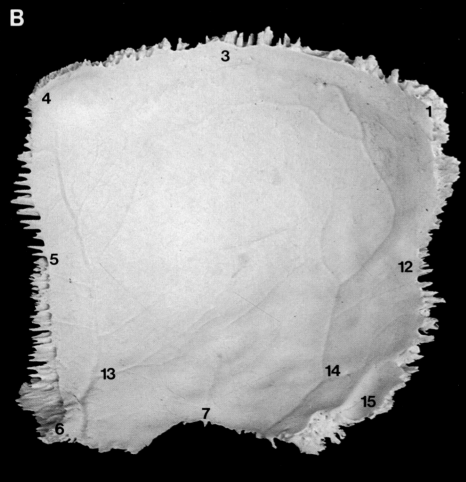

Right parietal bone, A external surface, B internal surface

1 Occipital (posterosuperior) angle
2 Parietal foramen
3 Sagittal (superior) border
4 Frontal (anterosuperior) angle
5 Frontal (anterior) border
6 Sphenoidal (antero-inferior) angle
7 Squamosal (inferior) border
8 Parietal tuberosity
9 Superior temporal line
10 Inferior temporal line
11 Mastoid (postero-inferior) angle
12 Occipital (posterior) border
13 Furrows for frontal branch of middle meningeal vessels
14 Furrows for parietal branch of middle meningeal vessels
15 Groove for sigmoid sinus at mastoid angle

Right zygomatic bone, C lateral surface, D from the medial side, E from behind

1 Frontal process
2 Orbital border
3 Zygomaticofacial foramen
4 Maxillary border
5 Temporal process
6 Temporal border
7 Orbital surface
8 Zygomatico-orbital foramen
9 Temporal surface
10 Zygomaticotemporal foramen
● The zygomatic process of the temporal bone and the temporal process of the zygomatic bone form the zygomatic arch.

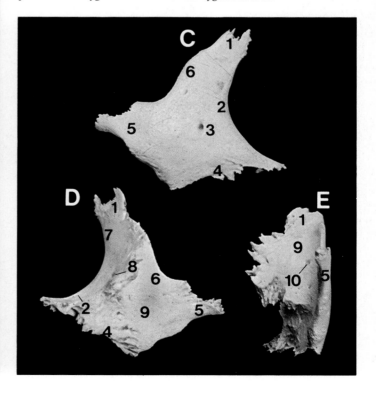

Sphenoid bone, A from the front, B from behind, C from above and behind, D from below, E from the left

1 Temporal surface ⎫
2 Infratemporal crest ⎬ of greater wing
3 Orbital surface
4 Superior orbital fissure
5 Lesser wing
6 Body with openings of sphenoidal sinuses
7 Rostrum
8 Vaginal process
9 Pterygoid canal
10 Foramen rotundum
11 Pterygoid process
12 Medial pterygoid plate
13 Pterygoid hamulus
14 Pterygoid notch
15 Lateral pterygoid plate
16 Spine
17 Cerebral surface of greater wing
18 Anterior ⎫
19 Posterior ⎬ clinoid process
20 Dorsum sellae
21 Scaphoid fossa
22 Ethmoidal spine
23 Jugum
24 Chiasmatic sulcus
25 Optic canal
26 Tuberculum sellae
27 Sella turcica (pituitary fossa)
28 Foramen ovale
29 Foramen spinosum
30 Carotid groove
31 Infratemporal surface of greater wing

Vomer, F from the right, G from behind

32 Ala
33 Posterior border
34 Groove for nasopalatine nerve and vessels

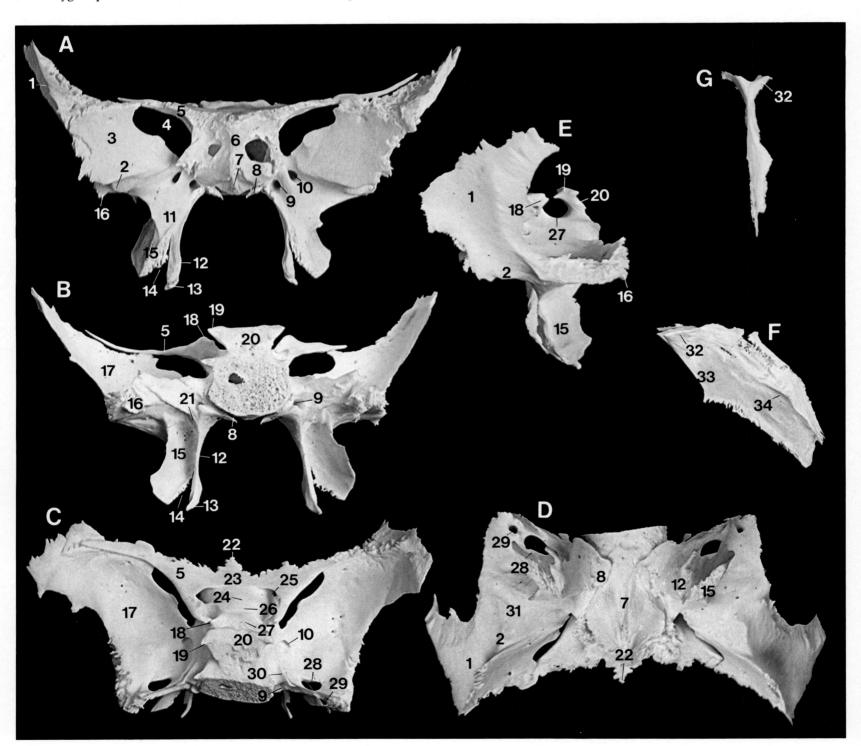

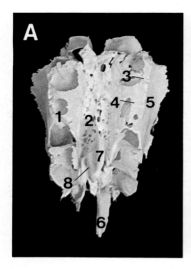
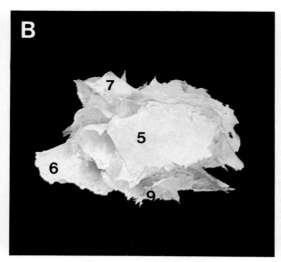
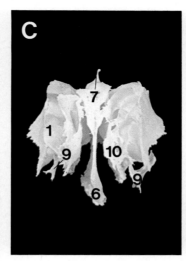
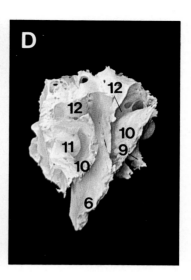

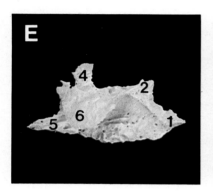
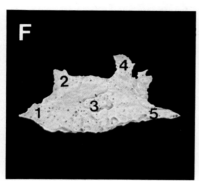
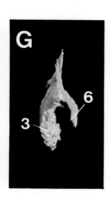

Ethmoid bone, A from above, B from the left, C from the front, D from the left, below and behind

1 Ethmoidal labyrinth (containing ethmoidal air cells)
2 Cribriform plate
3 Posterior ⎫
4 Anterior ⎬ ethmoidal groove
5 Orbital plate
6 Perpendicular plate
7 Crista galli
8 Ala of crista galli
9 Uncinate process
10 Middle concha
11 Ethmoidal bulla
12 Superior concha

Right inferior concha, E from the lateral side, F from the medial side, G from the front

1 Anterior end
2 Lacrimal process
3 Medial surface
4 Ethmoidal process
5 Posterior end
6 Maxillary process

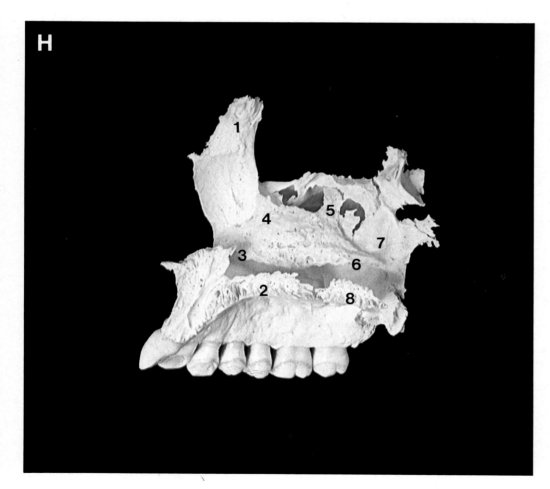

H Articulation of right maxilla, palatine bone and inferior concha, from the medial side

1 Frontal process ⎫
2 Palatine process ⎬ of maxilla
3 Anterior end ⎫
4 Lacrimal process ⎪
5 Ethmoidal process ⎬ of inferior concha
6 Posterior end ⎪
7 Perpendicular ⎫
8 Horizontal ⎬ plate of palatine

● Compare with fig. G on page 27.

31

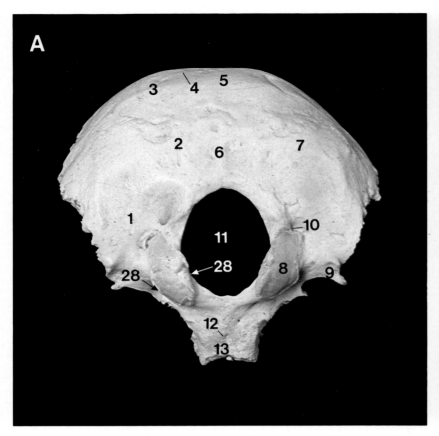

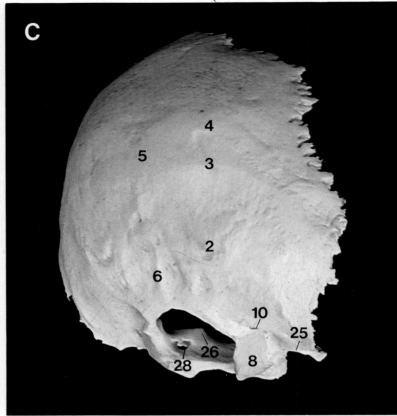

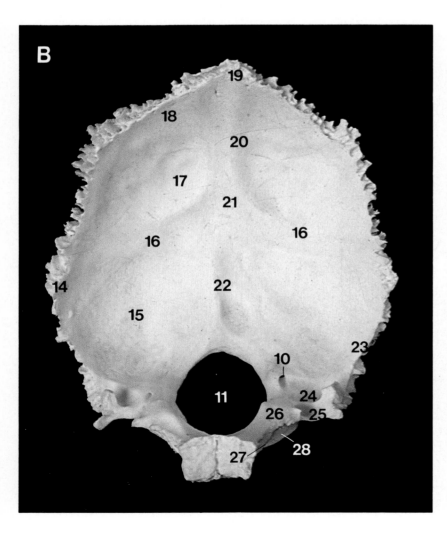

Occipital bone, A external surface from below, B internal surface, C external surface from the right and below

1 Lateral part
2 Inferior nuchal line
3 Superior nuchal line
4 Highest nuchal line
5 External occipital protuberance
6 External occipital crest
7 Squamous part
8 Condyle
9 Jugular process
10 Condylar fossa (and condylar canal in B and C)
11 Foramen magnum
12 Pharyngeal tubercle
13 Basilar part
14 Lateral angle
15 Cerebellar fossa
16 Groove for transverse sinus
17 Cerebral fossa
18 Lambdoid margin
19 Superior angle
20 Groove for superior sagittal sinus
21 Internal occipital protuberance
22 Internal occipital crest
23 Mastoid margin
24 Groove for sigmoid sinus
25 Jugular notch
26 Jugular tubercle
27 Groove for inferior petrosal sinus
28 Hypoglossal canal

Right side of the neck. Some surface markings

(External jugular vein, interrupted line; spinal part of accessory nerve, dotted line)

1 Anterior border of trapezius
2 Sternocleidomastoid
3 Bifurcation of common carotid artery
4 Hypoglossal nerve
5 Tip of greater horn of hyoid bone
6 Internal laryngeal nerve
7 Body of hyoid bone
8 Laryngeal prominence (Adam's apple)
9 Vocal folds
10 Lower border of lamina of thyroid cartilage
11 Arch of cricoid cartilage
12 Isthmus of thyroid gland
13 Jugular notch
14 Sternal head of sternocleidomastoid
15 Sternoclavicular joint and union of internal jugular and subclavian veins to form brachiocephalic vein
16 Upper trunk of brachial plexus

● As it crosses the posterior triangle, the spinal root of the accessory nerve is embedded in the investing layer of deep cervical fascia that forms the roof of the triangle. This and other parts of the deep cervical fascia (prevertebral and pretracheal fasciae and the carotid sheath) have been largely removed in the dissections that follow.

● The nerve usually called in English *the* accessory nerve is in official terminology the ramus externus of the nervus accessorius, and is often known as the *spinal part* or (in some texts) the *spinal root* of the accessory nerve. The spinal part or root (singular) is formed by the union of the spinal *roots* (plural) that emerge from the upper five or six cervical segments of the spinal medulla. (The cranial root or part of the accessory nerve, the ramus internus, arises from the medulla oblongata and joins the vagus nerve.)

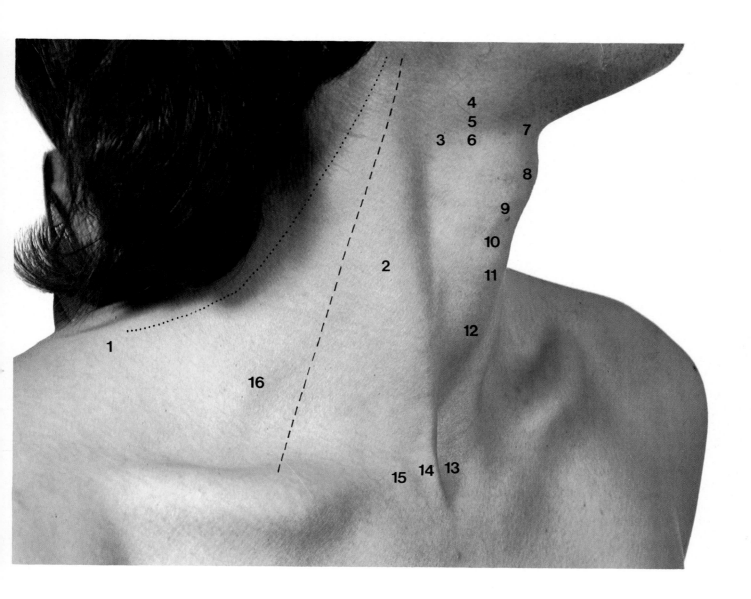

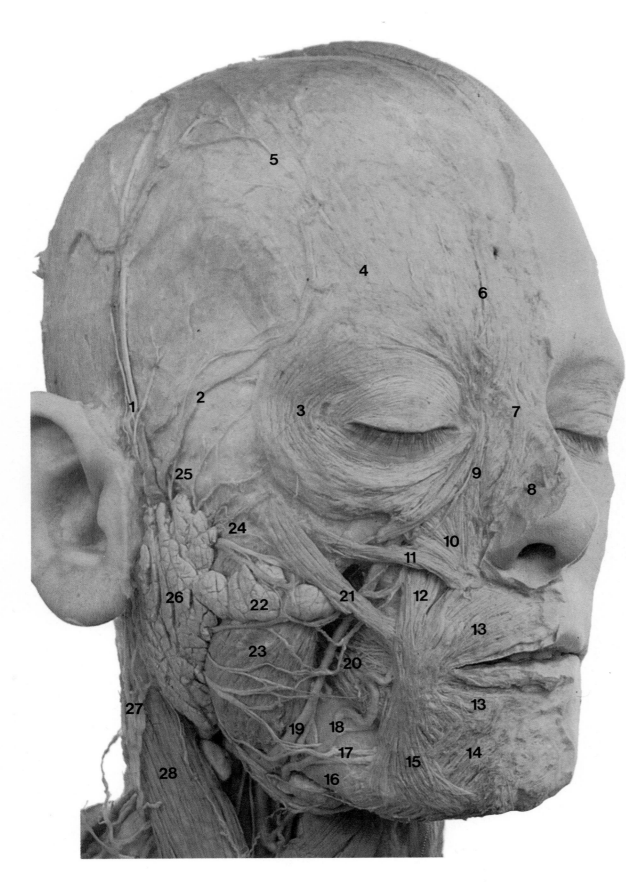

The face, from the front and the right

1 Auriculotemporal nerve and superficial temporal vessels
2 Anterior branch of superficial temporal artery
3 Orbicularis oculi
4 Frontalis part of occipitofrontalis
5 Supra-orbital nerve
6 Supratrochlear nerve
7 Procerus
8 Nasalis
9 Levator labii superioris alaeque nasi
10 Levator labii superioris
11 Zygomaticus minor
12 Levator anguli oris
13 Orbicularis oris
14 Depressor labii inferioris
15 Depressor anguli oris
16 Body of mandible
17 Marginal mandibular branch of facial nerve
18 Facial artery
19 Facial vein
20 Buccinator and buccal branches of facial nerve
21 Zygomaticus major
22 Accessory parotid gland overlying parotid duct
23 Masseter
24 Zygomatic ⎫ branches of
25 Temporal ⎭ facial nerve
26 Parotid gland
27 Great auricular nerve
28 Sternocleidomastoid
● The facial artery is tortuous and lies anterior to the facial vein which is straight. Both vessels pass deep to the zygomaticus muscles.
● The facial expression group of muscles (which includes the buccinator) is supplied by the facial nerve. (The muscles of mastication – temporalis, masseter, medial and lateral pterygoids – are supplied by the mandibular nerve).

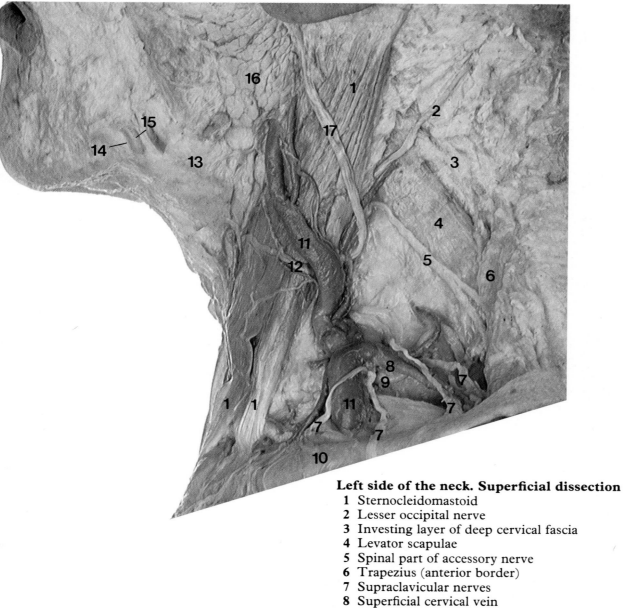

Left side of the neck. Superficial dissection
1 Sternocleidomastoid
2 Lesser occipital nerve
3 Investing layer of deep cervical fascia
4 Levator scapulae
5 Spinal part of accessory nerve
6 Trapezius (anterior border)
7 Supraclavicular nerves
8 Superficial cervical vein
9 Superficial cervical artery
10 Clavicle
11 External jugular vein
12 Transverse cutaneous nerve of neck
13 Submandibular gland
14 Facial artery
15 Facial vein
16 Parotid gland
17 Great auricular nerve

● In this dissection the investing layer of deep cervical fascia is mostly intact but has been partly removed, e.g. from the superficial surface of sternocleidomastoid and the parotid gland. The spinal part of the accessory nerve is normally embedded in the investing layer of fascia that forms the roof of the posterior triangle; here the nerve has been dissected out from the fascia.

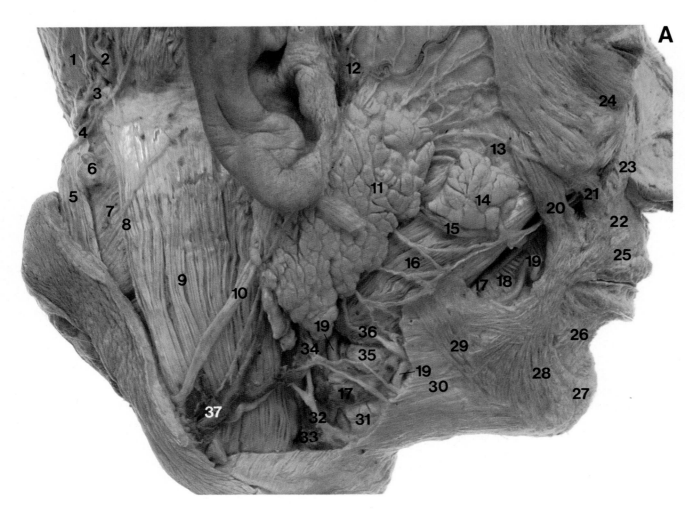

A Right parotid and upper cervical regions. Superficial dissection (with part of platysma muscle removed)

1 Occipital part of occipitofrontalis
2 Occipital artery
3 Greater occipital nerve
4 Third occipital nerve
5 Trapezius
6 Occipital lymph node
7 Splenius capitis
8 Lesser occipital nerve
9 Sternocleidomastoid
10 Great auricular nerve
11 Parotid gland and facial nerve branches at anterior border
12 Superficial temporal vessels and auriculotemporal nerve
13 Transverse facial vessels
14 Accessory parotid gland
15 Parotid duct
16 Masseter
17 Facial vein
18 Buccinator
19 Facial artery
20 Zygomaticus major
21 Zygomaticus minor
22 Levator labii superioris

● The risorius muscle has no bony attachment. It normally passes from the parotid fascia to the skin at the angle of the mouth, but is at a lower level in this specimen.

● The five branches (groups of branches) of the facial nerve on the face fan out from the anterior border of the parotid gland.

● Embedded within the parotid gland are the facial nerve, the retromandibular vein (page 38), the external carotid artery and its terminal branches (maxillary and superficial temporal – page 40), filaments from the auriculotemporal nerve (which convey to the gland secretomotor fibres from the otic ganglion – page 49), and lymph nodes.

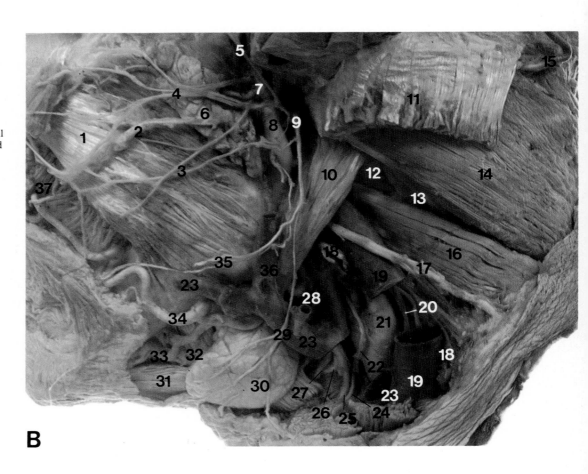

B

23 Levator labii superioris alaeque nasi
24 Orbicularis oculi
25 Orbicularis oris
26 Depressor labii inferioris
27 Mentalis
28 Depressor anguli oris
29 Risorius (aberrant)
30 Platysma
31 Submandibular gland
32 Transverse cutaneous nerve of neck
33 Internal jugular vein
34 Cervical branch of facial nerve
35 Submandibular lymph nodes
36 Marginal mandibular branch of facial nerve
37 External jugular vein

C The neck, from the front. Superficial dissection

(On the left the omohyoid has been displaced upwards and the sternocleidomastoid removed)

 1 Great auricular nerve
 2 Sternocleidomastoid
 3 Transverse cutaneous nerve of neck
 4 Internal jugular vein
 5 Upper root of ansa cervicalis (descending hypoglossal nerve)
 6 Nerve to superior belly of omohyoid
 7 External carotid artery
 8 Superior thyroid artery
 9 Superior laryngeal artery
10 Superior belly of omohyoid
11 Sternothyroid
12 Sternohyoid
13 Accessory thyroid gland
14 Laryngeal prominence

15 Lower root of ansa cervicalis (descending cervical nerve)
16 Levator scapulae
17 Scalenus medius
18 Suprascapular nerve
19 Trunks of brachial plexus
20 Scalenus anterior
21 Nerve to subclavius
22 Phrenic nerve
23 Clavicle
24 Subclavius
25 Anterior jugular vein
26 Manubrium of sternum
27 Jugular arch
28 Inferior thyroid vein
29 Right lateral lobe of thyroid gland
30 Cricoid cartilage

● For the left side of the neck in this specimen see the next page.

B Left parotid and upper cervical regions, after removal of most of the parotid gland

 1 Masseter
 2 Parotid duct
 3 Buccal }
 4 Zygomatic } branch of facial nerve
 5 Temporal }
 6 Deep part of parotid gland
 7 Superficial temporal artery
 8 External carotid artery
 9 Facial nerve
10 Posterior belly of digastric
11 Sternocleidomastoid
12 Inferior oblique
13 Longissimus capitis
14 Splenius capitis
15 Occipital artery
16 Levator scapulae
17 Spinal part of accessory nerve
18 Branches of cervical plexus
19 Internal jugular vein
20 Vagus nerve
21 Carotid sinus on internal carotid artery
22 Upper root of ansa cervicalis (descending hypoglossal nerve)
23 Facial vein
24 External laryngeal nerve
25 Superior thyroid artery
26 Internal laryngeal nerve
27 Superior laryngeal artery
28 Common origin of lingual and facial arteries
29 Cervical branch of facial nerve
30 Submandibular gland
31 Anterior belly of digastric
32 Mylohyoid
33 Submental artery
34 Facial artery
35 Marginal mandibular branch of facial nerve
36 Anterior branch of retromandibular vein
37 Buccinator

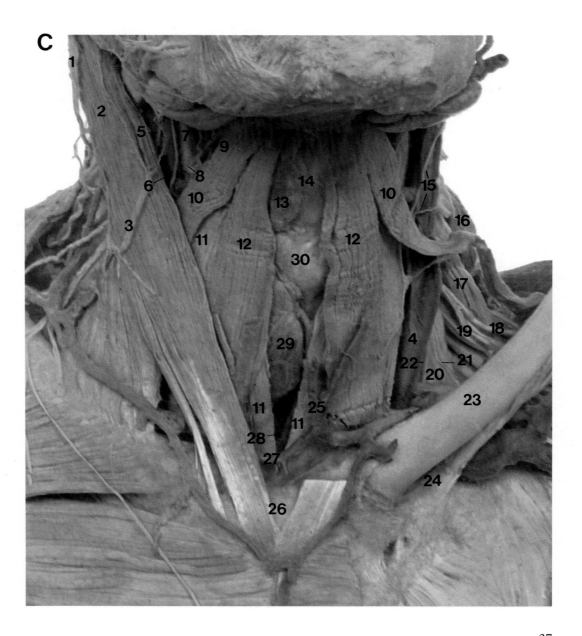

Left infratemporal fossa and the side of the neck

(After removal of much of the zygomatic arch, temporalis muscle, ramus of the mandible, parotid gland and sternocleidomastoid)

1 Temporalis
2 Maxillary nerve
3 Maxillary artery
4 Upper head of lateral pterygoid (partly removed)
5 Deep temporal nerve
6 Buccal nerve
7 Lower head of lateral pterygoid
8 Lateral (temporomandibular) ligament
9 Auriculotemporal nerve
10 Superficial temporal artery
11 Facial nerve
12 Retromandibular vein
13 Parotid gland
14 Splenius capitis
15 Deep cervical lymph nodes
16 Levator scapulae
17 Spinal part of accessory nerve
18 Cervical plexus
19 Scalenus medius
20 Long thoracic nerve
21 Inferior belly of omohyoid (displaced upwards)
22 Nerve to subclavius and phrenic nerve
23 Internal jugular vein
24 Ansa cervicalis
25 Sternothyroid
26 Sternohyoid
27 Superior belly of omohyoid
28 Upper root of ansa cervicalis (descending hypoglossal nerve)
29 Superior thyroid artery
30 Superior thyroid vein
31 External laryngeal nerve
32 Lower root of ansa cervicalis (descending cervical nerve)
33 External carotid artery
34 Inferior constrictor
35 Submandibular gland
36 Submandibular lymph nodes
37 Facial vein
38 Facial artery
39 Nerve to mylohyoid
40 Inferior alveolar nerve and artery
41 Medial pterygoid
42 Lingual nerve
43 Lingual branch of inferior alveolar artery
44 Buccinator
45 Parotid duct

● In the infratemporal fossa the lingual and inferior alveolar nerves emerge between the two pterygoid muscles, the lingual nerve lying about 1 cm anterior to the inferior alveolar.

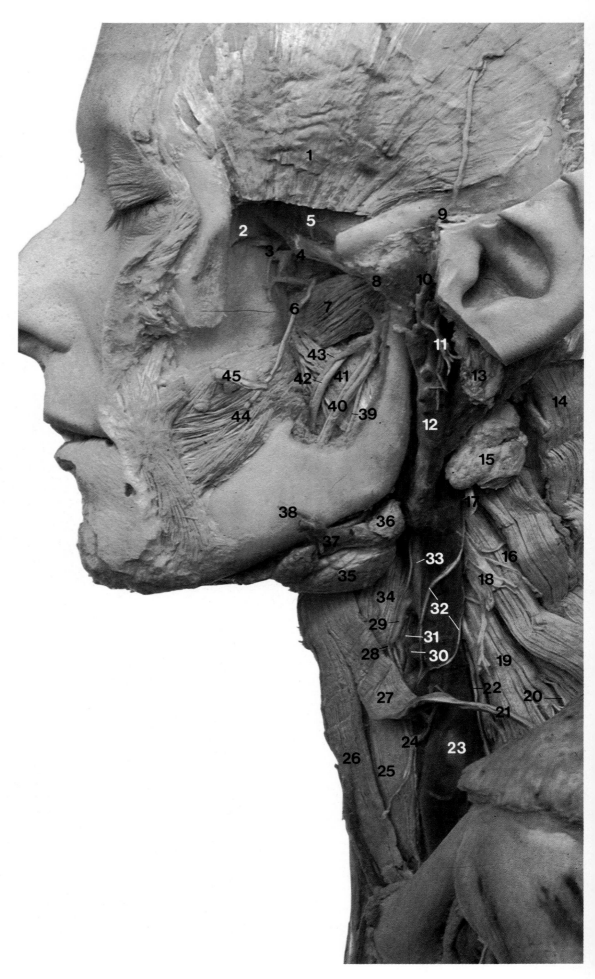

The neck and thoracic inlet from the front.
Deep dissection

(After removal of superficial muscles, major vessels, sternum, clavicles and costal cartilages)

1 Mandible
2 Anterior belly of digastric
3 Mylohyoid
4 Geniohyoid
5 Lingual nerve
6 Hypoglossal nerve
7 Hyoglossus
8 Internal laryngeal nerve
9 External laryngeal nerve
10 Sympathetic trunk
11 Vagus nerve
12 Phrenic nerve
13 Scalenus anterior
14 Ventral ramus of fifth cervical nerve
15 Ventral ramus of sixth cervical nerve
16 Ventral ramus of seventh cervical nerve
17 Ventral ramus of eighth cervical nerve
18 First rib
19 Cervicothoracic (stellate) ganglion
20 Apex of lung
21 Internal thoracic artery
22 Subclavian artery and ansa subclavia
23 Recurrent laryngeal nerve
24 Common carotid artery
25 Trachea
26 Brachiocephalic vein
27 Thyroidea ima artery
28 Brachiocephalic trunk
29 Isthmus ⎫
30 Lateral lobe ⎬ of thyroid gland
31 Pyramidal lobe ⎭
32 Suprascapular artery
33 Superficial cervical artery
34 Cricothyroid
35 Thyrohyoid
36 Levator glandulae thyroideae
37 Laryngeal prominence
38 Body of hyoid bone
39 Sternohyoid
40 Superior thyroid artery
41 External carotid artery
42 Lingual artery
43 Facial artery

● As in this specimen, a pyramidal lobe of the thyroid gland is often present. The occasional thyroidea ima artery is here unusually large.

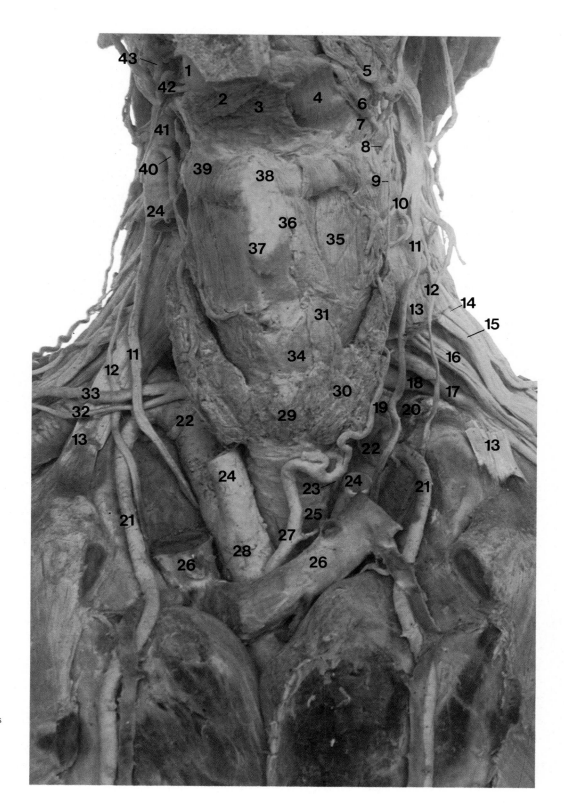

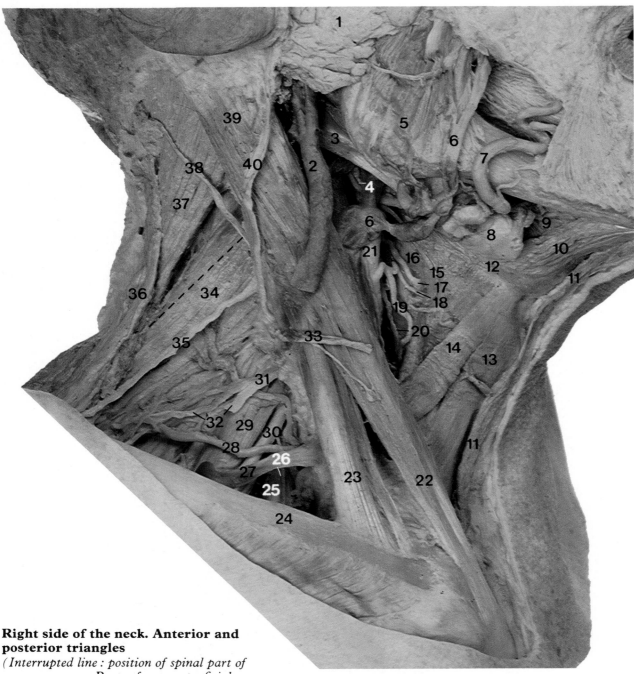

Right side of the neck. Anterior and posterior triangles

(Interrupted line: position of spinal part of accessory nerve. Parts of some superficial nerves and the external jugular vein have been removed)

1 Parotid gland
2 External jugular vein
3 Posterior belly of digastric
4 Hypoglossal nerve
5 Masseter
6 Facial vein
7 Facial artery
8 Submandibular gland
9 Mylohyoid
10 Anterior belly of digastric
11 Anterior jugular vein
12 Greater horn of hyoid bone
13 Sternohyoid
14 Superior belly of omohyoid
15 Thyrohyoid and nerve
16 Thyrohyoid membrane

17 Internal laryngeal nerve
18 Superior laryngeal artery
19 Superior thyroid artery
20 External laryngeal nerve
21 External carotid artery
22 Sternal head of sternocleidomastoid
23 Clavicular head of sternocleidomastoid
24 Clavicle
25 Scalenus anterior
26 Branch of fifth cervical nerve to phrenic nerve
27 Inferior belly of omohyoid
28 Superficial cervical artery
29 Scalenus medius
30 Ventral ramus of fifth cervical nerve
31 Ventral ramus of fourth cervical nerve
32 Supraclavicular nerves
33 Transverse cutaneous nerve of neck

34 Levator scapulae
35 Cervical nerve to trapezius
36 Trapezius
37 Splenius capitis
38 Lesser occipital nerve
39 Sternocleidomastoid
40 Great auricular nerve

● The spinal part of the accessory nerve that crosses the posterior triangle has been removed with the deep cervical fascia; its position overlying levator scapulae is indicated by the interrupted line.

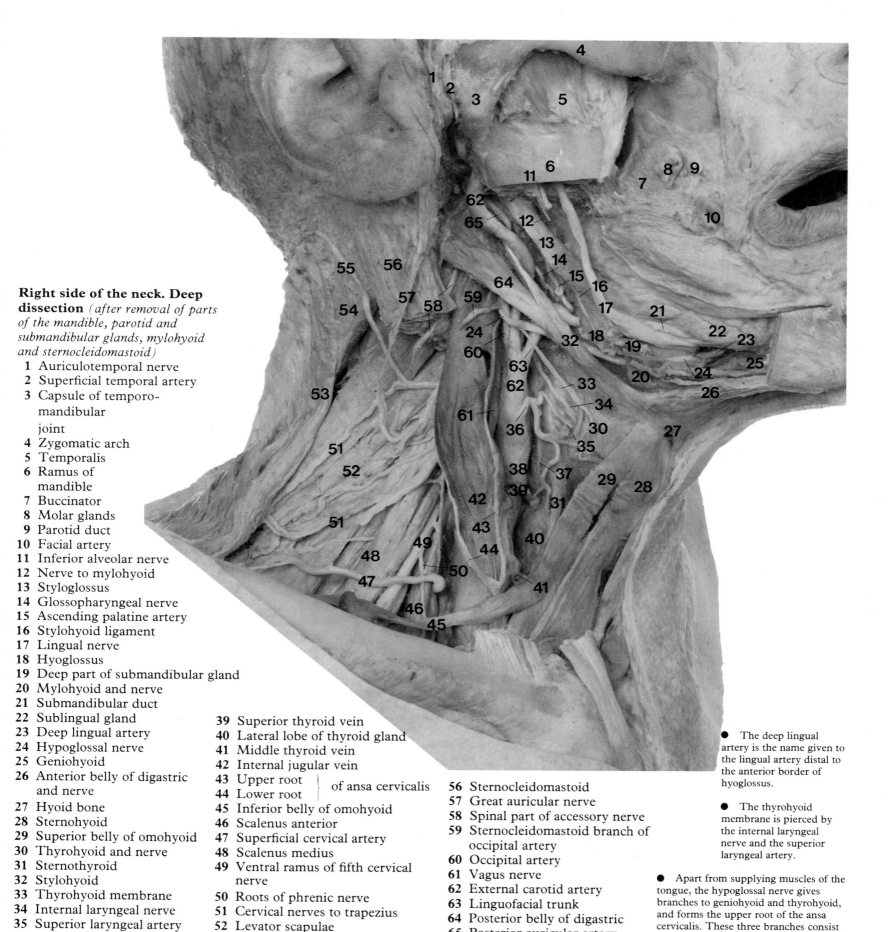

Right side of the neck. Deep dissection *(after removal of parts of the mandible, parotid and submandibular glands, mylohyoid and sternocleidomastoid)*

1 Auriculotemporal nerve
2 Superficial temporal artery
3 Capsule of temporo-mandibular joint
4 Zygomatic arch
5 Temporalis
6 Ramus of mandible
7 Buccinator
8 Molar glands
9 Parotid duct
10 Facial artery
11 Inferior alveolar nerve
12 Nerve to mylohyoid
13 Styloglossus
14 Glossopharyngeal nerve
15 Ascending palatine artery
16 Stylohyoid ligament
17 Lingual nerve
18 Hyoglossus
19 Deep part of submandibular gland
20 Mylohyoid and nerve
21 Submandibular duct
22 Sublingual gland
23 Deep lingual artery
24 Hypoglossal nerve
25 Geniohyoid
26 Anterior belly of digastric and nerve
27 Hyoid bone
28 Sternohyoid
29 Superior belly of omohyoid
30 Thyrohyoid and nerve
31 Sternothyroid
32 Stylohyoid
33 Thyrohyoid membrane
34 Internal laryngeal nerve
35 Superior laryngeal artery
36 Superior thyroid artery
37 External laryngeal nerve
38 Common carotid artery

39 Superior thyroid vein
40 Lateral lobe of thyroid gland
41 Middle thyroid vein
42 Internal jugular vein
43 Upper root ⎱ of ansa cervicalis
44 Lower root ⎰
45 Inferior belly of omohyoid
46 Scalenus anterior
47 Superficial cervical artery
48 Scalenus medius
49 Ventral ramus of fifth cervical nerve
50 Roots of phrenic nerve
51 Cervical nerves to trapezius
52 Levator scapulae
53 Trapezius
54 Splenius capitis
55 Lesser occipital nerve

56 Sternocleidomastoid
57 Great auricular nerve
58 Spinal part of accessory nerve
59 Sternocleidomastoid branch of occipital artery
60 Occipital artery
61 Vagus nerve
62 External carotid artery
63 Linguofacial trunk
64 Posterior belly of digastric
65 Posterior auricular artery

● The deep lingual artery is the name given to the lingual artery distal to the anterior border of hyoglossus.

● The thyrohyoid membrane is pierced by the internal laryngeal nerve and the superior laryngeal artery.

● Apart from supplying muscles of the tongue, the hypoglossal nerve gives branches to geniohyoid and thyrohyoid, and forms the upper root of the ansa cervicalis. These three branches consist of the fibres from the first cervical nerve that have joined the hypoglossal nerve higher in the neck; they are not derived from the hypoglossal nucleus.

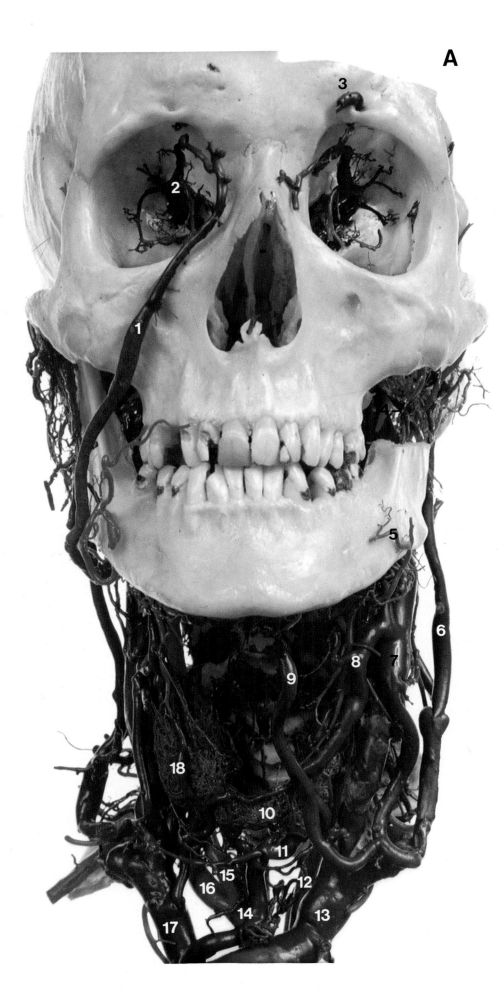

A Cast of vessels of the head and neck, from the front

1 Facial vein
2 Ophthalmic veins
3 Supra-orbital vein
4 Maxillary artery and pterygoid venous plexus
5 Facial artery
6 External jugular vein
7 Internal jugular vein
8 Superior thyroid vessels
9 Anterior jugular vein
10 Vessels of isthmus of thyroid gland
11 Inferior thyroid veins
12 Left common carotid artery
13 Left brachiocephalic vein
14 Brachiocephalic trunk
15 Right common carotid artery
16 Right subclavian artery
17 Right brachiocephalic vein
18 Vessels of lateral lobe of thyroid

B Cast of vessels of the head and neck, from the right

1 Posterior external jugular vein
2 Occipital vessels
3 External vertebral venous plexus
4 Posterior auricular vessels
5 Retromandibular vein
6 Transverse facial branch of superficial temporal artery
7 Pterygoid venous plexus
8 Facial vein
9 Facial artery
10 Submental artery
11 Anterior jugular vein
12 Superior thyroid vessels
13 Internal jugular vein
14 External jugular vein
15 Subclavian vein
16 Brachiocephalic vein
17 Subclavian artery
18 First rib
19 Internal thoracic artery

C Cast of the head and neck arteries of a full-term fetus, from the left

● The tongue and the thyroid gland are clearly outlined.

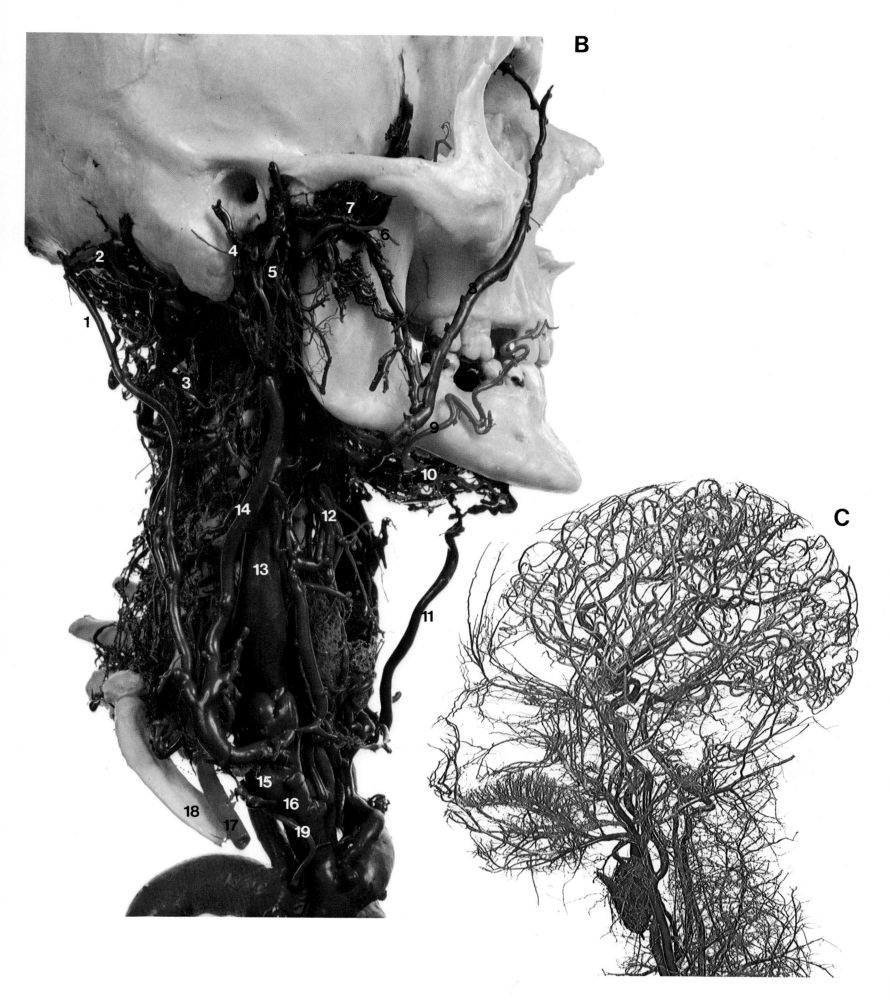

43

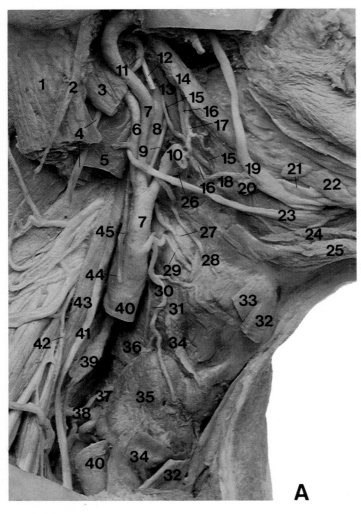

A

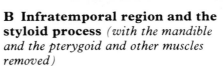

B

A Right side of the neck. Deep dissection and lateral lobe of the thyroid gland
1 Sternocleidomastoid
2 Great auricular nerve
3 Posterior belly of digastric
4 Spinal part of accessory nerve
5 Internal jugular vein
6 Occipital artery
7 External carotid artery
8 Internal carotid artery
9 Ascending pharyngeal artery
10 Facial artery
11 Posterior auricular artery
12 Stylohyoid (cut end displaced medially)
13 Stylopharyngeus
14 Styloglossus
15 Glossopharyngeal nerve
16 Stylohyoid ligament
17 Ascending palatine artery
18 Hyoglossus
19 Lingual nerve
20 Submandibular ganglion
21 Submandibular duct
22 Sublingual gland
23 Hypoglossal nerve
24 Mylohyoid
25 Anterior belly of digastric
26 Lingual artery

27 Internal laryngeal nerve
28 Thyrohyoid and nerve
29 Superior laryngeal artery
30 Superior thyroid artery
31 External laryngeal nerve
32 Sternothyroid
33 Superior belly of omohyoid
34 Sternohyoid
35 Lateral lobe of thyroid gland
36 Inferior constrictor
37 Recurrent laryngeal nerve
38 Inferior thyroid artery
39 Middle cervical sympathetic ganglion
40 Common carotid artery
41 Vagus nerve
42 Phrenic nerve
43 Scalenus anterior
44 Carotid sinus
45 Lower root of ansa cervicalis

B Infratemporal region and the styloid process *(with the mandible and the pterygoid and other muscles removed)*
1 Posterior wall of maxilla
2 Maxillary artery
3 Lateral pterygoid plate
4 Tensor veli palatini
5 Nerve to medial pterygoid
6 Mandibular nerve
7 Lingual nerve
8 Chorda tympani
9 Roots of auriculotemporal nerve
10 Accessory meningeal artery
11 Middle meningeal artery
12 Superficial temporal artery
13 External acoustic meatus
14 External carotid artery
15 Styloid process
16 Stylohyoid
17 Internal jugular vein
18 Spinal part of accessory nerve
19 Styloglossus
20 Stylopharyngeus
21 Ascending palatine artery
22 Glossopharyngeal nerve
23 Pharyngeal branch of glossopharyngeal nerve
24 Internal carotid artery

25 Superior laryngeal nerve
26 Ascending pharyngeal artery
27 Vagus nerve
28 Hypoglossal nerve
29 Occipital artery
30 Sternocleidomastoid artery
31 Upper root of ansa cervicalis
32 Lingual artery
33 Stylohyoid ligament
34 Facial artery
35 Hyoglossus
36 Submandibular gland (deep part)
37 Mylohyoid and nerve
38 Periosteum of mandible
39 Buccinator
40 Superior constrictor
41 Parotid duct
42 Molar glands
43 Levator veli palatini

● The roots of the auriculotemporal nerve embrace the middle meningeal artery.
● In this specimen the ascending palatine artery, normally a branch of the facial, is large and has an unusually low origin from the external carotid. The sternocleidomastoid branch of the occipital artery here has a direct origin from the external carotid.

Branches of the right trigeminal nerve and related structures, from the left

1 Nasal septum
2 Inferior ⎤
3 Middle ⎥
4 Superior ⎬ concha
5 Supreme ⎦
6 Optic nerve
7 Internal carotid artery
8 Oculomotor nerve
9 Trochlear nerve
10 Abducent nerve
11 Ophthalmic ⎤ branches of
12 Maxillary ⎬ trigeminal
13 Mandibular ⎦ nerve
14 Motor root of trigeminal nerve
15 Trigeminal ganglion
16 Petrous part of temporal bone
17 Trigeminal nerve
18 Pons
19 Jugular bulb
20 Posterior belly of digastric
21 Parotid gland
22 External carotid artery
23 Sphenomandibular ligament and maxillary artery
24 Roots of auriculotemporal nerve
25 Chorda tympani
26 Middle meningeal artery
27 Marker in auditory tube
28 Nerve to medial pterygoid
29 Tensor veli palatini
30 Medial pterygoid
31 Lingual nerve
32 Inferior alveolar nerve
33 Nerve to mylohyoid
34 Submandibular ganglion
35 Submandibular gland
36 Stylohyoid ligament
37 Lingual artery
38 Hyoglossus
39 Body of hyoid bone
40 Mylohyoid
41 Geniohyoid
42 Genioglossus
43 Sublingual gland
44 Submandibular duct
45 Hypoglossal nerve

● In this specimen much of the right petrous temporal bone has been removed, and the right cavernous sinus has been opened from the medial side, so revealing from this aspect the nerves that normally lie in the sinus – the ophthalmic, maxillary, oculomotor, trochlear and abducent.
● The occasional supreme (highest) concha is present in this specimen.
● The chorda tympani leaves the skull through the petrotympanic fissure and joins the posterior aspect of the lingual nerve about 2 cm below the skull.

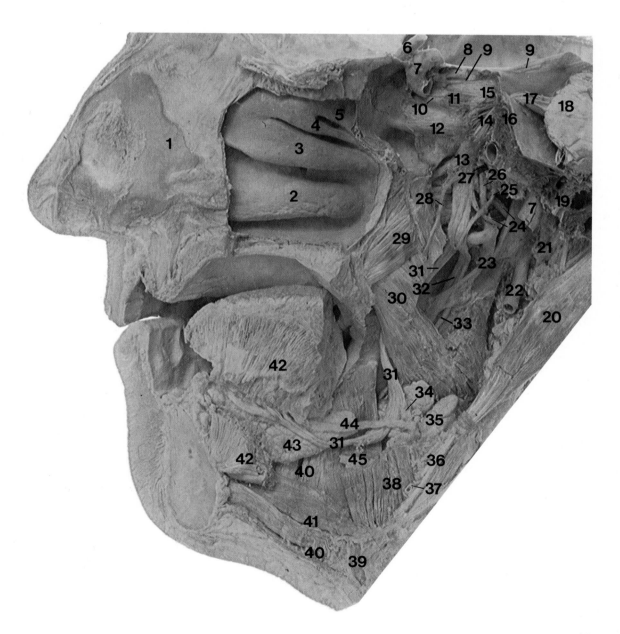

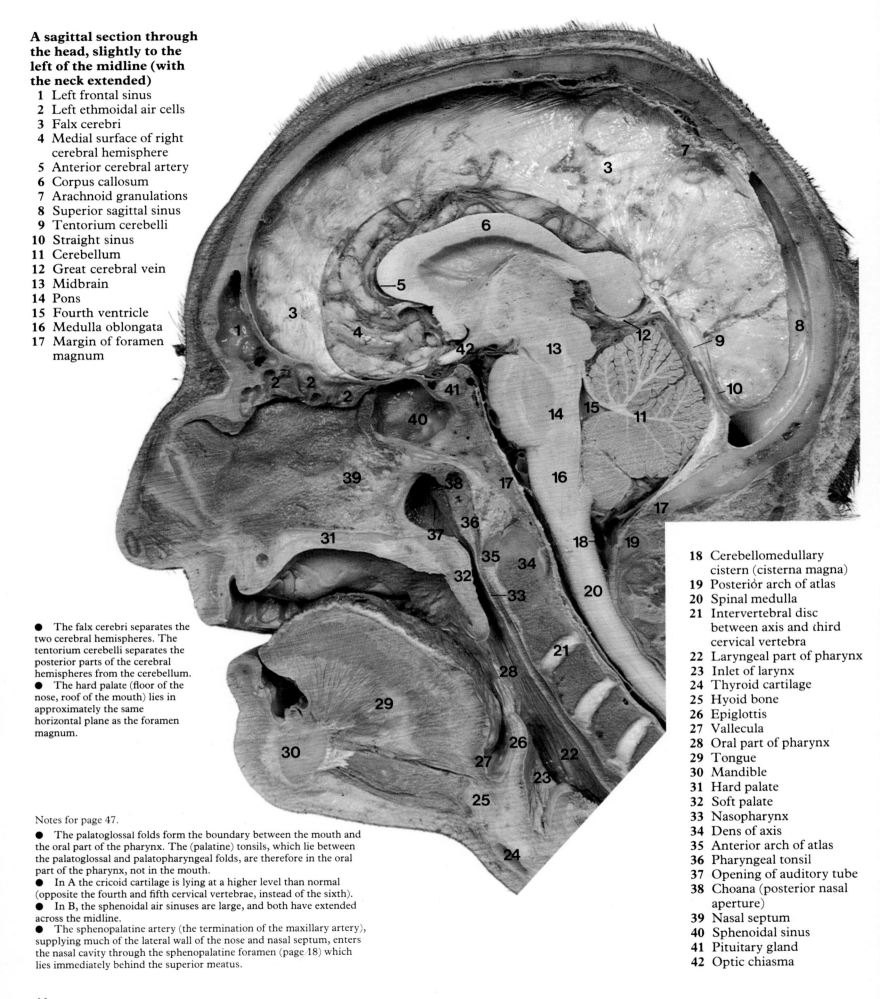

A sagittal section through the head, slightly to the left of the midline (with the neck extended)

1 Left frontal sinus
2 Left ethmoidal air cells
3 Falx cerebri
4 Medial surface of right cerebral hemisphere
5 Anterior cerebral artery
6 Corpus callosum
7 Arachnoid granulations
8 Superior sagittal sinus
9 Tentorium cerebelli
10 Straight sinus
11 Cerebellum
12 Great cerebral vein
13 Midbrain
14 Pons
15 Fourth ventricle
16 Medulla oblongata
17 Margin of foramen magnum

● The falx cerebri separates the two cerebral hemispheres. The tentorium cerebelli separates the posterior parts of the cerebral hemispheres from the cerebellum.
● The hard palate (floor of the nose, roof of the mouth) lies in approximately the same horizontal plane as the foramen magnum.

Notes for page 47.

● The palatoglossal folds form the boundary between the mouth and the oral part of the pharynx. The (palatine) tonsils, which lie between the palatoglossal and palatopharyngeal folds, are therefore in the oral part of the pharynx, not in the mouth.
● In A the cricoid cartilage is lying at a higher level than normal (opposite the fourth and fifth cervical vertebrae, instead of the sixth).
● In B, the sphenoidal air sinuses are large, and both have extended across the midline.
● The sphenopalatine artery (the termination of the maxillary artery), supplying much of the lateral wall of the nose and nasal septum, enters the nasal cavity through the sphenopalatine foramen (page 18) which lies immediately behind the superior meatus.

18 Cerebellomedullary cistern (cisterna magna)
19 Posterior arch of atlas
20 Spinal medulla
21 Intervertebral disc between axis and third cervical vertebra
22 Laryngeal part of pharynx
23 Inlet of larynx
24 Thyroid cartilage
25 Hyoid bone
26 Epiglottis
27 Vallecula
28 Oral part of pharynx
29 Tongue
30 Mandible
31 Hard palate
32 Soft palate
33 Nasopharynx
34 Dens of axis
35 Anterior arch of atlas
36 Pharyngeal tonsil
37 Opening of auditory tube
38 Choana (posterior nasal aperture)
39 Nasal septum
40 Sphenoidal sinus
41 Pituitary gland
42 Optic chiasma

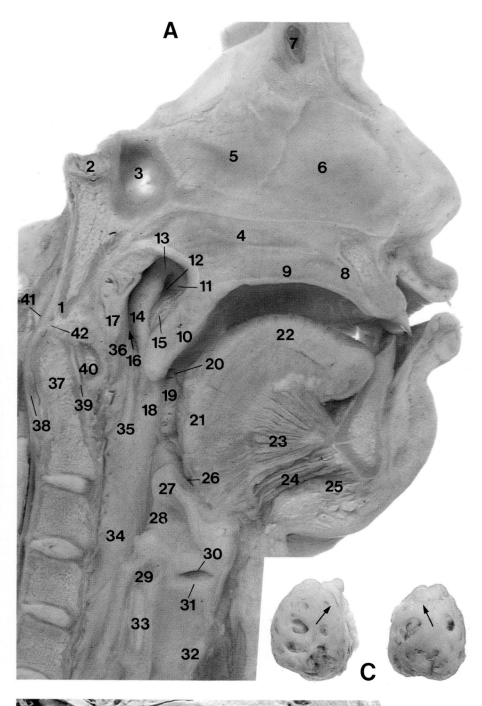

A

The nose, mouth, pharynx and larynx in a midline sagittal section, from the right, A with the nasal septum intact, B the left nasal cavity with the nasal septum removed

1 Anterior margin of foramen magnum
2 Pituitary gland
3 Left sphenoidal sinus
4 Vomer
5 Perpendicular plate of ethmoid
6 Septal cartilage
7 Frontal sinus
8 Incisive canal
9 Hard palate
10 Soft palate
11 Salpingopalatal fold
12 Opening of auditory tube
13 Tubal elevation
14 Salpingopharyngeal fold
15 Levator elevation
16 Pharyngeal recess
17 Pharyngeal tonsil
18 Palatopharyngeal fold
19 Palatine tonsil
20 Palatoglossal fold
21 Pharyngeal ⎫
22 Oral ⎬ part of dorsum of tongue
23 Genioglossus
24 Geniohyoid
25 Mylohyoid
26 Vallecula
27 Epiglottis
28 Aryepiglottic fold
29 Arytenoid cartilage
30 Vestibular fold
31 Vocal fold
32 Arch ⎫
33 Lamina ⎬ of cricoid cartilage
34 Laryngeal ⎫
35 Oral ⎬ part of pharynx
36 Nasal ⎭
37 Dens of axis
38 Transverse ligament of atlas
39 Median atlanto-axial joint
40 Anterior arch of atlas
41 Tectorial membrane
42 Apical ligament of dens
43 Intercavernous venous sinus
44 Optic nerve
45 Right sphenoidal sinus
46 Spheno-ethmoidal recess

47 Superior concha
48 Superior meatus
49 Middle concha
50 Middle meatus
51 Inferior concha
52 Inferior meatus
53 Atrium
54 Vestibule

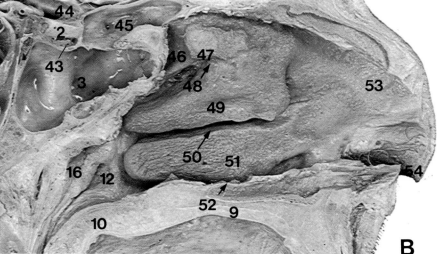

B

C The palatine tonsils. Medial surface (operation specimens from a child aged 14)

● The openings of the tonsillar crypts are seen on the surface. The arrow indicates the intratonsillar cleft (the remains of the embryonic second pharyngeal pouch).

● The palatine tonsils (commonly called simply 'the tonsils') are masses of lymphoid tissue that are frequently enlarged in childhood but become much reduced in size in later life. Together with the lymphoid tissue in the posterior part of the tongue (lingual tonsil) and in the posterior wall of the nasopharynx (pharyngeal tonsil), they form a protective 'ring' of lymphoid tissue at the upper end of the respiratory and alimentary tracts.

A

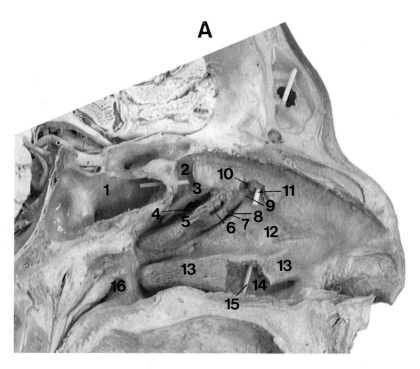

A Lateral wall of the left nasal cavity in a midline sagittal section of the head. Openings of the paranasal sinuses
(The middle concha and part of the inferior concha have been removed)

1 Left sphenoidal sinus
2 Spheno-ethmoidal recess
3 Superior concha
4 Superior meatus
5 Cut edge of middle concha
6 Ethmoidal bulla and opening of middle ethmoidal air cells
7 Semilunar hiatus
8 Marker in opening of maxillary sinus
9 Ethmoidal infundibulum
10 Opening of anterior ethmoidal air cells
11 Marker in frontonasal duct (opening of frontal sinus)
12 Middle meatus
13 Inferior concha
14 Inferior meatus
15 Marker in opening of nasolacrimal duct
16 Opening of auditory tube

● The sphenoidal sinus opens into the spheno-ethmoidal recess.
● The posterior ethmoidal air cells open into the superior meatus, the middle cells on or above the ethmoidal bulla, and the anterior cells into the infundibulum or frontonasal duct.
● The frontal sinus opens into the middle meatus by the frontonasal duct or via the infundibulum, which is the upward and anterior continuation of the semilunar hiatus.
● The maxillary sinus opens into the semilunar hiatus of the middle meatus; occasionally there are two openings, one of which may be below the hiatus (as in the specimen on the page opposite).
● The nasolacrimal duct opens into the inferior meatus.

● The olfactory area of the nasal mucosa occupies the mucosa overlying the superior concha, the corresponding part of the septum and the adjacent part of the roof of the nose.
● The nerve of the pterygoid canal is formed by the union of the greater petrosal nerve (from the facial) and the deep petrosal nerve (from the sympathetic plexus round the internal carotid artery – the internal carotid nerve).

B

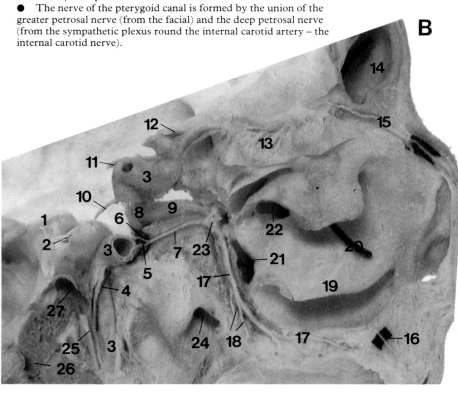

B Left nasal cavity and pterygopalatine ganglion, from the right
(See note opposite for an explanation of this dissection)

1 Arcuate eminence
2 Internal acoustic meatus and facial nerve
3 Internal carotid artery
4 Internal carotid (sympathetic) nerve
5 Deep petrosal nerve
6 Greater petrosal nerve
7 Nerve of pterygoid canal
8 Trigeminal ganglion
9 Maxillary nerve
10 Abducent nerve
11 Oculomotor nerve
12 Optic nerve
13 Olfactory nerve filaments
14 Frontal sinus and marker
15 Anterior ethmoidal nerve
16 Left nasopalatine nerve
17 Greater palatine nerve
18 Lesser palatine nerves
19 Inferior concha
20 Marker emerging from frontonasal duct in middle meatus
21 Artificial opening into maxillary sinus and marker
22 Opening of maxillary sinus and marker
23 Pterygopalatine ganglion
24 Opening of auditory tube and marker
25 Inferior ganglion of vagus nerve
26 Vertebral artery
27 Internal jugular vein

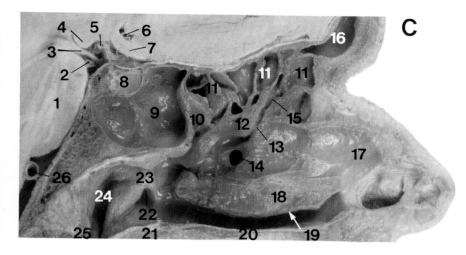

C Lateral wall of the left nasal cavity. Ethmoidal air cells and bulla

(In a midline sagittal section of the head after removal of the superior and middle conchae)

1 Pons	**15** Ethmoidal infundibulum
2 Superior cerebellar artery	**16** Frontal sinus
3 Oculomotor nerve	**17** Atrium
4 Mamillary body	**18** Inferior concha
5 Posterior cerebral artery	**19** Inferior meatus
6 Anterior cerebral artery	**20** Hard palate
7 Optic nerve	**21** Soft palate
8 Pituitary gland	**22** Opening of auditory tube
9 Sphenoidal sinus	**23** Tubal elevation
10 Spheno-ethmoidal recess	**24** Pharyngeal recess
11 Ethmoidal air cells	**25** Pharyngeal tonsil
12 Ethmoidal bulla	**26** Basilar artery (tortuous)
13 Semilunar hiatus	
14 Opening of maxillary sinus (unusually low)	

● When enlarged the lymphoid tissue of the pharyngeal tonsil constitutes the adenoids.

● The opening of the auditory tube lies just over 1 cm behind the posterior end of the inferior concha.

● The *greater* petrosal nerve is a branch of the facial nerve. The *lesser* petrosal nerve, although having a communication with the facial nerve (and appearing in D to be a branch of the facial), is derived from the tympanic branch of the glossopharyngeal nerve via the tympanic plexus (on the medial wall of the middle ear, which has been removed in D).

● In the dissection on page 48, the whole of the right half of the skull and part of the left side of the skull have been removed so that the left pterygoid canal could be opened up and the left pterygopalatine ganglion viewed from the medial side. In the dissection on this page, part of the right side of the skull has been removed; the medial sides of the orbit and maxillary sinus remain, and the right trigeminal nerve and right pterygopalatine ganglion are displayed from the lateral side.

D Right trigeminal nerve, petrosal nerves and associated ganglia

(See note for an explanation of this dissection)

1 Genicular ganglion of facial nerve
2 Greater ⎫
3 Lesser ⎬ petrosal nerve
4 Trigeminal ganglion
5 Mandibular nerve
6 Maxillary nerve
7 Ophthalmic nerve
8 Free margin of tentorium cerebelli
9 Oculomotor nerve
10 Frontal nerve
11 Nasociliary nerve
12 Bristle in lacrimal canaliculus
13 Medial wall of orbit
14 Medial rectus
15 Optic nerve
16 Inferior rectus
17 Ciliary ganglion
18 Lacrimal nerve
19 Pterygopalatine ganglion
20 Nerve of pterygoid canal
21 Greater and lesser palatine nerves
22 Medial wall of maxillary sinus and opening
23 Muscular branches of mandibular nerve
24 Lower head of lateral pterygoid and lateral pterygoid plate
25 Lingual nerve
26 Medial pterygoid
27 Tensor veli palatini
28 Chorda tympani
29 Otic ganglion
30 Facial nerve
31 Position of tympanic membrane
32 Glossopharyngeal nerve
33 Internal carotid artery
34 Occipital artery
35 External carotid artery
36 Hypoglossal nerve
37 Internal jugular vein and spinal part of accessory nerve
38 Transverse process of atlas
39 Rectus capitis lateralis

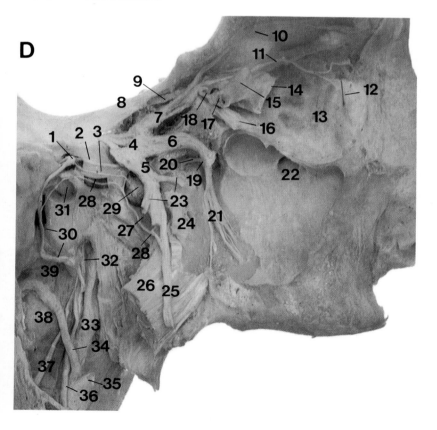

A The pharynx, from behind with the posterior part of the skull removed

1 Internal acoustic meatus with facial and vestibulocochlear nerves
2 Trigeminal nerve
3 Abducent nerve
4 Trochlear nerve
5 Optic nerve
6 Oculomotor nerve
7 Dura mater overlying clivus
8 Pharyngobasilar fascia
9 Glossopharyngeal nerve
10 Styloid process and stylopharyngeus
11 Posterior border of ramus of mandible
12 Masseter
13 Medial pterygoid

14 Thyropharyngeal ⎤ part of inferior
15 Cricopharyngeal ⎦ constrictor
16 Oesophagus
17 Middle constrictor
18 Superior constrictor
19 Pharyngeal raphe

● For the pharynx from the side see pages 41 and 44.
● The pharynx extends from the base of the skull to the level of the sixth cervical vertebra. The nasal part (nasopharynx), as far down as the lower border of the soft palate, contains the opening of the auditory tube, the pharyngeal tonsil and the pharyngeal recesses and opens anteriorly into the nasal cavity. The oral part, between the soft palate and the upper border of the epiglottis, contains the (palatine) tonsils, and opens into the mouth. The laryngeal part, below the upper border of the epiglottis, contains the piriform recess and opens anteriorly into the larynx, becoming continuous below with the oesophagus.

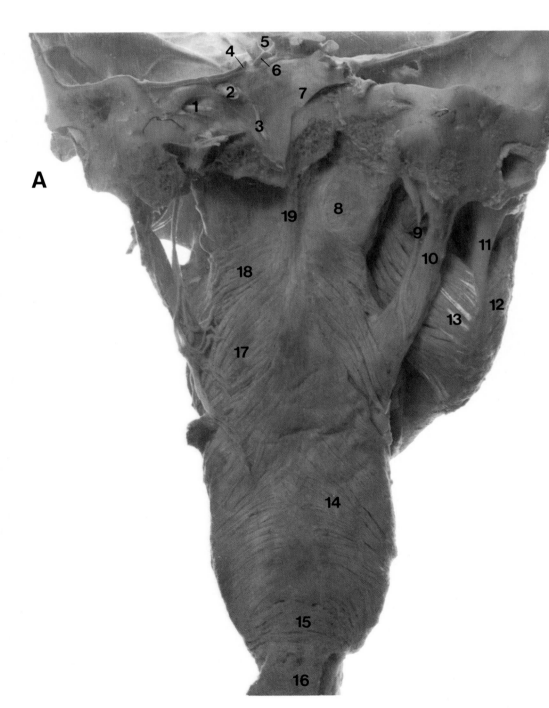

A

C The soft palate, from behind
(After removal of the pharynx and part of the base of the skull)

1 Groove for sigmoid sinus
2 Tympanic membrane
3 Apex of petrous part of temporal bone
4 Internal carotid artery
5 Clivus
6 Vomer (nasal septum)
7 Soft palate
8 Uvula
9 Marker in auditory tube
10 Levator veli palatini
11 Tensor veli palatini (superficial to marker)
12 Pterygoid hamulus
13 Tendon of tensor veli palatini
14 Styloid process
15 Part of stylomandibular ligament
16 Sphenomandibular ligament
17 Angle of mandible

● All the muscles of the pharynx and soft palate are supplied by the cranial part of the accessory nerve through the branches of the vagus that join the pharyngeal plexus, except for the stylopharyngeus which is supplied by the glossopharyngeal nerve and the tensor veli palatini by a branch from the nerve to the medial pterygoid muscle (mandibular nerve).

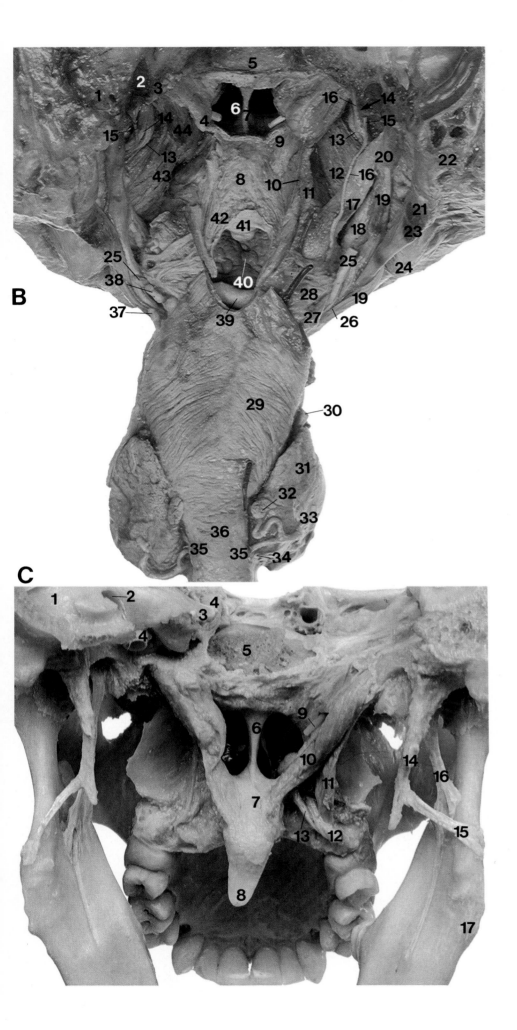

51

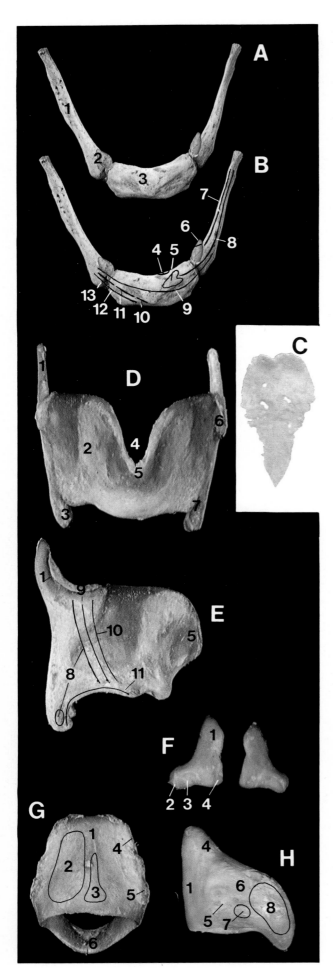

The hyoid bone, A from above and in front, B with muscle attachments
1 Greater horn
2 Lesser horn
3 Body
4 Genioglossus
5 Geniohyoid
6 Stylohyoid ligament
7 Middle constrictor
8 Hyoglossus
9 Mylohyoid
10 Sternohyoid
11 Omohyoid
12 Thyrohyoid
13 Stylohyoid

C The cartilage of the epiglottis, from the front. D The thyroid cartilage from the front, E from the right with attachments
1 Superior horn
2 Lamina
3 Inferior horn
4 Thyroid notch
5 Laryngeal prominence (Adam's apple)
6 Superior ⎱ tubercle
7 Inferior ⎰
8 Inferior constrictor
9 Sternothyroid
10 Thyrohyoid
11 Cricothyroid

F The arytenoid cartilages, from behind
1 Apex
2 Muscular process
3 Articular surface for cricoid cartilage
4 Vocal process

The cricoid cartilage and muscle attachments, G from behind and below, H from the right
1 Lamina
2 Posterior crico-arytenoid
3 Tendon of oesophagus
4 Articular surface for arytenoid cartilage
5 Articular surface for inferior horn of thyroid cartilage
6 Arch
7 Inferior constrictor
8 Cricothyroid

J The larynx from behind, with most of the posterior pharyngeal wall removed
(The left lamina of the thyroid cartilage has been reflected forwards, and a glass rod holds part of the pharynx open)
1 Epiglottis
2 Posterior pharyngeal wall
3 Cuneiform cartilage ⎱ in aryepi-
4 Corniculate cartilage ⎰ glottic fold
5 Transverse arytenoid muscle
6 Branch of internal laryngeal nerve
7 Branches of recurrent laryngeal nerve
8 Tendon of oesophagus
9 Circular fibres of oesophagus
10 Anastomosis between internal and recurrent laryngeal nerves
11 Cricothyroid muscle (reflected forwards with lamina of thyroid cartilage)

K The tongue and the inlet of the larynx, from above
1 Posterior wall of pharynx
2 Corniculate cartilage ⎱ in aryepi-
3 Cuneiform cartilage ⎰ glottic fold
4 Epiglottis
5 Median glosso-epiglottic fold
6 Vallecula
7 Lateral glosso-epiglottic fold
8 Pharyngeal part of dorsum of tongue
9 Foramen caecum
10 Sulcus terminalis
11 Vallate papilla
12 Fungiform papilla
13 Vestibular fold
14 Vocal fold

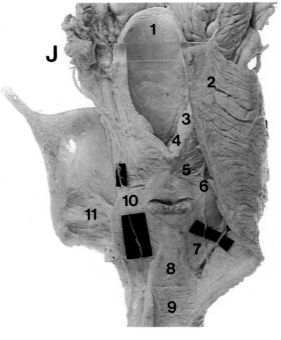

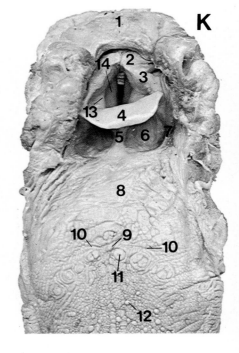

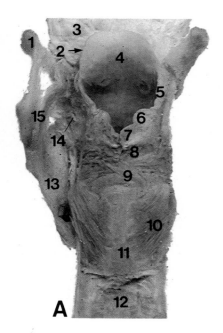
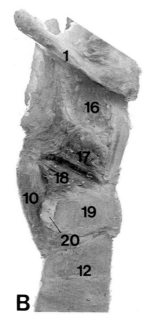
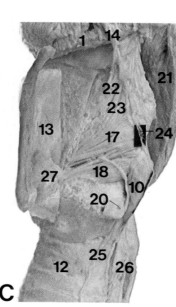

A

B

C

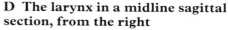

D The larynx in a midline sagittal section, from the right

1 Pharyngeal wall
2 Aryepiglottic fold and inlet of larynx
3 Epiglottis
4 Vallecula
5 Tongue
6 Body of hyoid bone
7 Lamina of thyroid cartilage
8 Vestibular fold
9 Sinus of larynx
10 Vocal fold
11 Arch of cricoid cartilage
12 Isthmus of thyroid gland
13 Trachea
14 Lamina of cricoid cartilage
15 Branches of recurrent laryngeal nerve
16 Transverse arytenoid muscle
17 Branches of internal laryngeal nerve anastomosing with recurrent laryngeal nerve
18 Corniculate cartilage and apex of arytenoid cartilage
19 Internal laryngeal nerve entering piriform recess
20 Vestibule of larynx

Intrinsic muscles of the larynx, A from behind, B from the right (with the right lamina of the thyroid cartilage removed), C from the left (with part of the thyroid lamina reflected forwards)

1 Greater horn of hyoid bone
2 Vallecula
3 Dorsum of tongue
4 Epiglottis
5 Aryepiglottic fold
6 Cuneiform ⎫
7 Corniculate ⎬ cartilage
8 Transverse ⎫
9 Oblique ⎬ arytenoid muscle
10 Posterior crico-arytenoid muscle
11 Area on lamina of cricoid cartilage for tendon of oesophagus
12 Trachea

13 Lamina of thyroid cartilage
14 Internal laryngeal nerve
15 Thyrohyoid membrane
16 Quadrangular membrane
17 Thyro-arytenoid muscle
18 Lateral crico-arytenoid muscle
19 Arch of cricoid cartilage
20 Cricothyroid joint
21 Posterior wall of pharynx
22 Aryepiglottic ⎫
23 Thyro-epiglottic ⎬ muscle
24 Anastomosis of internal and recurrent laryngeal nerves
25 Recurrent laryngeal nerve
26 Oesophagus
27 Cricothyroid muscle (reflected from cricoid attachment)

● In K (opposite) the V-shaped sulcus terminalis, behind the row of vallate papillae, is not well marked in this tongue.
● The fissure between the two vestibular folds is the rima of the vestibule. The fissure between the vocal folds (vocal cords) is the rima of the glottis.
● The vestibular folds are sometimes called the false vocal cords.

● The space between the vestibular and vocal folds is the sinus of the larynx, and this is continuous with the saccule, a small pouch that extends upwards for a few millimetres between the vestibular fold and the inner surface of the thyro-arytenoid muscle.

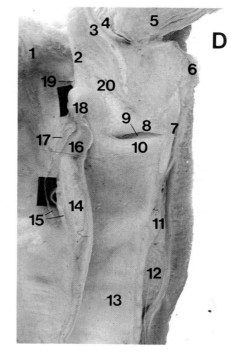

D

E Ligaments and membranes of the right side of the larynx. Internal surfaces, from the left

(After removal of most of the left side of the larynx but with the cricoid cartilage intact)

1 Hyoid bone
2 Hyo-epiglottic ligament
3 Epiglottis
4 Quadrangular membrane
5 Apex ⎫
6 Vocal process ⎬ of arytenoid cartilage
7 Lamina ⎫
8 Arch ⎬ of cricoid cartilage
9 Cricovocal membrane
10 Lamina of thyroid cartilage
11 Thyro-epiglottic ligament

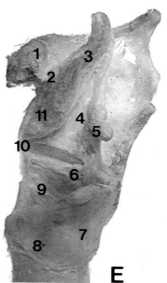

E

● The intrinsic muscles of the larynx are supplied by the recurrent laryngeal nerve, except the cricothyroid which is supplied by the external laryngeal nerve.
● The mucous membrane of the larynx above the level of the vocal folds is supplied by the internal laryngeal nerve, and below the vocal folds by the recurrent laryngeal nerve.
● The recurrent laryngeal nerve enters the larynx by passing beneath the lower border of the inferior constrictor of the pharynx, and here it lies immediately behind the cricothyroid joint.
● The vocal fold (vocal cord) is formed by the upper margin of the cricovocal membrane, which is triangular.
● The vestibular fold (false vocal cord) is formed by the lower margin of the quadrangular membrane, whose upper margin forms the aryepiglottic fold.
● The central (anterior) part of the cricothyroid membrane is usually known as the conus elasticus.

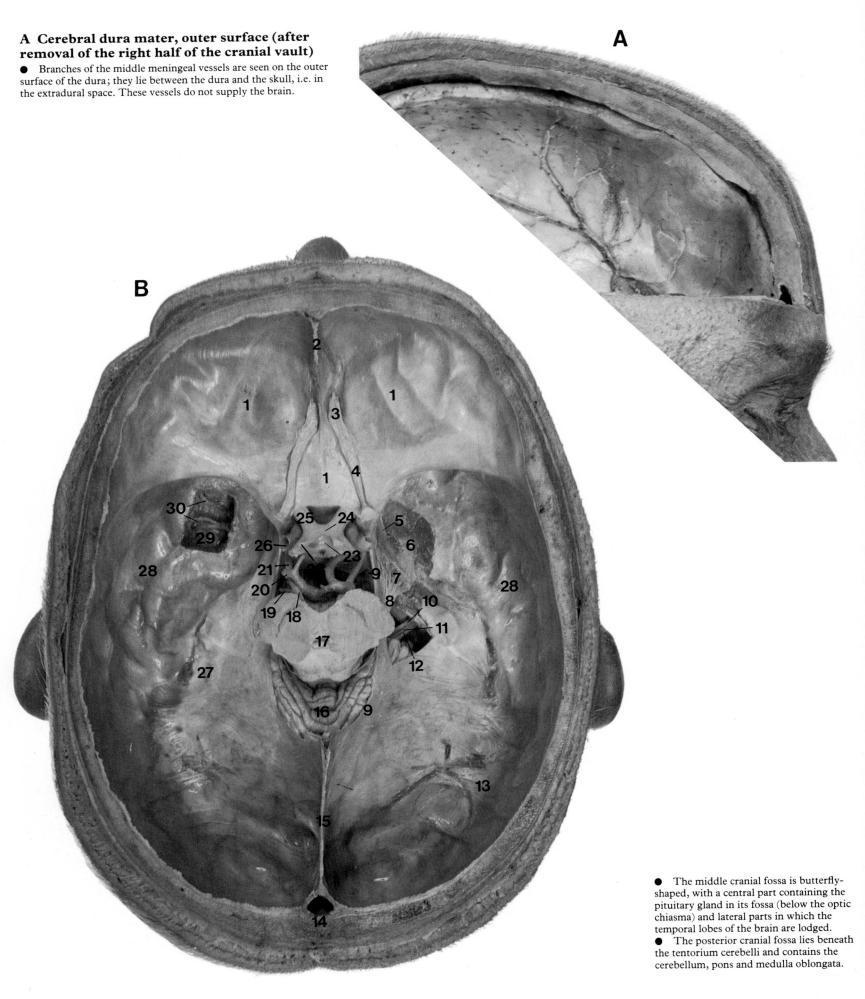

A Cerebral dura mater, outer surface (after removal of the right half of the cranial vault)

● Branches of the middle meningeal vessels are seen on the outer surface of the dura; they lie between the dura and the skull, i.e. in the extradural space. These vessels do not supply the brain.

A

B

● The middle cranial fossa is butterfly-shaped, with a central part containing the pituitary gland in its fossa (below the optic chiasma) and lateral parts in which the temporal lobes of the brain are lodged.
● The posterior cranial fossa lies beneath the tentorium cerebelli and contains the cerebellum, pons and medulla oblongata.

C Cerebral dura mater, falx cerebri, tentorium cerebelli and cranial nerves, on the right side of a midline sagittal section of the head
(After removal of the brain. A window has been cut in the posterior part of the falx)

1 Falx cerebri
2 Sphenoparietal sinus
3 Inferior sagittal sinus
4 Arachnoid granulations
5 Superior sagittal sinus
6 Transverse sinus
7 Tentorium cerebelli
8 Straight sinus
9 Margin of foramen magnum
10 Posterior arch of atlas
11 Spinal medulla
12 Dens of axis
13 Medulla oblongata
14 Rootlets of hypoglossal nerve
15 Spinal part of accessory nerve
16 Glossopharyngeal, vagus and accessory nerves

17 Vestibulocochlear nerve
18 Sensory root (nervus intermedius) ⎫ of facial nerve
19 Motor root ⎭
20 Abducent nerve
21 Trigeminal nerve
22 Free margin of tentorium cerebelli
23 Trochlear nerve
24 Oculomotor nerve
25 Internal carotid artery
26 Optic nerve
27 Olfactory tract
28 Pituitary gland
29 Sphenoidal sinus
30 Choana (posterior nasal aperture)
31 Nasal septum

B The cranial fossae and dura mater
(On the right part of the dura has been removed, and on the left a window has been cut in the base of the skull. The brainstem has been transected through the midbrain)

1 Anterior cranial fossa
2 Falx cerebri
3 Olfactory bulb
4 Olfactory tract
5 Maxillary nerve
6 Mandibular nerve
7 Trigeminal ganglion
8 Trigeminal nerve
9 Free margin of tentorium cerebelli
10 Motor root ⎫ of facial nerve
11 Sensory root (nervus intermedius) ⎭
12 Vestibulocochlear nerve
13 Attached margin of tentorium cerebelli (containing transverse sinus)
14 Superior sagittal sinus
15 Junction of falx cerebri and tentorium cerebelli (containing straight sinus)
16 Cerebellum
17 Midbrain
18 Oculomotor nerve
19 Superior cerebellar artery
20 Posterior cerebral artery
21 Posterior communicating artery
22 Optic tract
23 Infundibulum (pituitary stalk)
24 Optic chiasma
25 Optic nerve
26 Middle cerebral artery
27 Attached margin of tentorium cerebelli containing superior petrosal sinus
28 Lateral part of middle cranial fossa
29 Upper surface of lateral pterygoid
30 Deep temporal nerves and vessels

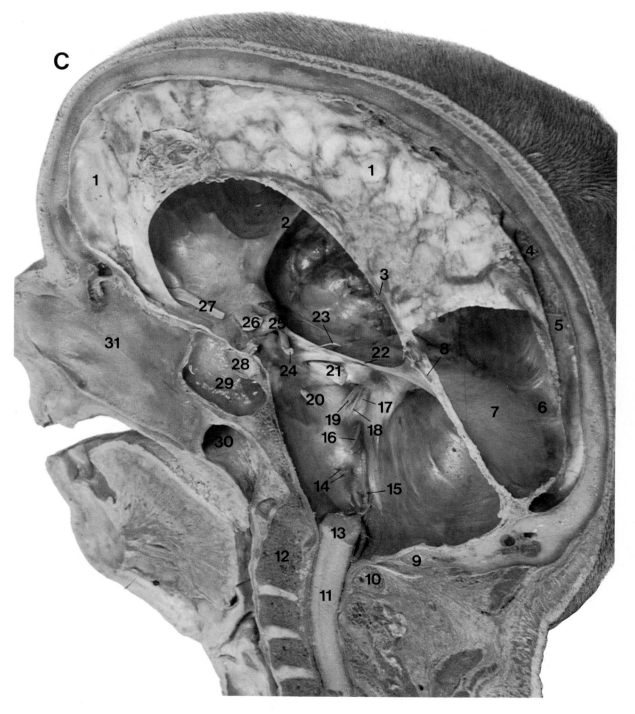

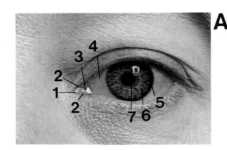

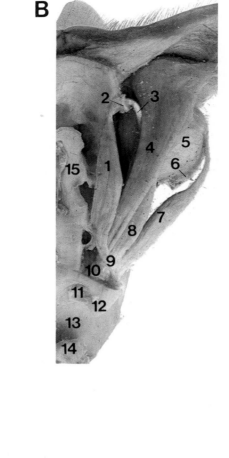

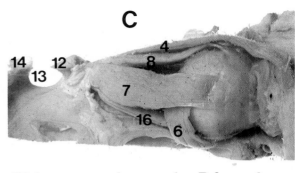

A Left eye

1 Lacrimal caruncle
2 Lacrimal papilla
3 Plica semilunaris
4 Sclera
5 Limbus (corneoscleral junction)
6 Iris
7 Pupil

● The cornea is the transparent anterior part of the outer coat of the eyeball and is continuous with the sclera at the limbus.
● The pupil is the central aperture of the iris, the circular pigmented diaphragm that lies in front of the lens.
● Each lacrimal papilla contains the lacrimal punctum, the minute opening of the lacrimal canaliculus which runs medially to open into the lacrimal sac, lying deep to the medial palpebral ligament and continuing downwards as the nasolacrimal duct within the nasolacrimal canal.

Right extra-ocular muscles, B from above, C from the right

1 Superior oblique
2 Trochlea
3 Tendon of superior oblique
4 Levator palpebrae superioris
5 Eyeball
6 Inferior oblique
7 Lateral rectus
8 Superior rectus
9 Tendinous ring
10 Optic nerve
11 Optic canal
12 Anterior clinoid process
13 Sella turcica (pituitary fossa)
14 Posterior clinoid process
15 Ethmoidal air cells
16 Inferior rectus

● Of the muscles that move the eyeball, the lateral rectus is supplied by the abducent nerve, the superior oblique by the trochlear nerve, and the others (medial, superior and inferior rectus and inferior oblique) by the oculomotor nerve. The levator palpebrae superioris is also supplied by the oculomotor nerve, but part of this muscle consists of visceral muscle fibres which receive a sympathetic supply.

Nerves of the left orbit, D from above, E from the left
(The roof and lateral wall of the orbit have been removed and the cavernous sinus opened. The lateral rectus muscle has been detached near the eyeball and reflected backwards)

● In E the lacrimal nerve passing to the lacrimal gland is double.

1 Lacrimal gland
2 Lacrimal nerve
3 Eyeball
4 Levator palpebrae superioris
5 Supra-orbital nerve
6 Supratrochlear nerve
7 Superior oblique
8 Frontal nerve
9 Trochlear nerve
10 Optic nerve
11 Ophthalmic artery
12 Internal carotid artery
13 Oculomotor nerve
14 Abducent nerve
15 Trigeminal ganglion
16 Lateral rectus (reflected backwards)
17 Superior rectus
18 Ophthalmic nerve
19 Ciliary ganglion
20 Short ciliary nerves (superficial to marker)
21 Nerve to medial rectus
22 Inferior rectus
23 Nerve to inferior oblique
24 Inferior oblique
25 Lateral rectus

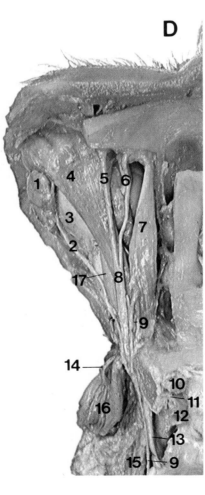

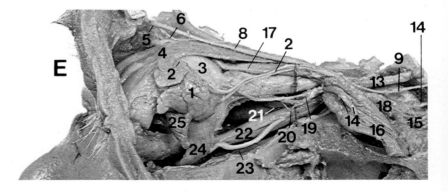

A The orbits opened from above, to show the principal vessels and nerves

(After partial removal of muscles and muscular branches of vessels)

1 Lacrimal gland
2 Levator palpebrae superioris
3 Superior rectus
4 Supra-orbital artery
5 Supra-orbital nerve
6 Supratrochlear nerve
7 Eyeball
8 Medial rectus
9 Nasociliary nerve
10 Superior oblique
11 Ophthalmic artery
12 Trochlear nerve
13 Frontal nerve
14 Lacrimal nerve
15 Lateral rectus
16 Optic nerve (with overlying short ciliary nerves in left orbit)
17 Internal carotid artery
18 Middle cerebral artery
19 Anterior cerebral artery
20 Optic chiasma
21 Anterior communicating artery
22 Cribriform plate of ethmoid
23 Lacrimal artery
24 Posterior ciliary artery
25 Infratrochlear nerve and ophthalmic artery
26 Anterior ethmoidal artery and nerve

● The most important branch of the ophthalmic artery – the central artery of the retina – is hidden below the optic nerve. It runs within the dural sheath of the nerve and pierces the inferomedial surface of the nerve 1.25 cm behind the eyeball, passing forwards in the centre of the nerve to reach the retina where its branches can be observed with the ophthalmoscope.
● In this specimen the supra-orbital artery is absent on the right and unusually small on the left.

B Right orbit, from the front with the eyeball removed

(The extra-ocular muscles and the optic nerve are intact)

1 Supra-orbital nerve
2 Supratrochlear nerve
3 Trochlea
4 Tendon of superior oblique
5 Superior oblique
6 Anterior ethmoidal nerve
7 Infratrochlear nerve
8 Medial rectus
9 Attachment of medial palpebral ligament
10 Inferior oblique
11 Inferior rectus
12 Optic nerve
13 Lateral rectus
14 Part of orbital septum
15 Lacrimal gland
16 Superior rectus
17 Levator palpebrae superioris

● The two oblique muscles (superior and inferior) both pass below the corresponding rectus muscles.
● The lateral palpebral ligament (connected to the tarsal plates of both eyelids) is attached to a small tubercle on the zygomatic bone (immediately in front of the part of the orbital septum seen in this specimen). The medial palpebral ligament is attached to the anterior lacrimal crest of the frontal process of the maxilla, and therefore lies anterior to the lacrimal sac.
● The orbital septum is the continuation into the eyelids of the orbital periosteum (properly called the orbital fascia).

C Right nasolacrimal duct *(with bristles in the puncta of the lacrimal canaliculi)*

1 Superior canaliculus
2 Dorsal nasal artery
3 Medial palpebral ligament overlying lacrimal sac
4 Nasolacrimal duct
5 Infra-orbital nerve
6 Inferior canaliculus

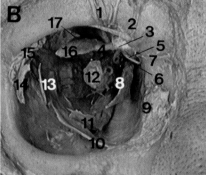

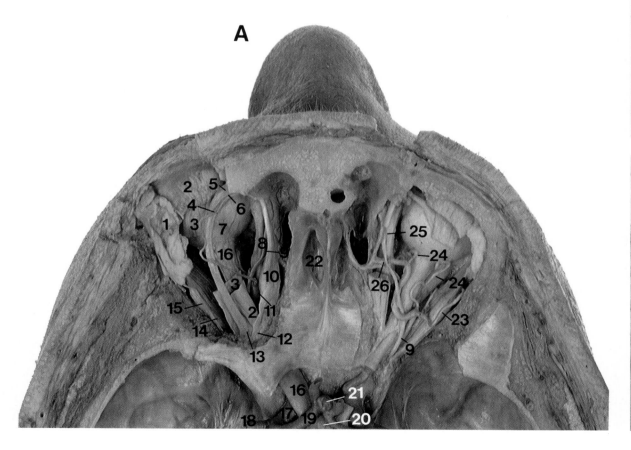

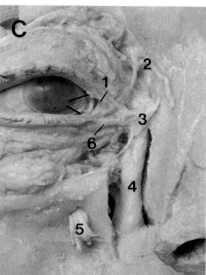

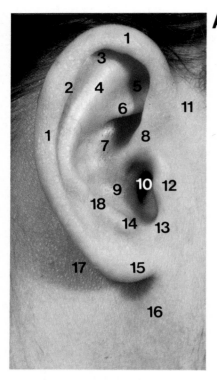

A Right external ear

1 Helix
2 Auricular tubercle
3 Scaphoid fossa
4 Upper crus of antihelix
5 Triangular fossa
6 Lower crus of antihelix
7 Upper part of concha
8 Crus of helix
9 Lower part of concha
10 External acoustic meatus
11 Superficial temporal vessels and auriculotemporal nerve
12 Tragus
13 Intertragic notch
14 Antitragus
15 Lobule
16 Transverse process of atlas
17 Mastoid process
18 Antihelix

● The external ear consists of the auricle (pinna) and external acoustic meatus.

● The concha is the deepest part of the external ear. The lower part of the concha leads into the external acoustic meatus; the suprameatal triangle and mastoid antrum lie behind the upper part.

C Cast of the mastoid air cells, within a transparent cast of their own right temporal bone, from the right

● This specimen is supported by a rod in the external acoustic meatus. The styloid process projects downwards immediately below the meatus, with the mastoid process behind it.

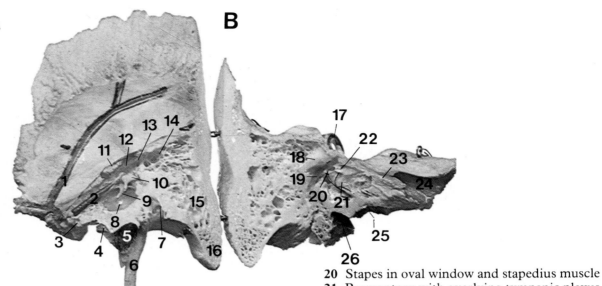

B Right temporal bone and middle ear

(The bone has been bisected, with some removal of the upper part of the petrous part. The section has opened up the tympanic (middle ear) cavity; on the left side of the figure the lateral wall, which includes the tympanic membrane, is seen from the medial side, while on the right the main features of the medial wall are in view)

1 Groove for middle meningeal vessels
2 Tensor tympani muscle in its canal
3 Bony part of auditory tube
4 Part of carotid canal (red)
5 Part of jugular bulb (blue)
6 Styloid process
7 Stylomastoid foramen
8 Tympanic membrane
9 Malleus
10 Incus
11 Tegmen tympani
12 Epitympanic recess
13 Aditus to mastoid antrum
14 Mastoid antrum
15 Mastoid air cells
16 Mastoid process
17 Superior ⎫
18 Lateral ⎬ semicircular canal
19 Canal for facial nerve (yellow)

20 Stapes in oval window and stapedius muscle
21 Promontory with overlying tympanic plexus
22 Lesser petrosal nerve
23 Groove for greater petrosal nerve (yellow)
24 Carotid canal (red)
25 Tympanic branch of glossopharyngeal nerve entering its canaliculus
26 Jugular bulb (blue)

● The middle ear or tympanic cavity is an irregular space within the temporal bone, containing the auditory ossicles and filled with air that communicates with the nasopharynx through the auditory tube.

● The epitympanic recess is the part of the tympanic cavity that lies above the tympanic membrane, and lodges the head of the malleus and the body of the incus. It leads backwards through the aditus into the mastoid antrum, which is an enlarged mastoid air cell.

● The medial wall of the middle ear contains (from below upwards) the promontory (due to the first turn of the cochlea), the canal for the facial nerve and the prominence due to the lateral semicircular canal. Below and behind the promontory (and just hidden by it in this view) is the round window (fenestra cochleae, closed by the secondary tympanic membrane), and above and behind it is the oval window (fenestra vestibuli, closed by the footplate of the stapes).

● The roof of the middle ear is the tegmen tympani; the jugular bulb lies below the floor, and the carotid canal in the anterior wall.

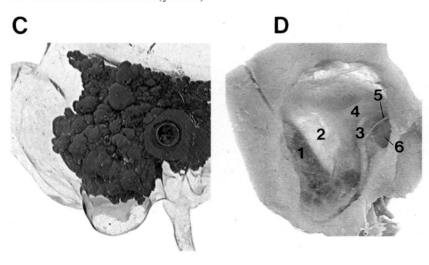

D Right temporal bone, from the right, after removal of mastoid air cells

(With the canal for the facial nerve opened up)

1 Sigmoid sinus
2 Dura mater of posterior cranial fossa
3 Facial nerve
4 Lateral semicircular canal
5 Chorda tympani
6 Tympanic membrane (upper part removed)

● The mastoid air cells are closely related to the sigmoid sinus and posterior cranial fossa posteromedially; above is the temporal lobe of the brain in the middle cranial fossa. The mastoid antrum and air cells can be approached surgically by opening up the bone through the suprameatal triangle (page 28).

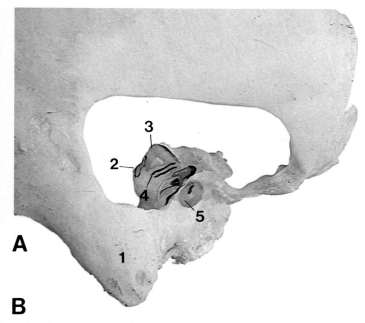

A

1

B

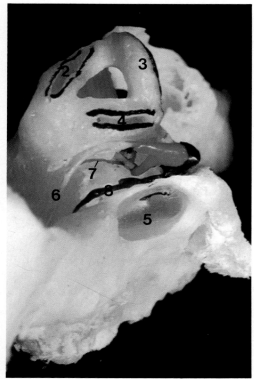

C

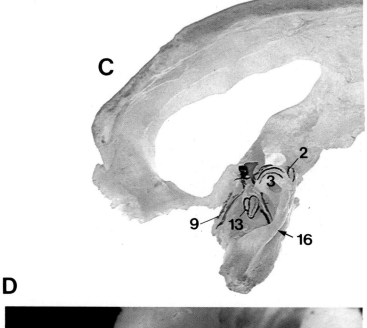

D

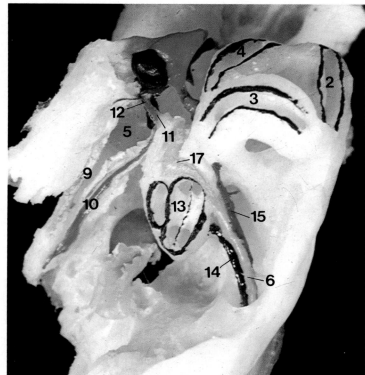

Right temporal bone, dissected to show parts of the external, middle and internal ear. A from the right, natural size, B from the right and slightly above and behind, magnified x 4, C and D from above and in front, natural size, and magnified x 4

(Auditory ossicles: dark blue, malleus; red, incus; green, stapes. Margins of opened semicircular canals and cochlea: black)

1 Mastoid process
2 Posterior ⎫
3 Superior   ⎬ semicircular canal
4 Lateral   ⎭
5 Tympanic membrane and (dark blue) handle of malleus
6 Facial nerve (yellow)
7 Stapedius muscle
8 Chorda tympani (purple)
9 Margins of auditory tube (mauve)

10 Tensor tympani muscle
11 Cochleariform process
12 Tendon of tensor tympani
13 Cochlea
14 Cochlear part ⎫
15 Vestibular part ⎬ of vestibulocochlear nerve
                   ⎭
16 Internal acoustic meatus
17 Genicular ganglion of facial nerve

● To assist orientation in A and C, part of the surrounding temporal bone has been preserved. Note the depth of the middle ear in relation to the mastoid process.
● The handle of the malleus is attached to the tympanic membrane.
● The chorda tympani passes between the fibrous and mucous layers of the tympanic membrane and crosses the handle of the malleus.
● From the genicular ganglion the facial nerve passes backwards in its canal above the promontory and then downwards in the medial wall of the aditus to reach the stylomastoid foramen.

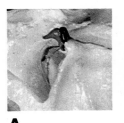

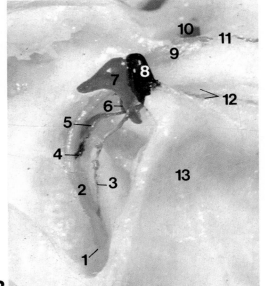

A

B

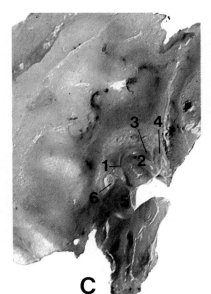

C

C Right temporal bone, from above, dissected to show the internal ear

1 Vestibule with stapes in oval window
2 Superior ⎫
3 Lateral ⎬ semicircular canal
4 Posterior ⎭
5 Cochlea
6 Tympanic membrane

● The internal ear consists of the bony labyrinth and the membranous labyrinth.
● The bony labyrinth consists of the vestibule, semicircular canals and cochlea.
● The membranous labyrinth is inside the bony labyrinth and consists of the utricle and saccule (within the vestibule), the semicircular ducts (within the semicircular canals) and the duct of the cochlea (within the cochlea).
● The membranous labyrinth contains endolymph and is separated from the bony labyrinth by perilymph. These two fluids do not communicate with one another, but the perilymph probably communicates with the subarachnoid space via the cochlear canaliculus (page 28).

Right temporal bone and middle ear, dissected to show the facial nerve and branches, A natural size, B magnified x 4

1 Facial canal leading to stylomastoid foramen
2 Facial nerve
3 Chorda tympani
4 Nerve to stapedius
5 Stapedius
6 Stapes
7 Incus
8 Malleus
9 Genicular ganglion of facial nerve
10 Internal acoustic meatus
11 Greater petrosal nerve
12 Margin of auditory tube
13 Paraffin wax (for support) overlying tympanic membrane

● The upper part of the facial canal has been opened up; the chorda tympani and nerve to stapedius branch from the facial nerve while it is in the canal. The greater petrosal nerve branches from the genicular ganglion.
● The stapedius tendon emerges from a small conical projection on the posterior wall of the tympanic cavity, the pyramid (here dissected away).

E Cast of the cerebral blood vessels, from the left

● The largest vessels on the lateral surface of the cerebral hemisphere are branches of the middle cerebral artery.

F Cast of cerebral veins and venous sinuses in the skull, from above and behind

(With the left half of the cranial vault removed)

1 Foramen caecum and vein from nasal cavity
2 Superior sagittal sinus
3 Superior cerebral veins
4 Middle meningeal veins
5 Inferior sagittal sinus
6 Internal cerebral vein
7 Great cerebral vein
8 Straight sinus
9 Transverse sinus
10 Inferior cerebral veins
11 Inferior petrosal sinus (right)
12 Superior petrosal sinus (left)
13 Petrosquamous vein
14 Basilar plexus
15 Cavernous sinus
16 Sphenoparietal sinus
17 Internal carotid artery
18 Middle cerebral artery
19 Anterior cerebral artery

● At the internal occipital protuberance the superior sagittal sinus usually turns to the right to become the right transverse sinus.
● The inferior sagittal sinus runs backwards in the free margin of the falx cerebri to join the straight sinus, which lies at the junction of the falx cerebri and tentorium cerebelli and turns to the left to become the left transverse sinus. The two transverse sinuses may communicate with one another.

D

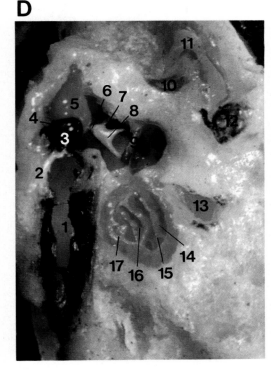

D Right temporal bone, dissected from above, magnified x 4

1 Auditory tube
2 Chorda tympani
3 Malleus
4 Incudomallear joint
5 Incus
6 Incudostapedial joint
7 Stapedius muscle
8 Stapes
9 Footplate of stapes in oval window of vestibule
10 Lateral ⎫
11 Posterior ⎬ semicircular canal
12 Superior ⎭
13 Internal acoustic meatus
14 Bony canal ⎫
15 Osseous spiral lamina ⎬ of
16 Modiolus ⎮ cochlea
17 Cupola ⎭

● The spiral organ (the end organ of hearing) lies on the basilar membrane, which stretches between the free edge of the osseous spiral lamina and the side of the bony canal.
● The modiolus is the central axis of the cochlea, and the cupola is its apex.

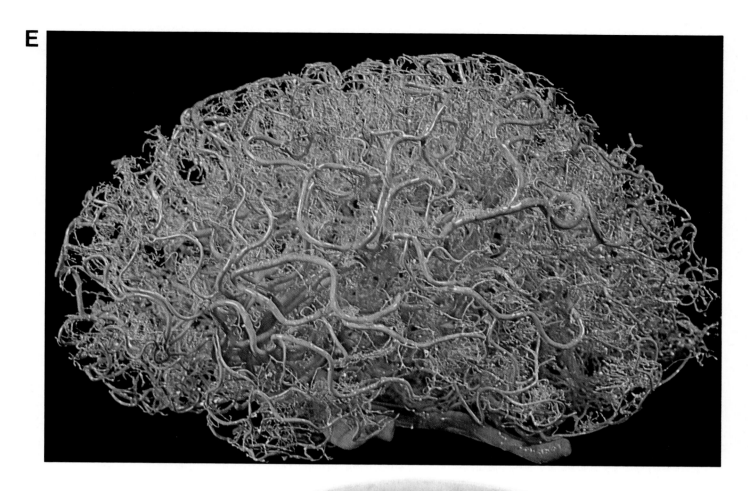

E

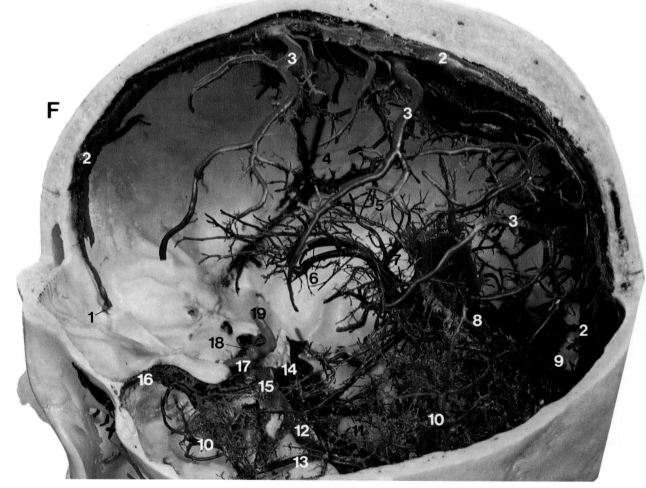

F

61

A The brain from above. The right cerebral hemisphere with the arachnoid mater
(A window has been cut in the arachnoid mater over the left cerebral hemisphere)

1 Longitudinal fissure
2 Frontal pole
3 Superolateral surface
4 Occipital pole
5 Arachnoid granulations

● When removed from the cranial cavity the brain is covered by the arachnoid mater which collapses on to the gyri of the cerebral hemispheres. In life the arachnoid mater is slightly separated from the brain surface by the cerebrospinal fluid in the subarachnoid space.

● The cerebral arteries and veins that appear to be on the brain surface are within the subarachnoid space.

B Gyri and sulci of the right cerebral hemisphere, from above after removal of the arachnoid mater

1 Superior frontal gyrus
2 Precentral sulcus
3 Precentral gyrus
4 Central sulcus
5 Postcentral gyrus
6 Postcentral sulcus
7 Parieto-occipital sulcus

C The brain from the right, with the arachnoid mater

1 Occipital pole
2 Superolateral surface of right cerebral hemisphere
3 Superior cerebral veins
4 Frontal pole
5 Temporal pole
6 Superficial middle cerebral vein overlying lateral sulcus
7 Inferior cerebral veins
8 Pons and basilar artery
9 Medulla oblongata and vertebral artery
10 Right cerebellar hemisphere

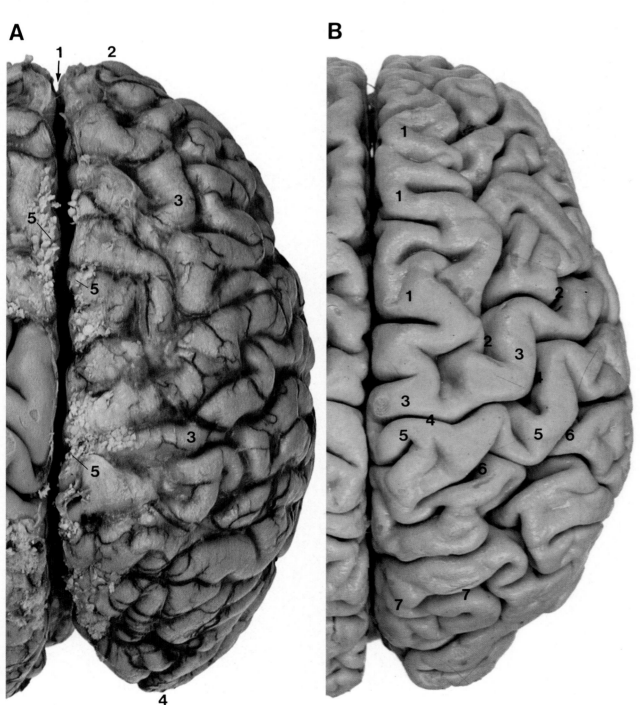

D Gyri and sulci of the superolateral surface of the right cerebral hemisphere

1 Lunate sulcus
2 Parieto-occipital sulcus
3 Pre-occipital notch
4 Inferior ⎫
5 Middle   ⎬ temporal gyrus
6 Superior ⎭
7 Middle   ⎫ temporal
8 Superior ⎭ sulcus
9 Supramarginal gyrus
10 Lateral sulcus (posterior ramus)
11 Postcentral sulcus
12 Postcentral gyrus
13 Central sulcus
14 Precentral gyrus
15 Precentral sulcus
16 Superior ⎫
17 Middle   ⎬ frontal gyrus
18 Inferior ⎭
19 Ascending ⎫ ramus of
20 Anterior ⎭ lateral sulcus
21 Pars triangularis

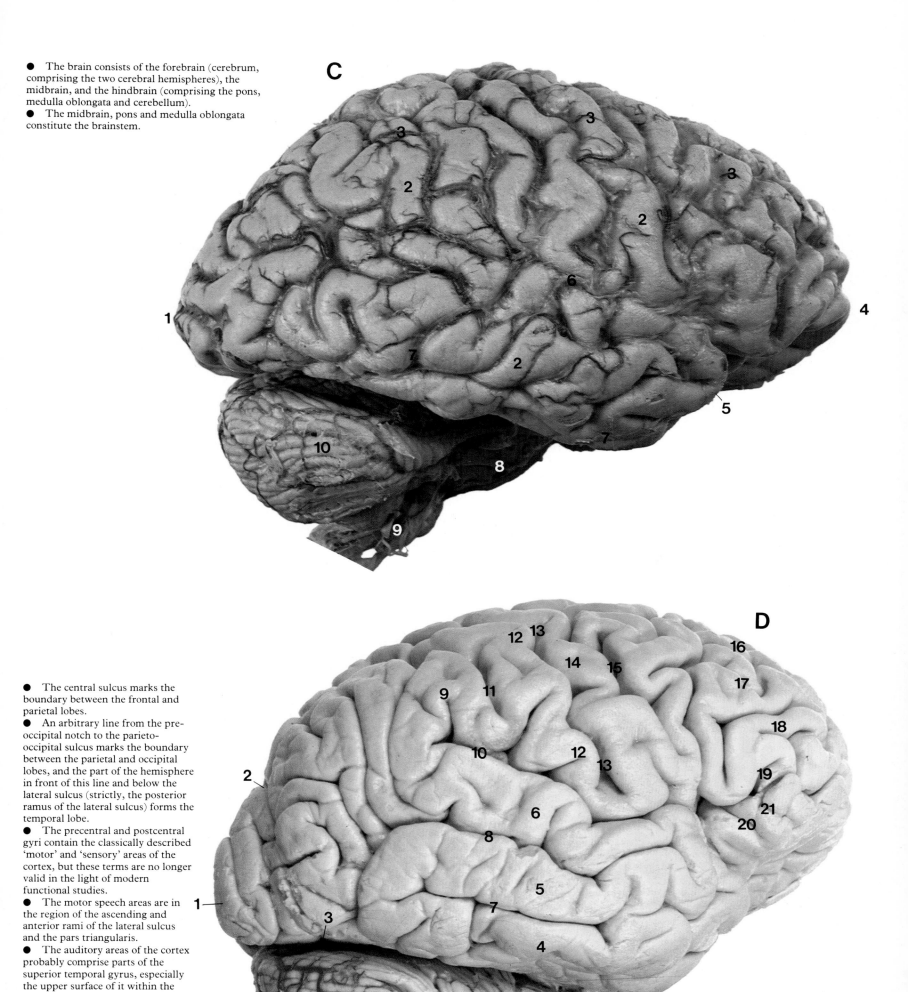

C

- The brain consists of the forebrain (cerebrum, comprising the two cerebral hemispheres), the midbrain, and the hindbrain (comprising the pons, medulla oblongata and cerebellum).
- The midbrain, pons and medulla oblongata constitute the brainstem.

D

- The central sulcus marks the boundary between the frontal and parietal lobes.
- An arbitrary line from the pre-occipital notch to the parieto-occipital sulcus marks the boundary between the parietal and occipital lobes, and the part of the hemisphere in front of this line and below the lateral sulcus (strictly, the posterior ramus of the lateral sulcus) forms the temporal lobe.
- The precentral and postcentral gyri contain the classically described 'motor' and 'sensory' areas of the cortex, but these terms are no longer valid in the light of modern functional studies.
- The motor speech areas are in the region of the ascending and anterior rami of the lateral sulcus and the pars triangularis.
- The auditory areas of the cortex probably comprise parts of the superior temporal gyrus, especially the upper surface of it within the lateral sulcus.

A The brain from below, with the arachnoid mater partially intact

(As typically seen when freshly removed from the cranial cavity and before dissection)

1 Inferior surface of frontal lobe
2 Frontal pole
3 Longitudinal fissure
4 Gyrus rectus
5 Olfactory bulb
6 Olfactory tract
7 Anterior perforated substance
8 Optic nerve
9 Optic chiasma
10 Infundibulum (pituitary stalk)
11 Internal carotid artery
12 Posterior communicating artery
13 Oculomotor nerve
14 Crus of cerebral peduncle (midbrain)
15 Basilar artery
16 Pons
17 Trigeminal nerve
18 Abducent nerve
19 Facial nerve
20 Vestibulocochlear nerve
21 Vertebral artery
22 Medulla oblongata
23 Spinal part of accessory nerve
24 Cerebellar hemisphere
25 Inferior surface of temporal lobe
26 Uncus
27 Arachnoid mater overlying mamillary bodies
28 Temporal pole

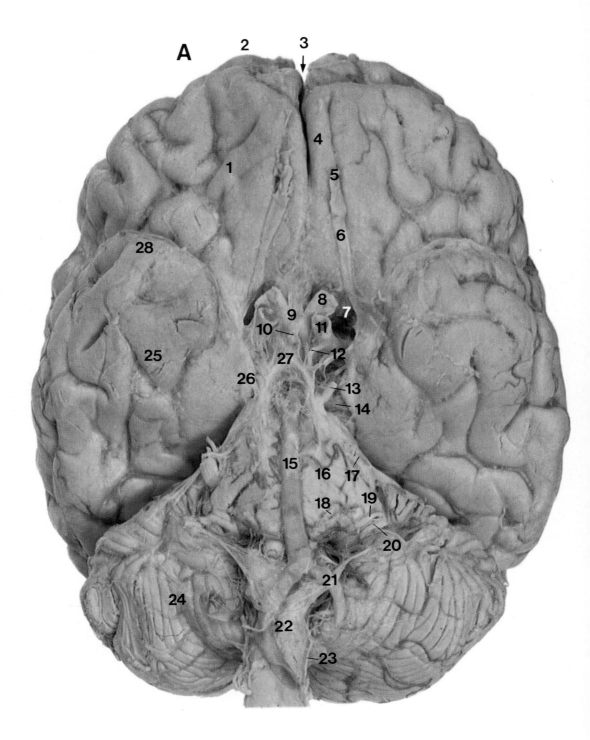

B The optic tract and geniculate bodies, from below

(After removal of part of the brainstem and cerebral hemispheres)

1 Olfactory tract
2 Anterior perforated substance
3 Optic nerve
4 Optic chiasma
5 Infundibulum (pituitary stalk)
6 Tuber cinereum
7 Mamillary body
8 Posterior perforated substance
9 Optic tract
10 Crus
11 Substantia nigra
12 Tegmentum   } of midbrain
13 Tectum
14 Aqueduct
15 Lateral   } geniculate body
16 Medial
17 Pulvinar of thalamus
18 Splenium of corpus callosum

● The lateral geniculate body is part of the visual pathway.
● The medial geniculate body is part of the acoustic pathway.

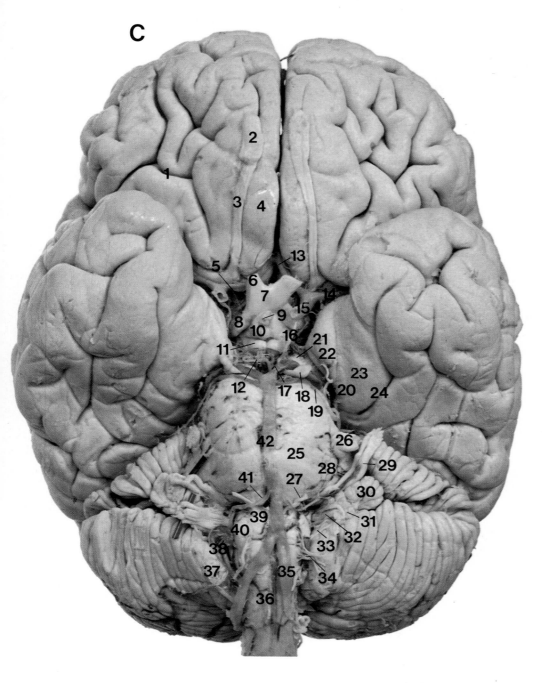

C

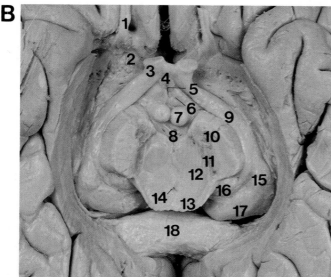

B

C The brain from below. Gyri, sulci and cranial nerves

(After removal of most of the arachnoid mater and minor blood vessels)

1 Orbital sulcus
2 Olfactory bulb
3 Olfactory tract
4 Gyrus rectus
5 Anterior perforated substance
6 Optic nerve
7 Optic chiasma
8 Optic tract
9 Infundibulum (pituitary stalk)
10 Tuber cinereum
11 Mamillary body
12 Posterior perforated substance
13 Anterior cerebral artery
14 Middle cerebral artery
15 Internal carotid artery
16 Posterior communicating artery
17 Posterior cerebral artery
18 Oculomotor nerve
19 Superior cerebellar artery
20 Trochlear nerve
21 Crus of cerebral peduncle
22 Uncus
23 Parahippocampal gyrus
24 Collateral sulcus
25 Pons
26 Trigeminal nerve
27 Abducent nerve
28 Facial nerve
29 Vestibulocochlear nerve
30 Flocculus of cerebellum
31 Choroid plexus from lateral recess of fourth ventricle
32 Roots of glossopharyngeal, vagus and accessory nerves
33 Spinal part of accessory nerve
34 Rootlets of hypoglossal nerve (superficial to marker)
35 Vertebral artery
36 Medulla oblongata
37 Tonsil of cerebellum
38 Posterior inferior cerebellar artery
39 Pyramid ⎤ of medulla
40 Olive ⎦ oblongata
41 Anterior inferior cerebellar artery
42 Basilar artery

● A blue marker has been placed behind the right flocculus and the overlying facial and vestibulocochlear nerves.
● A red marker has been placed behind the roots of the right glossopharyngeal, vagus and accessory nerves.

65

The medial surface of the right cerebral hemisphere and a midline sagittal section through the brainstem

1 Anterior cerebral artery
2 Rostrum
3 Genu
4 Body
} of corpus callosum
5 Cingulate gyrus
6 Precentral gyrus
7 Central sulcus
8 Postcentral gyrus
9 Parieto-occipital sulcus
10 Calcarine sulcus
11 Lingual gyrus
12 Cerebellum
13 Medulla oblongata
14 Median aperture of fourth ventricle
15 Fourth ventricle
16 Pons
17 Basilar artery
18 Tegmentum
19 Aqueduct
20 Inferior colliculus
21 Superior colliculus
} of mid-brain
22 Posterior commissure
23 Pineal body
24 Suprapineal recess
25 Great cerebral vein
26 Splenium of corpus callosum
27 Fornix
28 Cut edge of septum pellucidum
29 Body of lateral ventricle
30 Thalamus
31 Interthalamic connexion
32 Hypothalamic sulcus
33 Hypothalamus
34 Posterior perforated substance
35 Mamillary body
36 Tuber cinereum
37 Infundibular recess
38 Optic chiasma
39 Supra-optic recess
40 Lamina terminalis
41 Anterior commissure
42 Anterior column of fornix
43 Interventricular foramen and choroid plexus

● The interventricular foramen (between the third and lateral ventricles) is bounded in front by the anterior column of the fornix and behind by the thalamus.

● The aqueduct of the midbrain connects the third and fourth ventricles. The part of the midbrain dorsal to the aqueduct (and containing the superior and inferior colliculi) is the tectum, and ventral to it is the tegmentum.

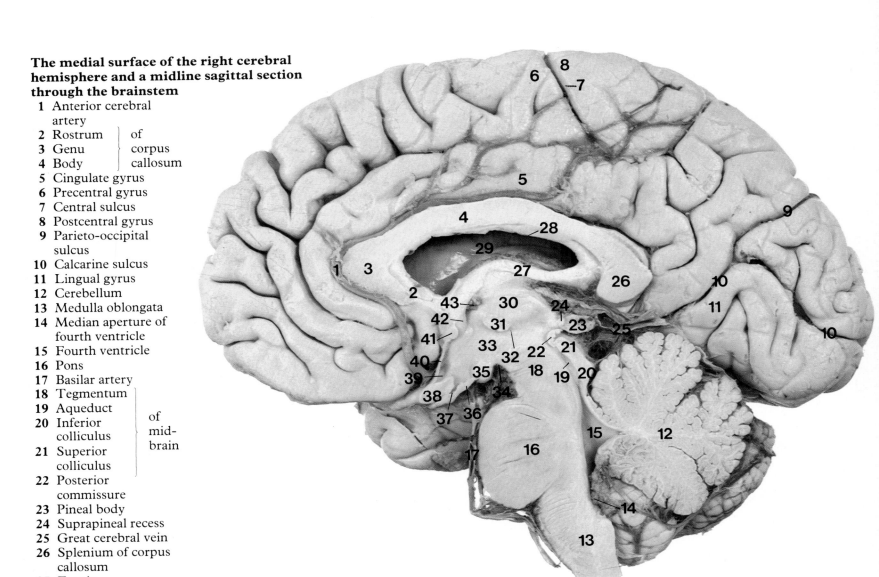

The cerebellum and cerebellomedullary cistern, from behind

1 Cerebellar hemisphere
2 Arachnoid mater

● The cerebellomedullary cistern (cisterna magna) is formed by arachnoid mater bridging the space between the medulla oblongata and the under surface of the cerebellum (see page 46 for the cistern in sagittal section).

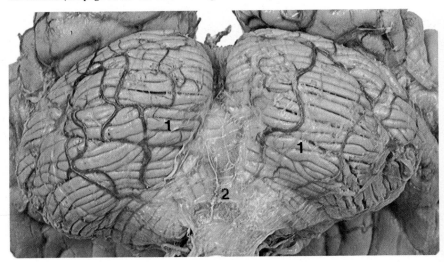

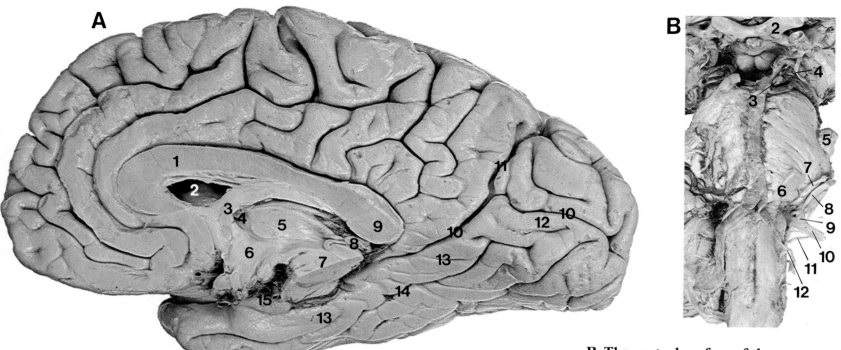

A

B

A The medial surface of the right cerebral hemisphere, with the brainstem removed through the midbrain

1 Corpus callosum
2 Anterior horn of lateral ventricle
3 Anterior column of fornix
4 Interventricular foramen
5 Thalamus ⎫ in lateral wall
6 Hypothalamus ⎭ of third ventricle
7 Midbrain
8 Pineal body
9 Splenium of corpus callosum
10 Calcarine sulcus
11 Parieto-occipital sulcus
12 Lingual gyrus
13 Parahippocampal gyrus
14 Collateral sulcus
15 Uncus

● The parahippocampal gyrus is continuous anteriorly with the hook-like uncus and posteriorly with the lingual gyrus.
● The visual area of the cerebral cortex occupies the upper and lower lips of the posterior part of the calcarine sulcus (behind the parieto-occipital sulcus), and part of the lower lip of the calcarine sulcus anterior to its junction with the parieto-occipital sulcus.

B The ventral surface of the brainstem. Cranial nerves

(The left cerebellar hemisphere has been removed. The cranial nerves are identified by their official numbers and names. The filaments of the first cranial nerve, the olfactory, run into the olfactory bulb and so are not seen with the brainstem)

2 Optic
3 Oculomotor
4 Trochlear
5 Trigeminal
6 Abducent
7 Facial
8 Vestibulocochlear
9 Glossopharyngeal
10 Vagus
11 Accessory
12 Hypoglossal

● For notes on the emergence of cranial nerves from the brainstem see page 68.

C The brainstem from the left, with the cerebellum in a midline sagittal section

(The left half of the cerebellum has been removed by transecting the cerebellar peduncles)

1 Pons
2 Trigeminal nerve
3 Superior cerebellar artery
4 Trochlear nerve
5 Basal cerebral vein
6 Crus of cerebral peduncle
7 Posterior cerebral artery
8 Inferior colliculus
9 Superior ⎫
10 Middle ⎬ cerebellar peduncle
11 Inferior ⎭
12 Superior medullary velum
13 Lingula
14 Anterior lobe
15 Primary fissure
16 Prepyramidal fissure
17 Pyramid
18 Postpyramidal fissure
19 Uvula
20 Nodule
21 Tonsil
22 Fourth ventricle
23 Choroid plexus in lateral recess
24 Medulla oblongata
25 Roots of glossopharyngeal, vagus and accessory nerves
26 Olive
27 Rootlets of hypoglossal nerve
28 Pyramid
29 Abducent nerve
30 Facial and vestibulocochlear nerves

● The central part of the cerebellum constitutes the vermis (nodule, uvula and pyramid), which is continuous laterally with the hemispheres.
● The folia of the cerebellar cortex are considerably narrower than the gyri of the cerebral cortex.
● The largest of the subcortical nuclei of the cerebellar hemisphere is the dentate nucleus, whose axons constitute the main efferent pathway from the cerebellum and leave in the superior peduncle.

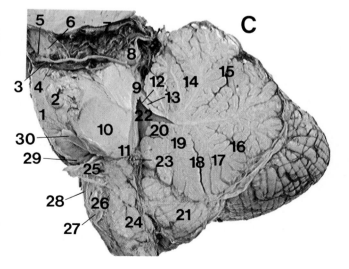

C

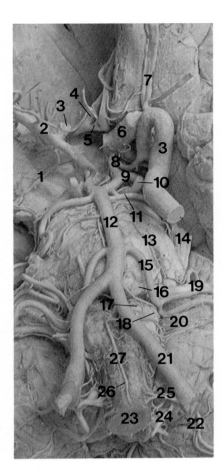

Injected arteries of the base of the brain
(With partial removal of the right side of the brain)

1 Anterior choroidal
2 Middle cerebral
3 Internal carotid
4 Anterior cerebral
5 Anterior communicating
6 Optic nerve
7 Olfactory tract
8 Posterior communicating
9 Posterior cerebral
10 Oculomotor nerve
11 Superior cerebellar
12 Basilar with pontine branches
13 Pons
14 Trigeminal nerve
15 Anterior inferior cerebellar
16 Abducent nerve
17 Pyramid
18 Olive
19 Facial and vestibulocochlear nerves
20 Filaments of glossopharyngeal, vagus and accessory nerves
21 Vertebral
22 Posterior inferior cerebellar
23 Spinal medulla
24 Spinal part of accessory nerve
25 Rootlets of first cervical nerve
26 Anterior spinal
27 Medulla oblongata

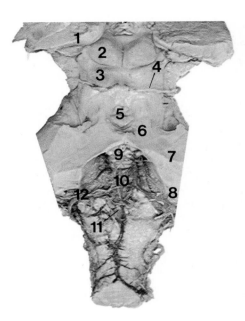

The dorsal surface of the roof of the fourth ventricle
(With most of the cerebellum removed by transecting the peduncles)

1 Pulvinar of thalamus
2 Superior colliculus
3 Inferior colliculus
4 Trochlear nerve
5 Superior medullary velum and lingula of cerebellum
6 Superior ⎫
7 Middle ⎬ cerebellar peduncle
8 Inferior ⎭
9 Nodule of cerebellum
10 Ependyma and pia mater forming roof
11 Median aperture
12 Lateral recess

● The median aperture in the posterior part of the roof of the fourth ventricle and the two lateral apertures (in the lateral recesses) are the only sites of communication between the ventricular system and the subarachnoid space.

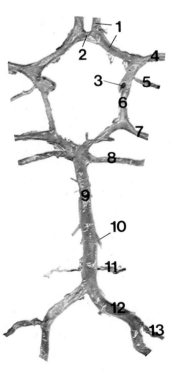

The arterial circle and basilar artery, after removal from the base of the brain

1 Anterior cerebral
2 Anterior communicating
3 Internal carotid
4 Middle cerebral
5 Anterior choroidal
6 Posterior communicating
7 Posterior cerebral
8 Superior cerebellar
9 Basilar
10 Labyrinthine
11 Anterior inferior cerebellar
12 Vertebral
13 Posterior inferior cerebellar

● The trochlear nerve is the only cranial nerve to emerge from the *dorsal* surface of the brainstem (from the midbrain, below the inferior colliculus).
● The oculomotor nerve emerges on the *medial* side of the crus of the cerebral peduncle, and the trochlear nerve winds round the *lateral* side of the peduncle. Both nerves pass between the posterior cerebral and superior cerebellar arteries.
● The trigeminal nerve emerges from the lateral side of the pons.
● The abducent nerve emerges between the pons and the pyramid.
● The facial and vestibulocochlear nerves emerge from the lateral pontomedullary angle.
● The glossopharyngeal and vagus nerves and the cranial root of the accessory nerve emerge from the medulla oblongata lateral to the olive.
● The spinal part of the accessory nerve emerges from the lateral surface of the upper five or six cervical segments of the spinal medulla, dorsal to the denticulate ligament.

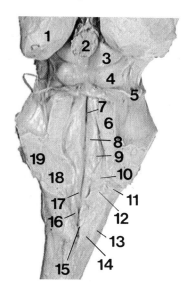

The floor of the fourth ventricle

1 Pulvinar of thalamus
2 Pineal body
3 Superior colliculus
4 Inferior colliculus
5 Trochlear nerve
6 Superior cerebellar peduncle
7 Median sulcus
8 Medial eminence
9 Facial colliculus
10 Vestibular area
11 Lateral recess
12 Medullary striae
13 Cuneate tubercle
14 Gracile tubercle
15 Obex
16 Vagal triangle
17 Hypoglossal triangle
18 Inferior ⎤
19 Middle ⎦ cerebellar peduncle

The brainstem and upper part of the spinal medulla, from behind

(After removal of the posterior part of the skull, cerebellum and vertebral arches)

1 Petrous part of temporal bone
2 Tentorium cerebelli
3 Inferior ⎤
4 Middle ⎥ cerebellar
5 Superior ⎦ peduncle
6 Superior medullary velum
7 Trochlear nerve
8 Inferior ⎤
9 Superior ⎦ colliculus
10 Straight sinus
11 Medial eminence
12 Facial colliculus
13 Medullary striae
14 Facial and vestibulocochlear nerves and internal acoustic meatus
15 Glossopharyngeal, vagus and accessory nerves and jugular foramen
16 Spinal part of accessory nerve
17 Rootlets of hypoglossal nerve and hypoglossal canal
18 Margin of foramen magnum
19 Vertebral artery
20 Lateral mass of atlas
21 Ventral ramus of first cervical nerve
22 Dorsal rootlets ⎤ of
23 Dorsal root ganglion ⎥ second
24 Ventral ramus ⎥ cervical
25 Dorsal ramus ⎦ nerve
26 Posterior belly of digastric
27 Internal jugular vein
28 Zygapophysial joint
29 Spinal medulla
30 Denticulate ligament
31 Dura mater
32 Sympathetic trunk
33 Common carotid artery
34 Vagus nerve
35 Internal carotid artery
36 Superior cervical sympathetic ganglion
37 Hypoglossal nerve

● Occasionally (as in this specimen) the dorsal root of the first cervical nerve is absent. The dorsal ramus of this nerve has been removed; the ventral ramus lies between the vertebral artery and the posterior arch of the atlas.

● After emerging from the foramen in the transverse process of the atlas the vertebral artery winds backwards round the lateral mass of the atlas before passing under the posterior atlanto-occipital membrane and piercing the dura and arachnoid mater to enter the skull.

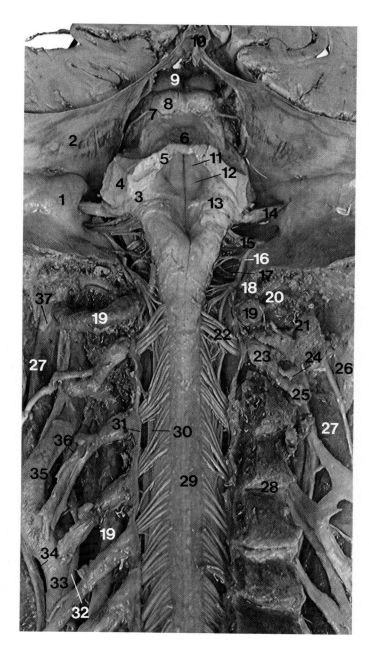

The cerebral hemispheres in horizontal sections

(The left hemisphere is cut on a level with the interventricular foramen, and the right 1 cm higher)

 1 Insula in lateral sulcus
 2 Claustrum
 3 Putamen ⎫ forming
 4 Globus pallidus ⎬ lentiform nucleus
 5 Head of caudate nucleus
 6 Anterior limb ⎫
 7 Genu ⎬ of internal capsule
 8 Posterior limb ⎭
 9 Thalamus
10 Third ventricle
11 Interventricular foramen
12 Anterior column of fornix
13 Anterior horn of lateral ventricle
14 Forceps minor (corpus callosum)
15 Thalamostriate vein
16 Choroid plexus
17 Forceps major
18 Inferior horn ⎫
19 Posterior horn ⎬ of lateral ventricle
20 Visual area of cortex
21 Lunate sulcus
22 Optic radiation
23 Tapetum
24 Collateral trigone
25 Calcar
26 Bulb
27 Hippocampus
28 Fimbria
29 Tail of caudate nucleus
30 Retrolentiform part of internal capsule

● The important corticonuclear and corticospinal fibres pass through the posterior limb of the internal capsule. The striate branches of the anterior and middle cerebral arteries supply this area, entering the brain through the anterior perforated substance (page 65). One of these vessels may constitute the 'artery of cerebral haemorrhage'.

● The choroid plexus of the third ventricle passes through the interventricular foramen into the body of the lateral ventricle and then into the inferior horn; there is no choroid plexus in the anterior or posterior horns.

● The optic radiation is alternatively known as the geniculocalcarine tract, and passes from the lateral geniculate body to the calcarine area of the cortex.

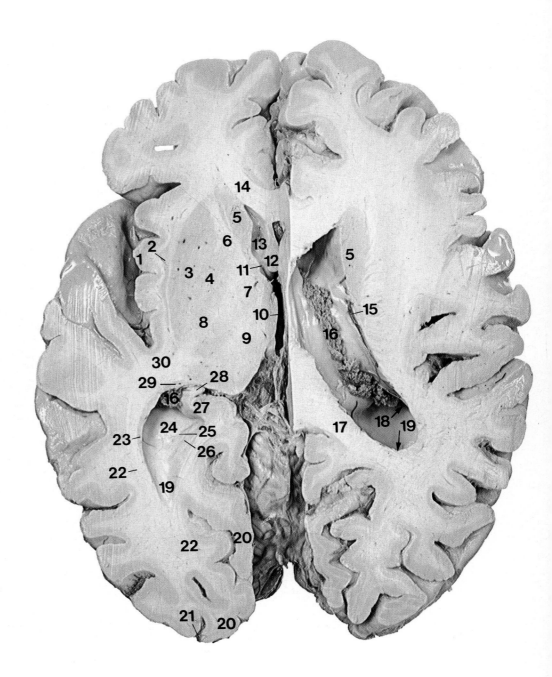

A The brain in oblique coronal section, from the front

(At a level through the interventricular foramen and the ventral junction of the pons and medulla oblongata)

1 Insula
2 Putamen
3 Globus pallidus
4 Internal capsule
5 Caudate nucleus
6 Corpus callosum
7 Lateral ventricle
8 Septum pellucidum
9 Fornix
10 Interventricular foramen
11 Choroid plexus
12 Thalamostriate vein
13 Thalamus
14 Third ventricle
15 Choroidal fissure
16 Inferior horn of lateral ventricle
17 Hippocampus
18 Pons
19 Pyramid
20 Olive
21 Substantia nigra
22 Red nucleus
23 Optic tract

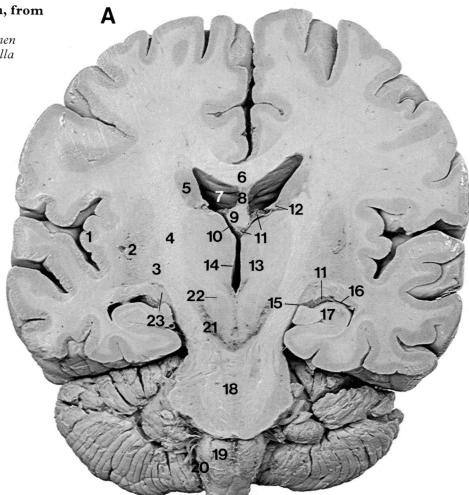

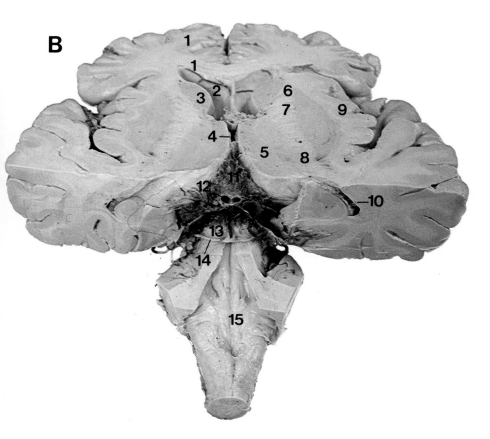

B The cerebral hemispheres in horizontal section, from above and behind

(With the posterior part of the hemispheres and the whole of the cerebellum removed)

1 Forceps minor
2 Anterior horn of lateral ventricle
3 Head of caudate nucleus
4 Third ventricle
5 Thalamus
6 Anterior limb ⎱
7 Genu   ⎬ of internal capsule
8 Posterior limb ⎰
9 Insula
10 Choroid plexus and junction of inferior and posterior horn
11 Tela choroidea of roof of third ventricle
12 Internal cerebral vein
13 Inferior colliculus
14 Trochlear nerve
15 Floor of fourth ventricle

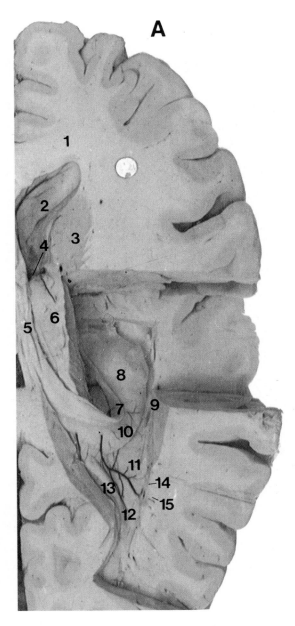

A

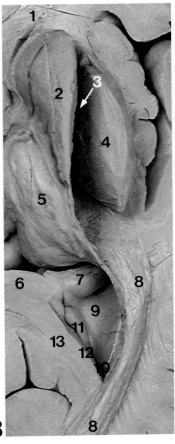

B The optic radiation and the caudate and lentiform nuclei, from above
(Partly dissected out from a horizontal section of the right cerebral hemisphere)

1 Forceps minor
2 Caudate nucleus
3 Internal capsule
4 Lentiform nucleus
5 Thalamus
6 Splenium of corpus callosum
7 Hippocampus
8 Optic radiation
9 Collateral trigone
10 Posterior horn of lateral ventricle
11 Calcar
12 Bulb
13 Forceps major

B

A Fornix, hippocampus and horns of the lateral ventricle of the right cerebral hemisphere, dissected from above

1 Forceps minor
2 Anterior horn of lateral ventricle
3 Head of caudate nucleus
4 Interventricular foramen
5 Fornix
6 Thalamus (floor of body of lateral ventricle)
7 Fimbria
8 Pes hippocampi ⎤ in floor of
9 Collateral eminence ⎦ inferior horn
10 Hippocampus
11 Collateral trigone
12 Posterior horn
13 Calcar
14 Tapetum
15 Optic radiation

C Cast of the cerebral ventricles, from the left

1 Anterior horn ⎤
2 Body ⎟ of lateral
3 Posterior horn ⎟ ventricle
4 Inferior horn ⎦
5 Interventricular foramen
6 Third ventricle (with gap for interthalamic connexion)
7 Supra-optic ⎤
8 Infundibular ⎟ recess of
9 Suprapineal ⎦ third ventricle
10 Aqueduct of midbrain
11 Fourth ventricle
12 Lateral recess

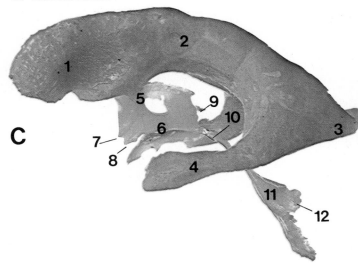

C

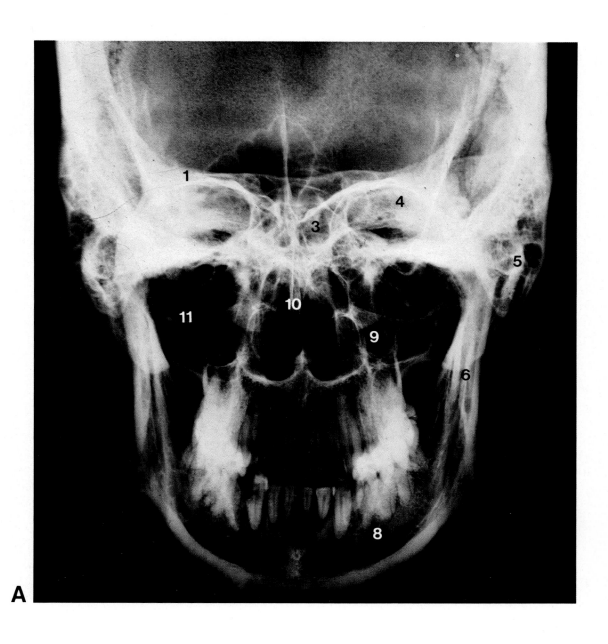

A

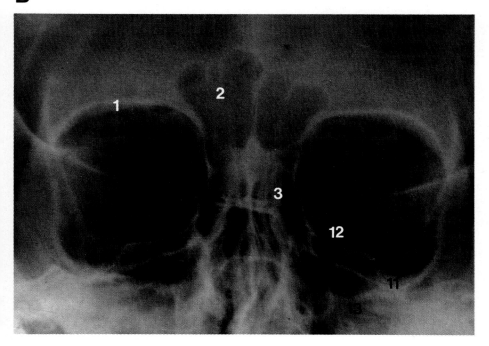

B

**Radiographs of the skull, from the front,
A general view, B orbital features**
   1 Superior orbital margin
   2 Frontal sinus
   3 Ethmoidal sinus
   4 Petrous part of temporal bone
   5 Mastoid process and air cells
   6 Ramus ⎫
   7 Angle ⎬ of mandible
   8 Body ⎭
   9 Maxillary sinus
  10 Nasal septum
  11 Inferior orbital margin
  12 Superior orbital fissure
  13 Foramen rotundum

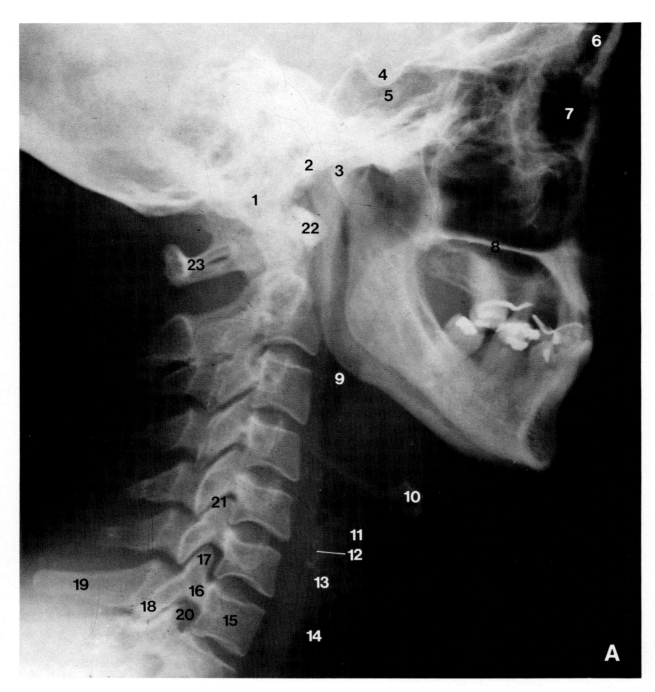

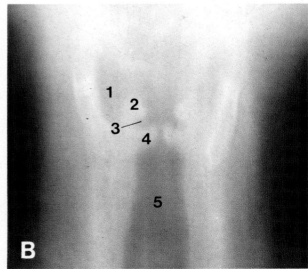

Vertebral Column & Spinal Medulla

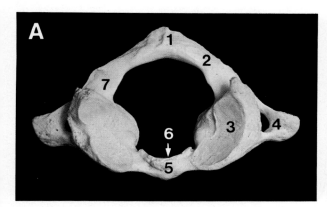

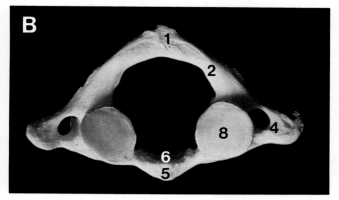

Atlas (first cervical vertebra), A from above, B from below
1 Posterior tubercle
2 Posterior arch
3 Lateral mass with superior articular facet
4 Transverse process and foramen
5 Anterior arch and tubercle
6 Facet for dens of axis
7 Groove for vertebral artery
8 Lateral mass with inferior articular facet

● The superior articular facets are concave and kidney-shaped.
● The inferior articular facets are round and almost flat.
● The anterior arch is straighter and shorter than the posterior arch, and contains on its posterior surface the facet for the dens of the axis.
● The atlas is the only vertebra that has no body.

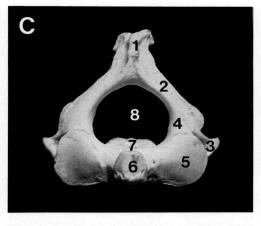

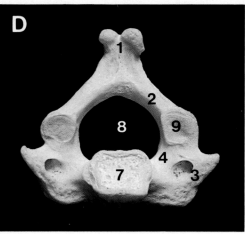

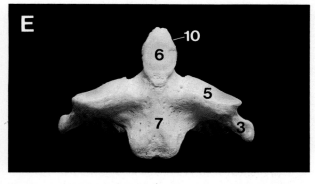

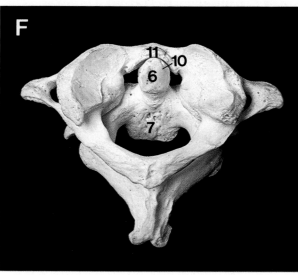

Axis (second cervical vertebra), C from above, D from below, E from the front, F articulated with the atlas, from above and behind
1 Bifid spinous process
2 Lamina
3 Transverse process and foramen
4 Pedicle
5 Superior articular surface
6 Dens
7 Body
8 Vertebral foramen
9 Inferior articular process
10 Impression for alar ligament
11 Anterior arch of atlas

● The axis is unique in having the dens which projects upwards from the body, and represents the body of the atlas.

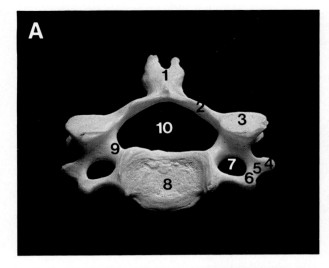

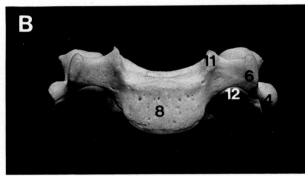

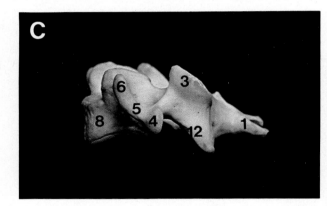

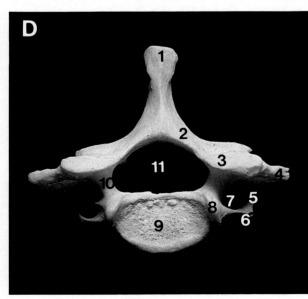

Fifth cervical vertebra (a typical cervical vertebra), A from above, B from the front, C from the left

1 Bifid spinous process
2 Lamina
3 Superior articular process
4 Posterior tubercle ⎤
5 Costotransverse bar ⎬ of transverse
6 Anterior tubercle ⎥ process
7 Foramen ⎦
8 Body
9 Pedicle
10 Vertebral foramen
11 Posterolateral lip
12 Inferior articular process

D Seventh cervical vertebra (vertebra prominens), from above

1 Spinous process with tubercle
2 Lamina
3 Superior articular process
4 Posterior tubercle ⎤
5 Costotransverse bar ⎬ of transverse
6 Anterior tubercle ⎥ process
7 Foramen ⎦
8 Posterolateral lip
9 Body
10 Pedicle
11 Vertebral foramen

● All cervical vertebrae (1–7) have a foramen in each transverse process.
● Typical cervical vertebrae (3–6) have superior articular processes that face backwards and upwards, posterolateral lips on the upper surface of the body, a triangular vertebral foramen and a bifid spinous process.
● The anterior tubercle of the transverse process of the sixth cervical vertebra is large and known as the carotid tubercle.
● The seventh cervical vertebra (vertebra prominens) has a spinous process that ends in a single tubercle.
● The rib element of a cervical vertebra is represented by the anterior root of the transverse process, the anterior tubercle, the costotransverse bar and the anterior part of the posterior tubercle.

Seventh thoracic vertebra (a typical thoracic vertebra), E from above, F from the left, G from behind

1 Spinous process
2 Lamina
3 Superior articular process
4 Transverse process
5 Pedicle
6 Body
7 Vertebral foramen
8 Superior costal facet
9 Superior vertebral notch
10 Costal facet of transverse process
11 Inferior articular process
12 Inferior vertebral notch
13 Inferior costal facet

● Typical thoracic vertebrae (2–9) are characterised by articular facets on the bodies, articular facets on the transverse processes, a round vertebral foramen, a spinous process that points downwards as well as backwards, and superior articular processes that are vertical, flat, and face backwards and laterally.

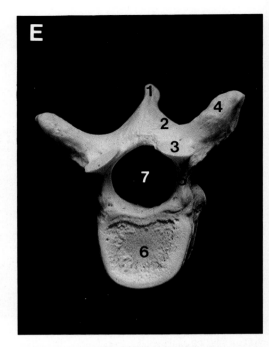

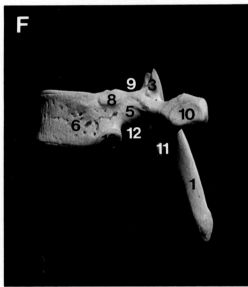

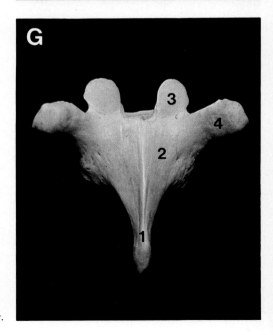

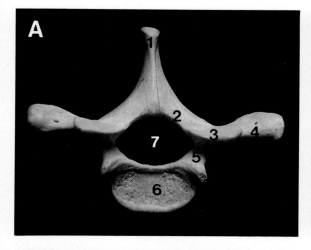

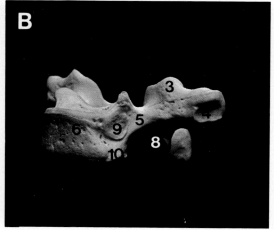

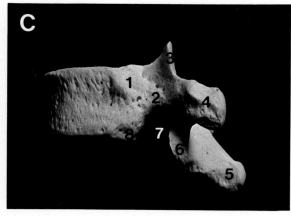

First thoracic vertebra, A from above, B from the front and the left

1 Spinous process
2 Lamina
3 Superior articular process
4 Transverse process with costal facet
5 Pedicle
6 Body with posterolateral lip
7 Vertebral foramen
8 Inferior articular process
9 Superior costal facet
10 Inferior costal facet

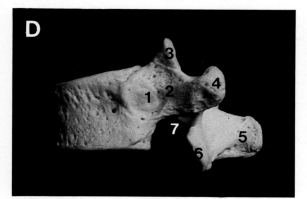

Tenth thoracic vertebra, C, and eleventh thoracic vertebra, D, from the left

1 Costal facet
2 Pedicle
3 Superior articular process
4 Transverse process
5 Spinous process
6 Inferior articular process
7 Inferior vertebral notch
8 Inferior costal facet (not usually present on this vertebra)

Twelfth thoracic vertebra, E from the left, F from above, G from behind

1 Body
2 Costal facet
3 Pedicle
4 Superior articular process
5 Superior tubercle
6 Inferior tubercle
7 Spinous process
8 Inferior articular process
9 Lateral tubercle

● The atypical thoracic vertebrae are the first, tenth, eleventh and twelfth.

● The first thoracic vertebra has a posterolateral lip on each side of the upper surface of the body and a triangular vertebral foramen (features like typical cervical vertebrae), and complete (round) superior articular facets on the sides of the body.

● The tenth, eleventh and twelfth thoracic vertebrae are characterised by a single complete articular facet on each side of the body that in the successive vertebrae comes to lie increasingly far from the upper surface of the body and encroaches increasingly on to the pedicle. There is also no articular facet on the transverse process.

● The transverse process of the twelfth thoracic vertebra is replaced by three tubercles – superior (corresponding to the mamillary process of a lumbar vertebra), lateral (corresponding to a true transverse process) and inferior (corresponding to the accessory process of a lumbar vertebra).

● The inferior articular processes of the twelfth thoracic vertebra are curved to articulate with the curved superior processes of the first lumbar vertebra.

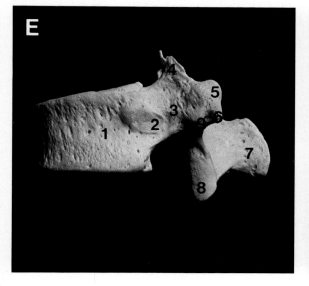

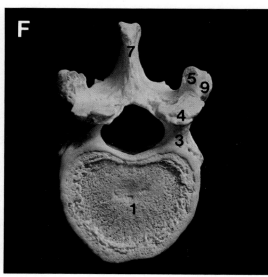

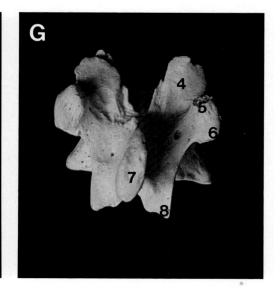

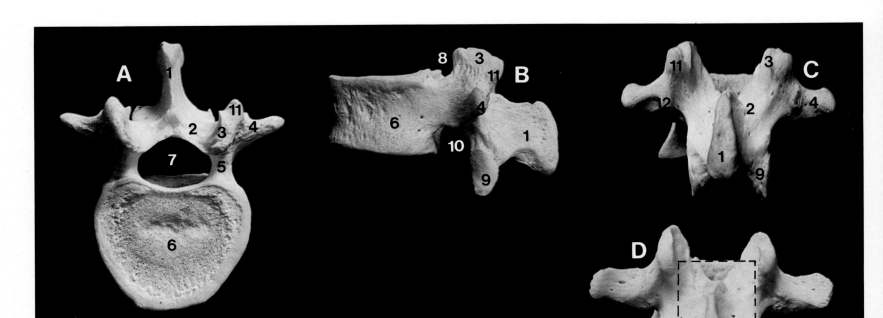

First lumbar vertebra, A from above, B from the left, C from behind

1 Spinous process
2 Lamina
3 Superior articular process
4 Transverse process
5 Pedicle
6 Body
7 Vertebral foramen
8 Superior vertebral notch
9 Inferior articular process
10 Inferior vertebral notch
11 Mamillary process
12 Accessory process

● Lumbar vertebrae are characterised by the large size of the bodies, the absence of costal facets on the bodies and the transverse processes, a triangular vertebral foramen, a spinous process that points backwards and is quadrangular or hatchet-shaped, and superior articular processes that are vertical, curved, face backwards and medially and possess a mamillary process at their posterior rim.

● The rib element of a lumbar vertebra is represented by the transverse process.

D Second lumbar vertebra, from behind; E Third lumbar vertebra, from behind; F Fourth lumbar vertebra, from behind; G Fifth lumbar vertebra, from behind

● Viewed from behind, the four articular processes of the first and second lumbar vertebrae make a pattern (indicated by the interrupted line) of a vertical rectangle; those of the third or fourth vertebra make a square, and those of the fifth lumbar vertebra make a horizontal rectangle.

H Fifth lumbar vertebra, from above

1 Spinous process
2 Lamina
3 Superior articular process
4 Transverse process fusing with pedicle and body
5 Body
6 Vertebral foramen

● The fifth lumbar vertebra is unique in that the transverse process unites directly with the side of the body as well as with the pedicle.

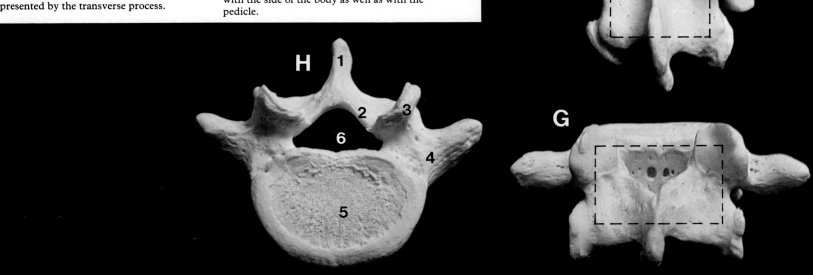

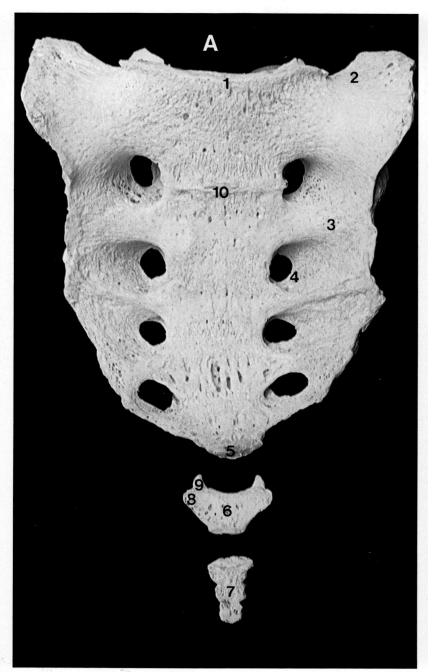

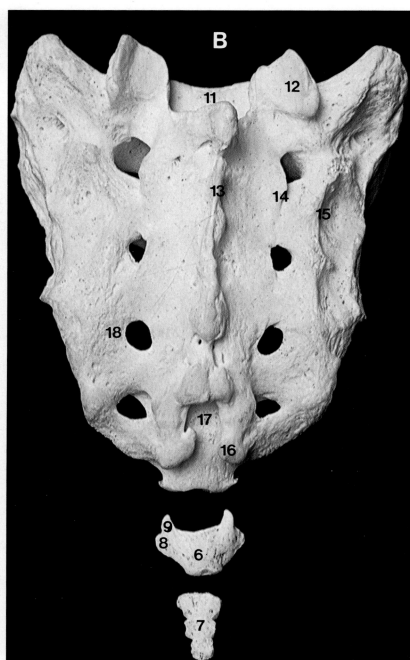

Sacrum and coccyx, A pelvic surface, B dorsal surface

 1 Promontory
 2 Upper surface of lateral part
 3 Lateral part
 4 Second pelvic sacral foramen
 5 Facet for coccyx
 6 First coccygeal vertebra
 7 Fused second to fourth vertebrae
 8 Transverse process
 9 Coccygeal cornu
10 Site of fusion of first and second sacral vertebrae
11 Sacral canal
12 Superior articular process

13 Median sacral crest
14 Intermediate sacral crest
15 Lateral sacral crest
16 Sacral cornu
17 Sacral hiatus
18 Third dorsal sacral foramen

● The sacrum is formed by the fusion of the five sacral vertebrae. The median sacral crest represents the fused spinous processes, the intermediate crest the fused articular processes, and the lateral crest the fused transverse processes.
● The sacral hiatus is the lower opening of the sacral canal.
● The coccyx is usually formed by the fusion of four rudimentary vertebrae but the number varies from three to five. In this specimen the first piece of the coccyx is not fused with the remainder.

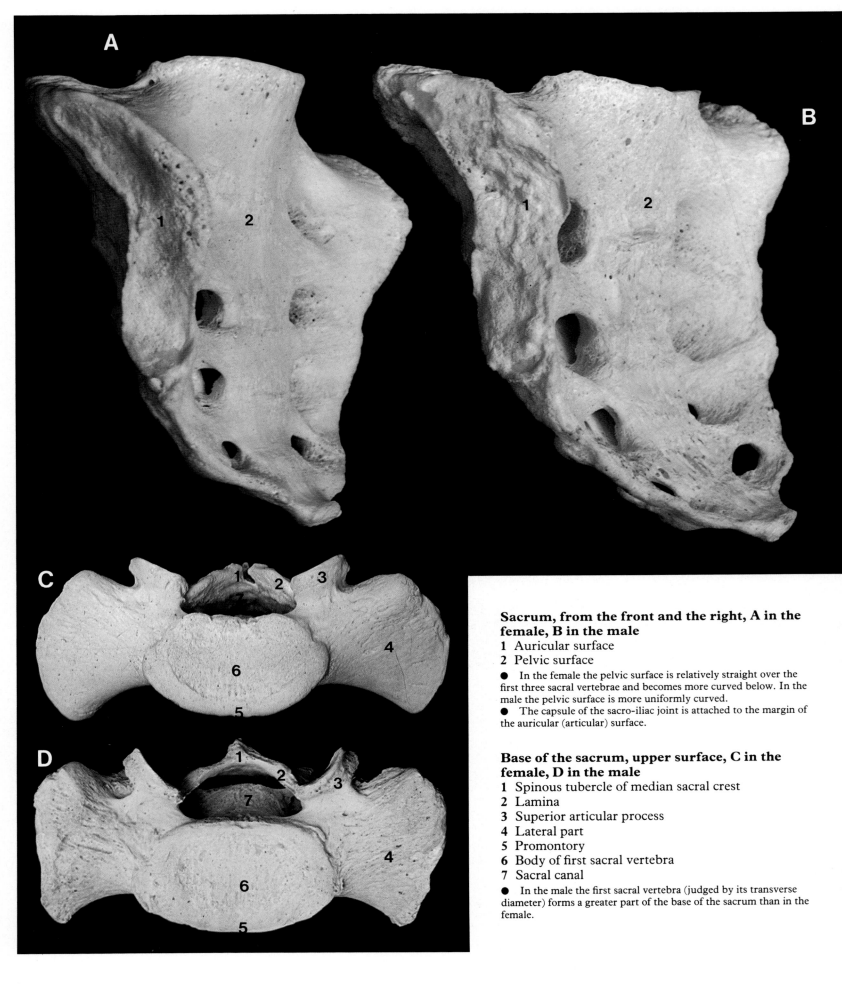

Sacrum, from the front and the right, A in the female, B in the male

1 Auricular surface
2 Pelvic surface

● In the female the pelvic surface is relatively straight over the first three sacral vertebrae and becomes more curved below. In the male the pelvic surface is more uniformly curved.

● The capsule of the sacro-iliac joint is attached to the margin of the auricular (articular) surface.

Base of the sacrum, upper surface, C in the female, D in the male

1 Spinous tubercle of median sacral crest
2 Lamina
3 Superior articular process
4 Lateral part
5 Promontory
6 Body of first sacral vertebra
7 Sacral canal

● In the male the first sacral vertebra (judged by its transverse diameter) forms a greater part of the base of the sacrum than in the female.

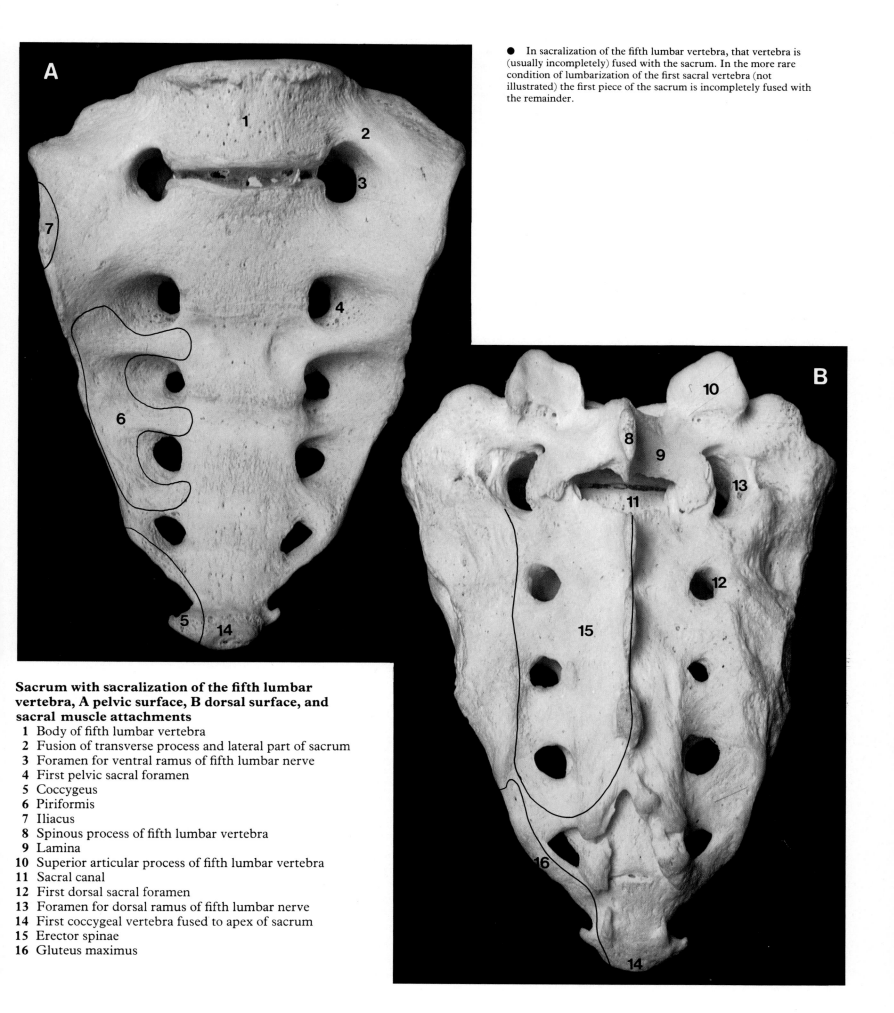

● In sacralization of the fifth lumbar vertebra, that vertebra is (usually incompletely) fused with the sacrum. In the more rare condition of lumbarization of the first sacral vertebra (not illustrated) the first piece of the sacrum is incompletely fused with the remainder.

Sacrum with sacralization of the fifth lumbar vertebra, A pelvic surface, B dorsal surface, and sacral muscle attachments

1 Body of fifth lumbar vertebra
2 Fusion of transverse process and lateral part of sacrum
3 Foramen for ventral ramus of fifth lumbar nerve
4 First pelvic sacral foramen
5 Coccygeus
6 Piriformis
7 Iliacus
8 Spinous process of fifth lumbar vertebra
9 Lamina
10 Superior articular process of fifth lumbar vertebra
11 Sacral canal
12 First dorsal sacral foramen
13 Foramen for dorsal ramus of fifth lumbar nerve
14 First coccygeal vertebra fused to apex of sacrum
15 Erector spinae
16 Gluteus maximus

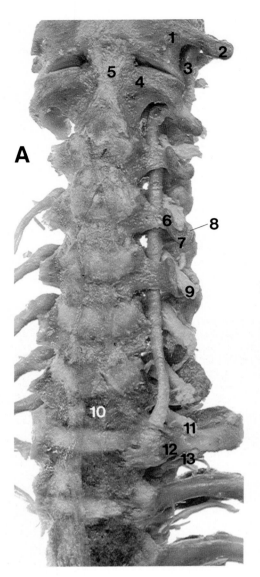

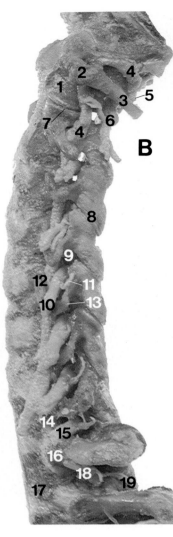

A Vertebral column, cervical region, from the front
(On the right the transverse processes have been partly removed)
1 Lateral mass ⎫
2 Transverse process ⎬ of atlas
3 Vertebral artery
4 Axis
5 Anterior longitudinal ligament
6 Anterior tubercle ⎫ of
7 Costotransverse bar ⎬ transverse process
8 Posterior tubercle ⎭ process
9 Ventral ramus of fifth cervical nerve
10 Body of seventh cervical vertebra
11 Ventral ramus of eighth cervical nerve
12 Head of first rib
13 Ventral ramus of first thoracic nerve

B Vertebral column, cervical and upper thoracic regions, from the left. Nerve roots and rami
1 Lateral mass ⎫
2 Transverse process ⎬ of atlas
3 Posterior arch ⎭
4 Vertebral artery
5 First cervical nerve
6 Dorsal root ganglion and rami of second cervical nerve
7 Atlanto-axial joint
8 Zygapophysial joint
9 Intervertebral foramen
10 Ventral ⎫ ramus of fifth
11 Dorsal ⎬ cervical nerve
12 Anterior tubercle ⎫ of transverse process of
13 Posterior tubercle ⎬ fifth cervical vertebra
14 Body of seventh cervical vertebra
15 Ventral ramus of eighth cervical nerve
16 Head of first rib
17 Body of first thoracic vertebra
18 Ventral ⎫ ramus of first
19 Dorsal ⎬ thoracic nerve

● The first and second cervical nerves pass respectively above and below the posterior arch of the atlas.
● On its upward course from the subclavian artery the vertebral artery enters the foramen of the transverse process of the sixth cervical vertebra.
● For the joints of the ribs with thoracic vertebrae see pages 196 and 197.

C Vertebral column, cervical region, from the left. Intervertebral foramina
1 Body of third cervical vertebra
2 Intervertebral disc
3 Pedicle
4 Intervertebral foramen
5 Zygapophysial joint
6 Posterior tubercle ⎫ of
7 Costotransverse bar ⎬ transverse process of fifth cervical vertebra
8 Anterior tubercle ⎭
● Each intervertebral foramen is bounded in front by a vertebral body and intervertebral disc, above and below by pedicles, and behind by a zygapophysial joint.

D Vertebral column, cervical region, from behind and slightly right, with the left half of the vertebral arches removed
1 Part of occipital bone of skull
2 Posterior arch ⎫ of
3 Transverse process ⎬ atlas
4 Spinous process of axis
5 Lamina of fifth cervical vertebra
6 Zygapophysial joint
7 Ligamentum flavum
8 Spinous process of seventh cervical vertebra
9 Dorsal root ganglion ⎫ of
10 Dorsal ramus ⎬ fifth cervical
11 Ventral ramus ⎭ nerve
● The ligamenta flava pass between the laminae of adjacent vertebrae. They are larger and thicker in the lumbar region (page 86) than elsewhere.

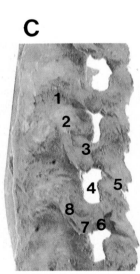

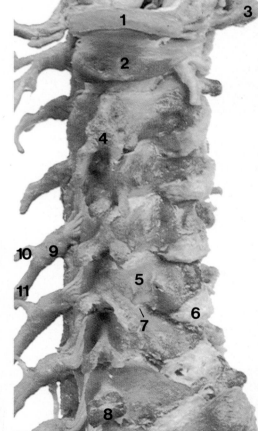

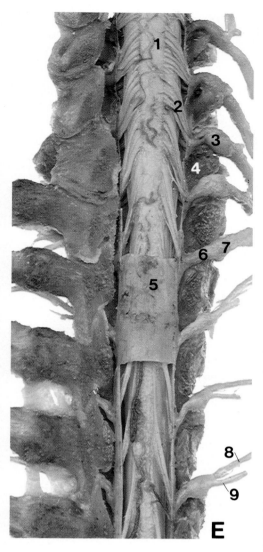

E Lower cervical and upper thoracic regions of the spinal medulla, from behind with vertebral arches and meninges removed

1 Spinal medulla and posterior spinal vessels
2 Dorsal rootlets ⎫ of eighth
3 Dorsal root ganglion ⎭ cervical nerve
4 Pedicle of first thoracic vertebra
5 Dura mater
6 Dural sheath ⎫ of second
7 Dorsal root ganglion ⎭ thoracic nerve
8 Ventral ⎫ ramus of fifth
9 Dorsal ⎭ thoracic nerve

- The spinal medulla is commonly called the spinal cord.
- Each nerve *root* is formed by the union of several *rootlets*.
- Each spinal nerve is formed by the union of ventral and dorsal nerve roots. The union occurs immediately distal to the dorsal root ganglion, within the intervertebral foramen, and the nerve at once divides into a ventral and a dorsal (primary) ramus. The spinal nerve proper is therefore only a few millimetres or so in length.
- The lowest cervical and upper thoracic nerve roots become acutely angled in order to enter their dural sheaths.
- For the upper cervical spinal medulla and its continuity with the brainstem see page 69.

F Vertebral column and spinal medulla, cervical and upper thoracic regions, from the left with parts of the vertebral arches and meninges removed

1 Spinal part of accessory nerve
2 Medulla oblongata
3 Foramen magnum
4 Occipital bone
5 Posterior arch of atlas
6 Spinous process of axis (abnormally large)
7 Spinal medulla
8 Dura mater
9 Denticulate ligament
10 Ventral rootlets ⎫
11 Dorsal rootlets ⎪ of fifth
12 Dorsal root ganglion ⎬ cervical
13 Dorsal ramus ⎪ nerve
14 Ventral ramus ⎭
15 Spinous process of seventh cervical vertebra
16 Dorsal root ganglion of eighth cervical nerve
17 Body of first thoracic vertebra
18 Arachnoid mater
19 Sympathetic trunk

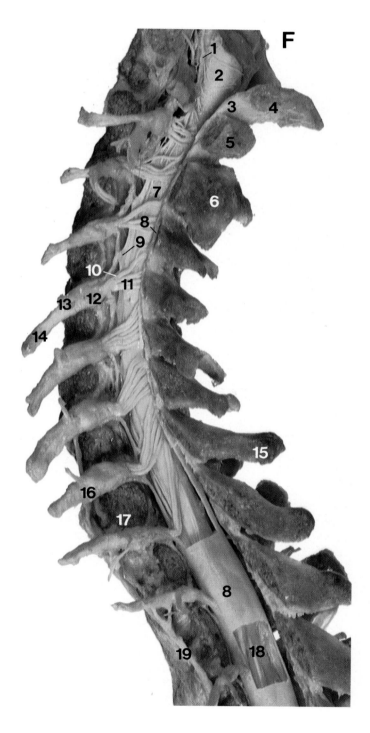

G Part of the cervical region of the spinal medulla, from behind. Dura mater and denticulate ligament

1 Dura mater and arachnoid mater
2 Dorsal rootlets of first cervical nerve
3 Spinal root of accessory nerve
4 Denticulate ligament

- The denticulate ligament is composed of pia mater.
- On the right some dorsal rootlets have been cut and turned medially and the ventral rootlets removed(they lie anterior to the denticulate ligament).

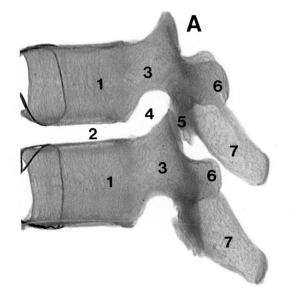

A

A Cleared specimens of thoracic vertebrae, from the left

1 Body
2 Space for intervertebral disc
3 Pedicle
4 Intervertebral foramen
5 Zygapophysial joint
6 Transverse process
7 Spinous process

● The intervertebral foramen is bounded in front by the lower part of the vertebral body and the intervertebral disc, above and below by the pedicles, and behind by the zygapophysial joint.

B Vertebral column, lumbar and sacral regions. Meninges and cauda equina from behind, with the vertebral arches removed

1 Conus medullaris
2 Cauda equina
3 Dura mater
4 Superior articular process of third lumbar vertebra
5 Filum terminale
6 Roots of fifth lumbar nerve
7 Fourth lumbar intervertebral disc
8 Pedicle of fifth lumbar vertebra
9 Dorsal root ganglion of fifth lumbar nerve
10 Fifth lumbar (lumbosacral) intervertebral disc
11 Dural sheath of first sacral nerve roots
12 Lateral part of sacrum
13 Second sacral vertebra

● The spinal medulla ends at the level of the first lumbar vertebra.

● The subarachnoid space ends at the level of the second sacral vertebra.

● For a similar specimen of this important region see page 86.

C Vertebral column and spinal medulla, lower thoracic and upper lumbar regions, from the left with parts of the vertebral arches and meninges removed

1 Greater splanchnic nerve
2 Sympathetic trunk
3 Sympathetic ganglion
4 Rami communicantes
5 Dorsal root ganglion of tenth thoracic nerve
6 Spinal medulla
7 Dura mater
8 Spinous process of tenth thoracic vertebra
9 Interspinous ligament
10 Supraspinous ligament
11 Cauda equina
12 Body of first lumbar vertebra
13 First lumbar intervertebral disc

C

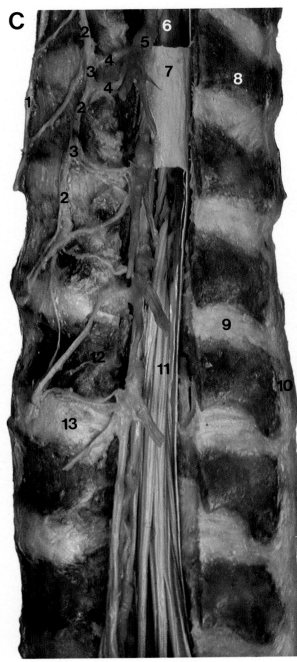

B

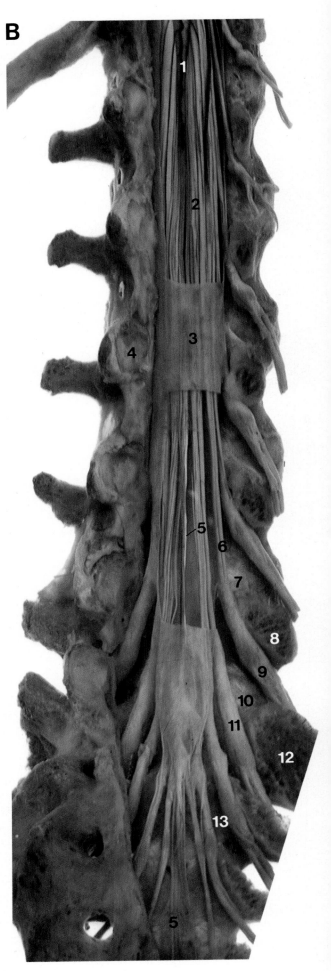

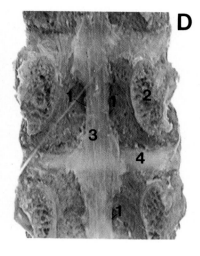

D **Vertebral column, lower thoracic region, from behind with the vertebral arches removed to show the posterior longitudinal ligament**
1 Vascular foramina in posterior surface of body
2 Pedicle
3 Posterior longitudinal ligament
4 Intervertebral disc

● The posterior longitudinal ligament is broad where it is firmly attached to the intervertebral discs, but narrow and less firmly attached to the vertebral bodies (to leave the vascular foramina patent).

● The anterior longitudinal ligament is broad and firmly attached to vertebral bodies and intervertebral discs.

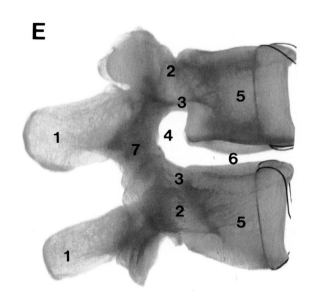
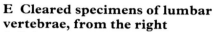

E Cleared specimens of lumbar vertebrae, from the right
1 Spinous process
2 Transverse process
3 Pedicle
4 Intervertebral foramen
5 Body
6 Space for intervertebral disc
7 Zygapophysial joint

● The boundaries of the intervertebral foramina in the lumbar region are similar to those in the cervical and thoracic regions (pages 83 and 84).

F Vertebral column, lower lumbar region, from the front. Anterior longitudinal ligament
1 Anterior longitudinal ligament (anterior to marker and reflected)
2 Body of fourth lumbar vertebra
3 Fourth lumbar intervertebral disc
4 Body of fifth lumbar vertebra
5 Ventral ramus of fifth lumbar nerve
6 Lateral part of sacrum

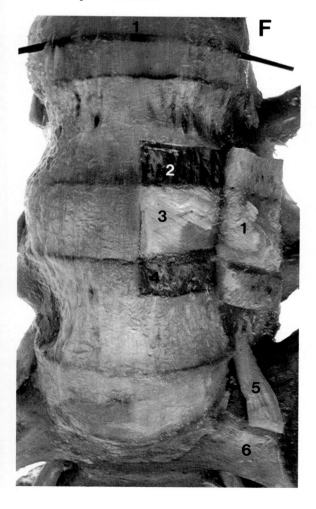

G Vertebral column, upper lumbar region, from the right. Intervertebral foramina and spinal nerves
1 Twelfth rib
2 Sympathetic trunk ganglion
3 Anterior longitudinal ligament
4 First lumbar vertebra
5 Rami communicantes
6 First lumbar nerve emerging from intervertebral foramen
7 Ventral   ramus of first
8 Dorsal   lumbar nerve
9 First lumbar intervertebral disc
10 Ventral   ramus of second
11 Dorsal   lumbar nerve
12 Zygapophysial joint
13 Spinous process of second lumbar vertebra
14 Interspinous ligament
15 Supraspinous ligament

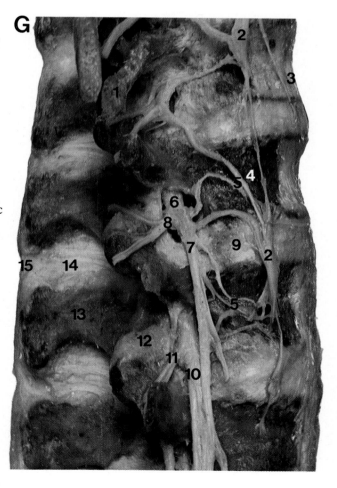

Nerve roots and meninges in the lumbar and sacral regions, from behind with the vertebral arches removed

1 Dura mater
2 Pedicle of fifth lumbar vertebra
3 Dural sheath containing roots and dorsal root ganglion of fifth lumbar nerve in intervertebral foramen
4 Fifth lumbar nerve
5 Fifth lumbar intervertebral disc
6 Filum terminale
7 Dural sheath containing roots and dorsal root ganglion of first sacral nerve
8 Second sacral vertebra

● If the fifth lumbar intervertebral disc protrudes backwards ('slipped disc') it may irritate the roots of the first sacral nerve. This is the general rule for any part of the vertebral column – a protruded disc may irritate the roots of the nerve numbered one below the disc. Note for example that the fifth lumbar nerve roots within their dural sheath pass laterally immediately below the pedicle of the fifth lumbar vertebra and so do not come to lie immediately behind the fifth lumbar disc; it is the first sacral roots that lie in this position.

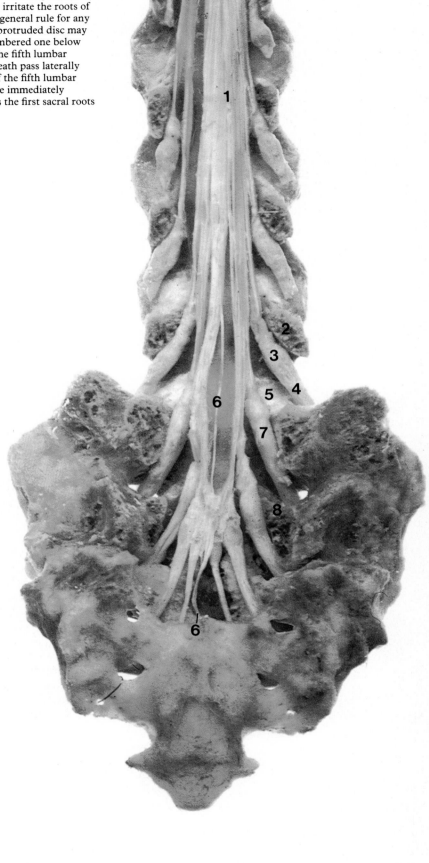

Vertebral column, lumbar region, from the right and behind. Ligamenta flava

1 Supraspinous ligament
2 Spinous process ⎫ of second
3 Lamina ⎬ lumbar vertebra
4 Interspinous ligament
5 Ligamentum flavum
6 Zygapophysial joint
7 Transverse process of third lumbar vertebra

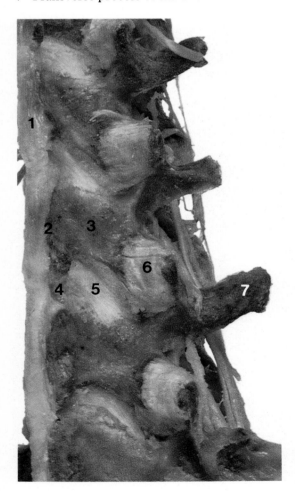

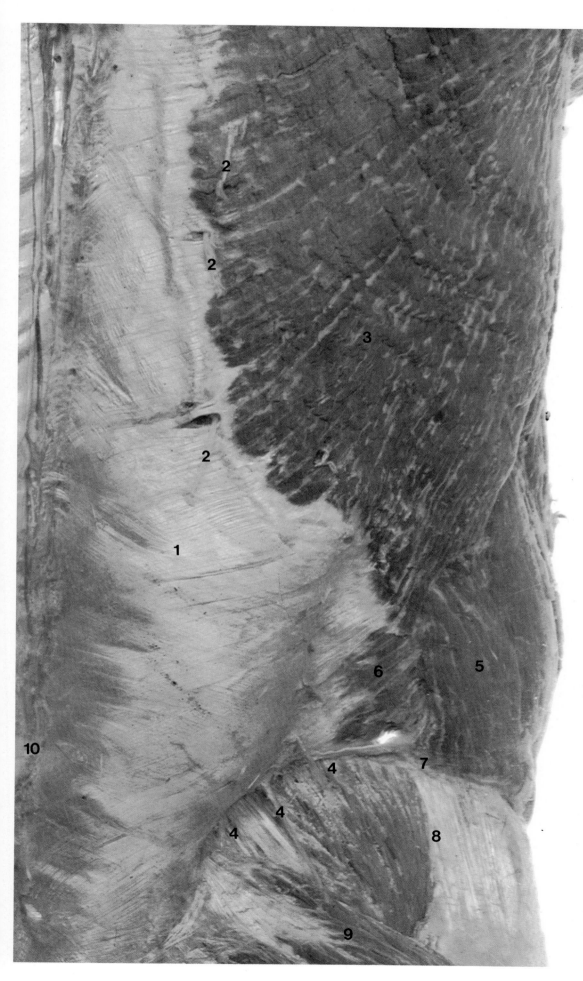

Muscles of the vertebral column. Erector spinae and the thoracolumbar fascia on the right

1 Posterior layer of lumbar part of thoracolumbar fascia overlying erector spinae
2 Branches of dorsal rami of thoracic nerves
3 Latissimus dorsi
4 Cutaneous branches of dorsal rami of first three lumbar nerves
5 External oblique
6 Internal oblique
7 Iliac crest
8 Gluteal fascia (partly removed) overlying gluteus medius
9 Gluteus maximus
10 Level of fourth lumbar spinous process

● For other parts of erector spinae see pages 88 and 157.

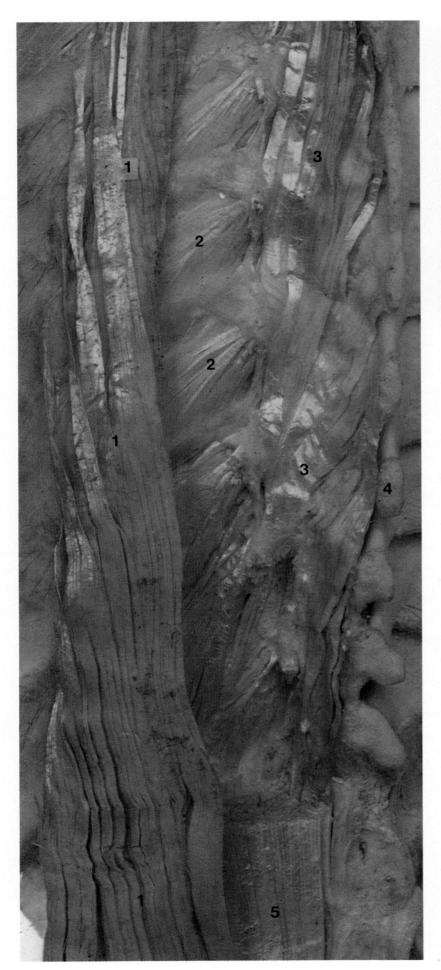

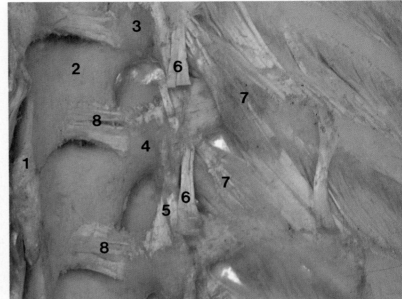

Muscles of the vertebral column. Rotator and intertransverse muscles of the thoracic region

1 Spinous process ⎱
2 Lamina   ⎰ of fourth thoracic vertebra
3 Transverse process
4 Transverse process of fifth thoracic vertebra
5 Intertransverse muscle and ligament
6 Tendons of longissimus
7 Levator costae
8 Rotator muscle

● The rotator muscles, only prominent in the thoracic region, pass from the transverse process of one vertebra to the lamina of the vertebra above.

Muscles of the vertebral column. Erector spinae in the thoracolumbar region

1 Iliocostalis
2 Levator costae
3 Spinalis
4 Spine of eighth thoracic vertebra
5 Erector spinae

● In the upper lumbar region the erector spinae divides into three muscle masses: iliocostalis laterally, an intermediate longissimus muscle (removed in this specimen), and spinalis medially. The details of the subdivision of each group and their precise attachments are not usually considered important.

● The levatores costarum muscles are classified as muscles of the thorax (see page 155) not of the vertebral column. They are revealed in this specimen because the longissimus muscle has been removed.

Radiograph of upper cervical vertebrae, from behind with the mouth open
1 Dens of axis
2 Lateral mass of atlas
3 Atlanto-axial joint
4 Body of axis
5 Third cervical vertebra

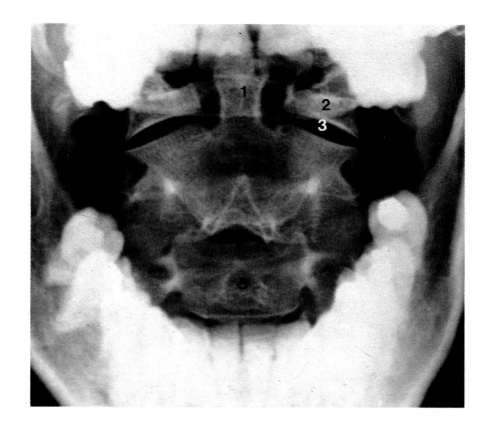

Radiograph of lower cervical and upper thoracic vertebrae, from the front
1 Body of sixth cervical vertebra
2 Margin of tracheal shadow
3 Body ⎫
4 Transverse process ⎬ of first thoracic vertebra
5 Head ⎫
6 Neck ⎬ of first rib
7 Tubercle ⎬ of first rib
8 Shaft ⎭
9 Head ⎫
10 Neck ⎬ of second rib
11 Tubercle ⎭

● For a radiograph of cervical vertebrae from the side see page 74, and of other thoracic vertebrae and ribs see page 202.

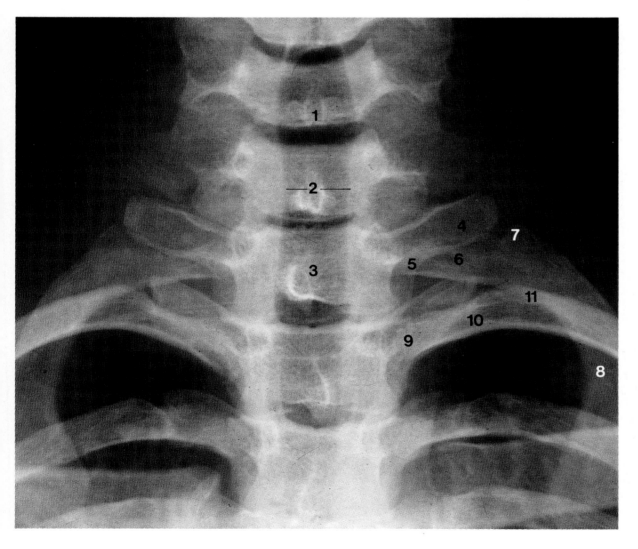

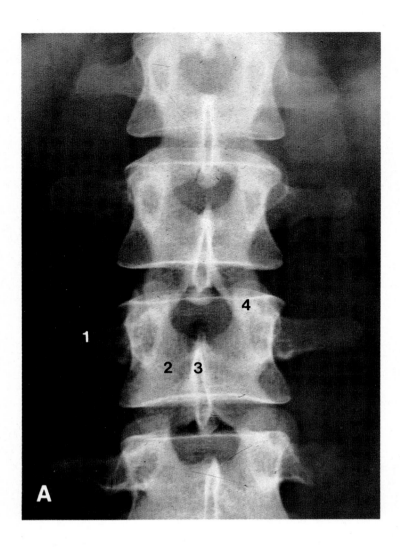

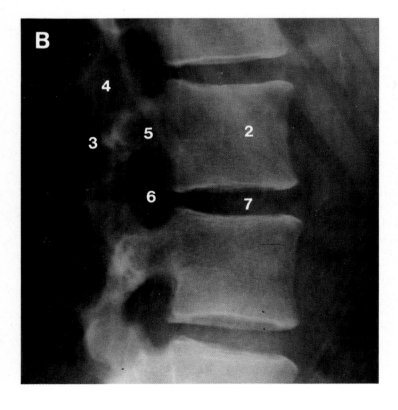

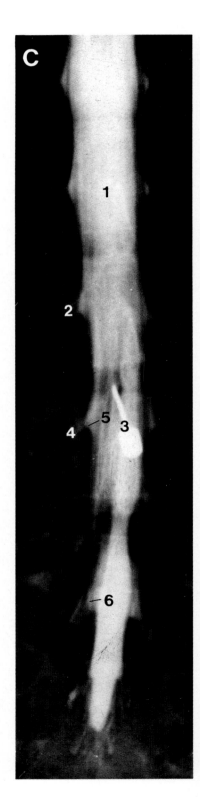

Radiographs of lumbar vertebrae, A from behind, B lateral view

1 Transverse process
2 Body
3 Spinous process
4 Superior articular process
5 Pedicle
6 Intervertebral foramen
7 Intervertebral disc

} of third lumbar vertebra

● Compare with the cleared specimens of vertebrae on page 85.

C Myelogram of the lumbrosacral region, from behind

(After injection of contrast medium into the subarachnoid space)

1 Subarachnoid space
2 Third lumbar vertebra
3 Needle for injection
4 Fourth lumbar vertebra
5 Dural sheath containing fourth lumbar nerve roots
6 Dural sheath containing first sacral nerve roots

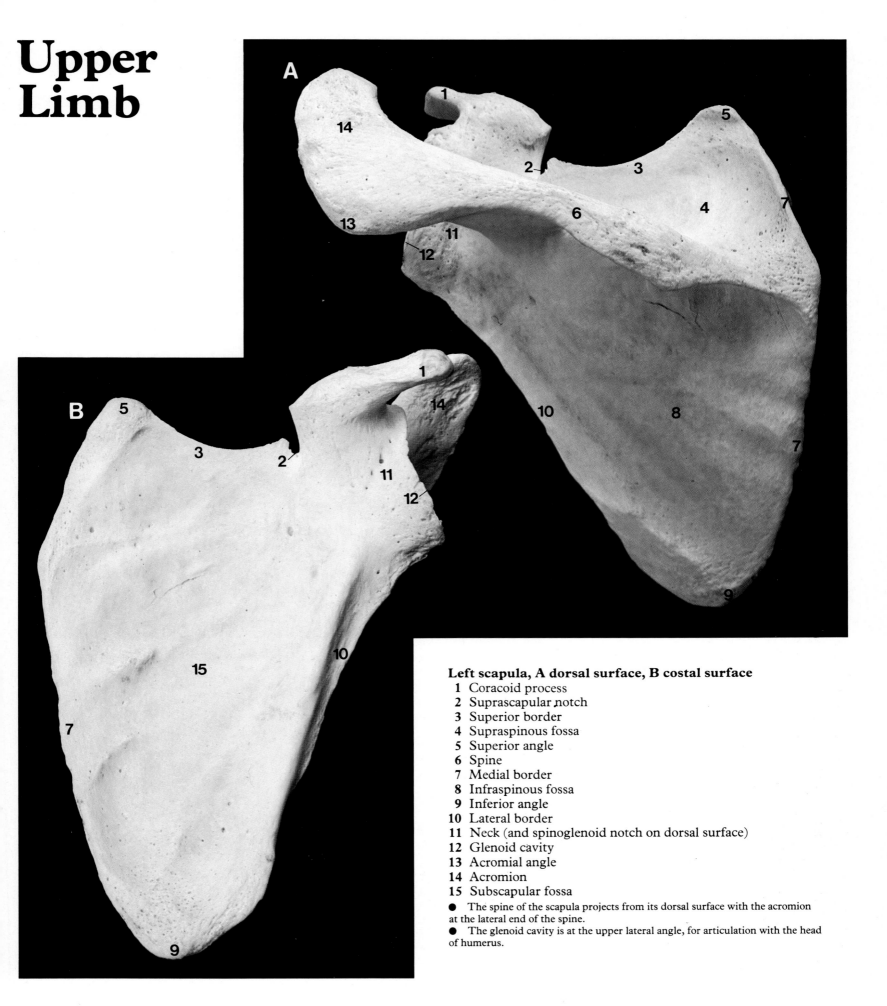

Left scapula, A dorsal surface, B costal surface
1 Coracoid process
2 Suprascapular notch
3 Superior border
4 Supraspinous fossa
5 Superior angle
6 Spine
7 Medial border
8 Infraspinous fossa
9 Inferior angle
10 Lateral border
11 Neck (and spinoglenoid notch on dorsal surface)
12 Glenoid cavity
13 Acromial angle
14 Acromion
15 Subscapular fossa

● The spine of the scapula projects from its dorsal surface with the acromion at the lateral end of the spine.
● The glenoid cavity is at the upper lateral angle, for articulation with the head of humerus.

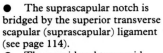

- The suprascapular notch is bridged by the superior transverse scapular (suprascapular) ligament (see page 114).
- The conoid and trapezoid ligaments together constitute the coracoclavicular ligament.
- The coracoclavicular ligament connects the clavicle to the coracoid process of the scapula. The coracohumeral ligament reinforces the upper part of the capsule of the shoulder joint. The coraco-acromial ligament connects the coracoid process with the acromion, forming with those bony processes an arch above the head of the humerus.

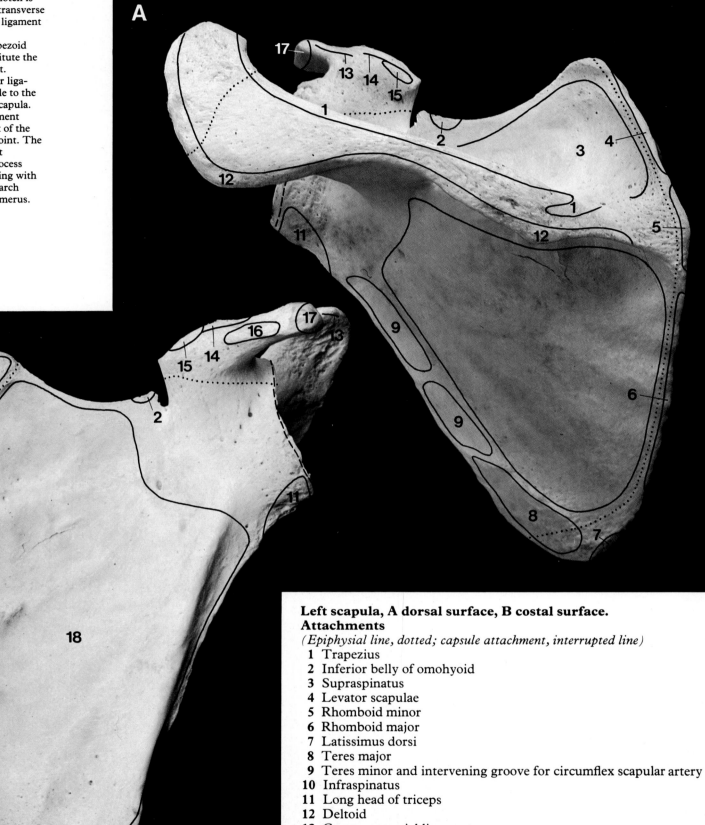

Left scapula, A dorsal surface, B costal surface.
Attachments
(Epiphysial line, dotted; capsule attachment, interrupted line)
1 Trapezius
2 Inferior belly of omohyoid
3 Supraspinatus
4 Levator scapulae
5 Rhomboid minor
6 Rhomboid major
7 Latissimus dorsi
8 Teres major
9 Teres minor and intervening groove for circumflex scapular artery
10 Infraspinatus
11 Long head of triceps
12 Deltoid
13 Coraco-acromial ligament
14 Trapezoid ligament
15 Conoid ligament
16 Pectoralis minor
17 Coracobrachialis and short head of biceps
18 Subscapularis
19 Serratus anterior

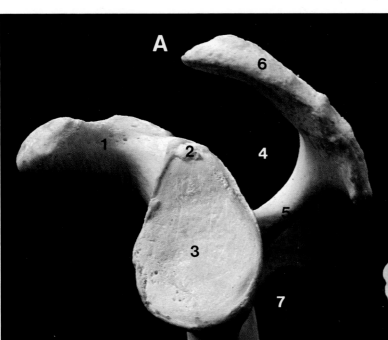

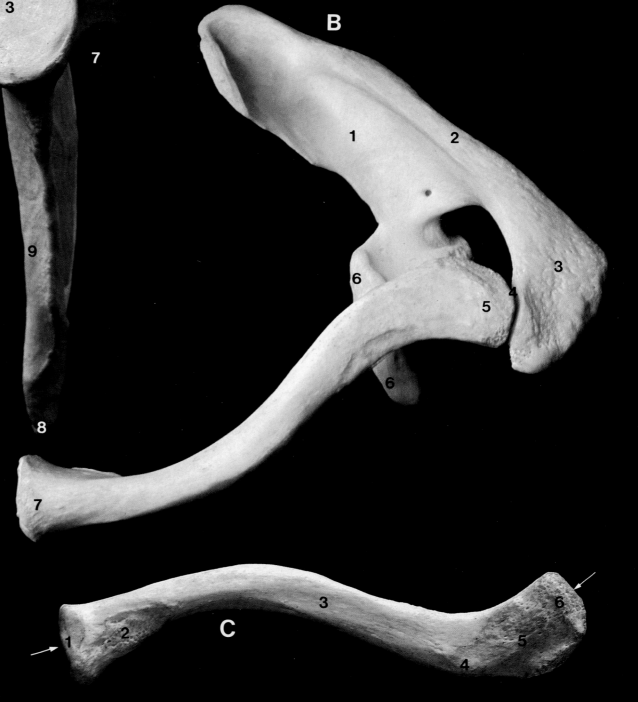

A Left scapula, from the lateral side
1 Coracoid process
2 Supraglenoid tubercle
3 Glenoid cavity
4 Supraspinous fossa
5 Spine
6 Acromion
7 Infraspinous fossa
8 Inferior angle
9 Lateral border
10 Infraglenoid tubercle

B Articulation of left scapula and clavicle, from above
1 Supraspinous fossa
2 Spine of scapula
3 Acromion
4 Acromioclavicular joint
5 Acromial end of clavicle
6 Coracoid process
7 Sternal end of clavicle

● The sternal end of the clavicle is bulbous; the acromial end is flattened. The shaft is convex anteriorly in its medial two-thirds, and the groove for the subclavius muscle is on the inferior surface.

C Left clavicle, from below
1 Sternal end with articular surface (arrow)
2 Impression for costoclavicular ligament
3 Groove for sub-clavius muscle
4 Conoid tubercle
5 Trapezoid line
6 Acromial end with articular surface (arrow)

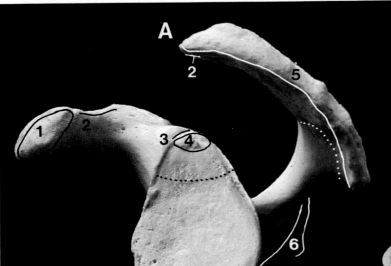

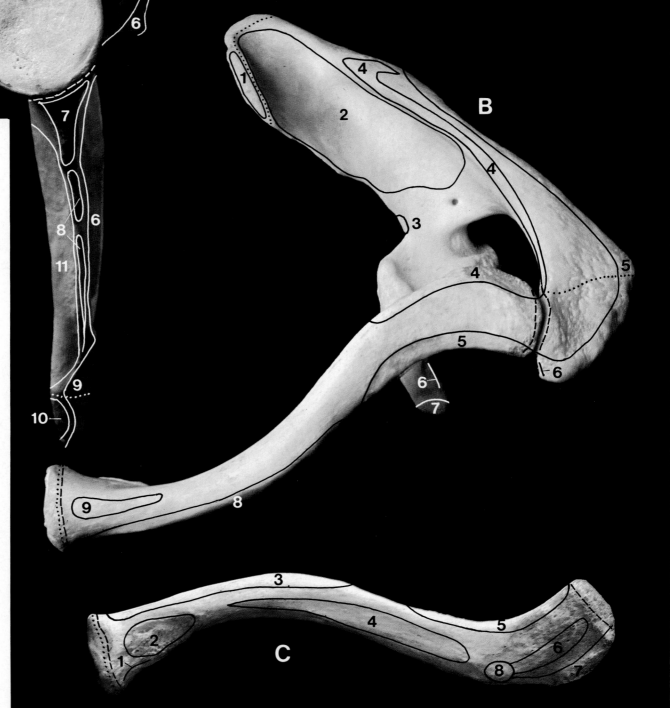

A Left scapula, from the lateral side. Attachments
(Epiphysial line, dotted; capsule attachment, interrupted line)
1 Coracobrachialis and short head of biceps
2 Coraco-acromial ligament
3 Coracohumeral ligament
4 Long head of biceps
5 Deltoid
6 Infraspinatus
7 Long head of triceps
8 Teres minor and intervening groove for circumflex scapular artery
9 Teres major
10 Serratus anterior
11 Subscapularis

B Articulation of left scapula and clavicle, from above
(Epiphysial line, dotted; capsule attachment, interrupted line)
1 Levator scapulae
2 Supraspinatus
3 Inferior belly of omohyoid
4 Trapezius
5 Deltoid
6 Coraco-acromial ligament
7 Coracobrachialis and short head of biceps
8 Pectoralis major
9 Sternocleidomastoid

C Left clavicle, from below. Attachments
(Epiphysial line, dotted; capsule attachment, interrupted line)
1 Sternohyoid
2 Costoclavicular ligament
3 Pectoralis major
4 Subclavius and clavipectoral fascia
5 Deltoid
6 Trapezoid ligament
7 Trapezius
8 Conoid ligament

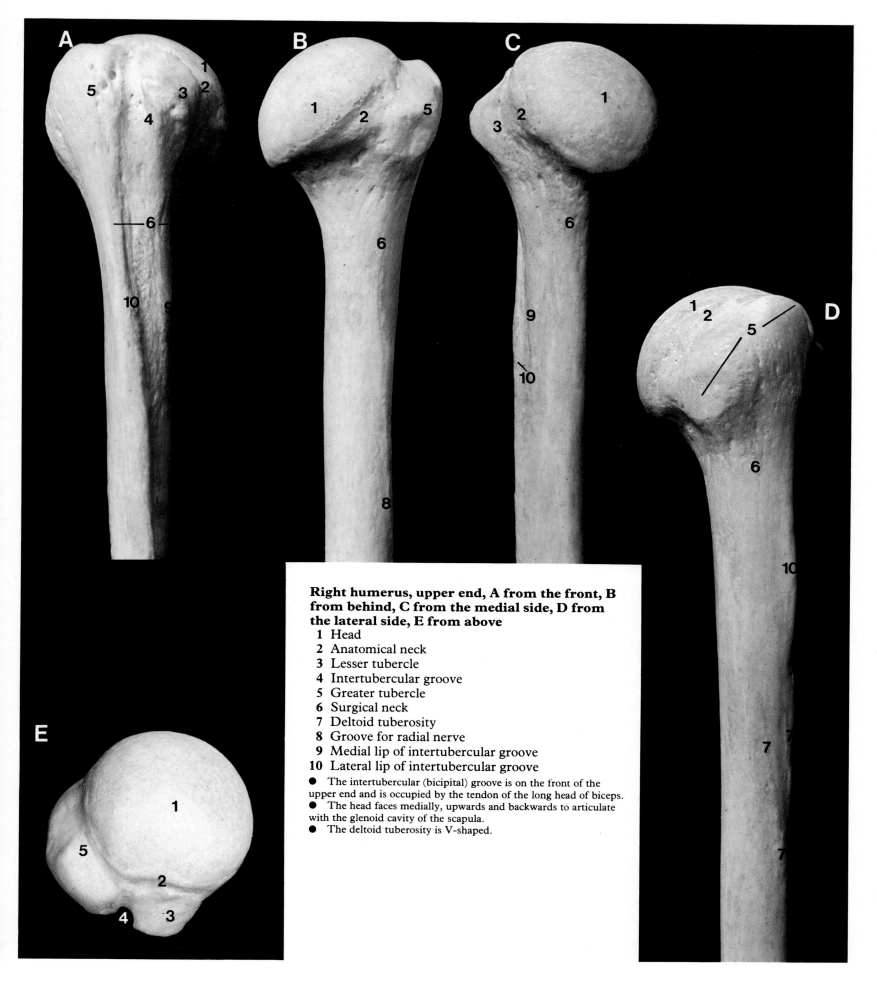

Right humerus, upper end, A from the front, B from behind, C from the medial side, D from the lateral side, E from above

  1 Head
  2 Anatomical neck
  3 Lesser tubercle
  4 Intertubercular groove
  5 Greater tubercle
  6 Surgical neck
  7 Deltoid tuberosity
  8 Groove for radial nerve
  9 Medial lip of intertubercular groove
  10 Lateral lip of intertubercular groove

● The intertubercular (bicipital) groove is on the front of the upper end and is occupied by the tendon of the long head of biceps.
● The head faces medially, upwards and backwards to articulate with the glenoid cavity of the scapula.
● The deltoid tuberosity is V-shaped.

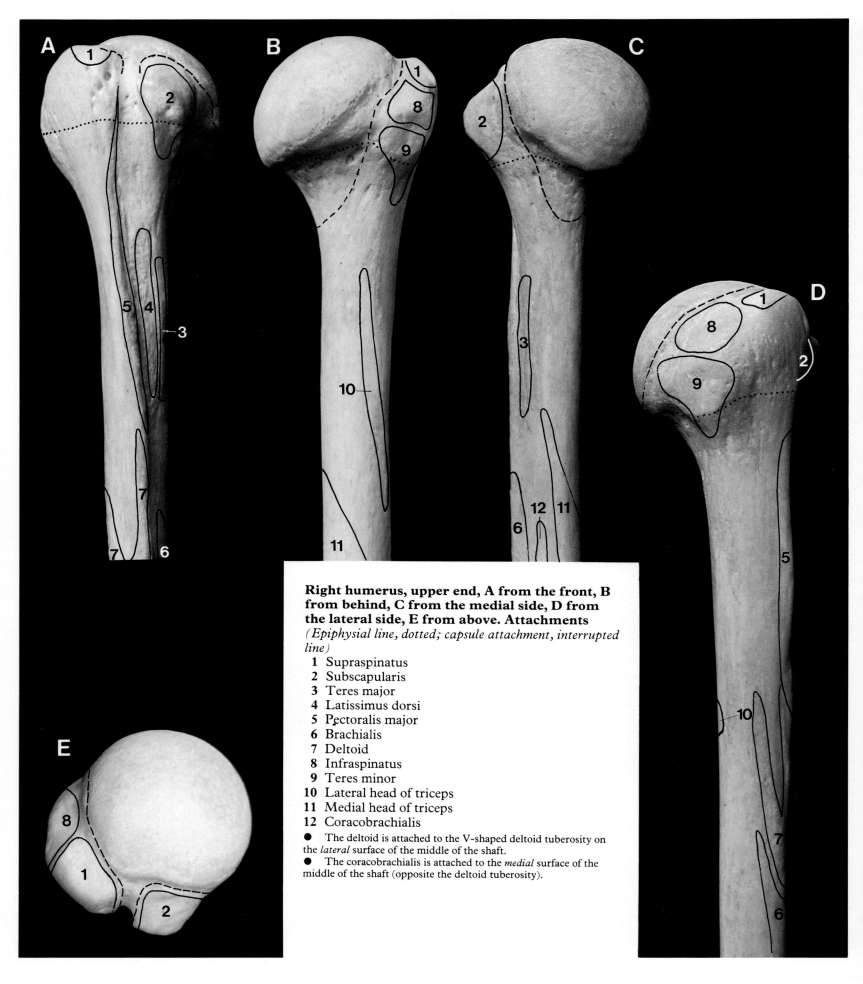

Right humerus, upper end, A from the front, B from behind, C from the medial side, D from the lateral side, E from above. Attachments
(Epiphysial line, dotted; capsule attachment, interrupted line)

1 Supraspinatus
2 Subscapularis
3 Teres major
4 Latissimus dorsi
5 Pectoralis major
6 Brachialis
7 Deltoid
8 Infraspinatus
9 Teres minor
10 Lateral head of triceps
11 Medial head of triceps
12 Coracobrachialis

● The deltoid is attached to the V-shaped deltoid tuberosity on the *lateral* surface of the middle of the shaft.
● The coracobrachialis is attached to the *medial* surface of the middle of the shaft (opposite the deltoid tuberosity).

Right humerus, lower end, A from the front, B from behind, C from below, D from the medial side, E from the lateral side

  1 Lateral supracondylar ridge
  2 Lateral epicondyle
  3 Capitulum
  4 Radial fossa
  5 Trochlea
  6 Coronoid fossa
  7 Medial epicondyle
  8 Medial supracondylar ridge
  9 Anterior surface
 10 Posterior surface
 11 Olecranon fossa
 12 Medial surface of trochlea
 13 Lateral edge of capitulum

● The medial epicondyle is more prominent than the lateral.

● The olecranon fossa (on the posterior surface) is deeper than the radial and coronoid fossae (on the anterior surface).

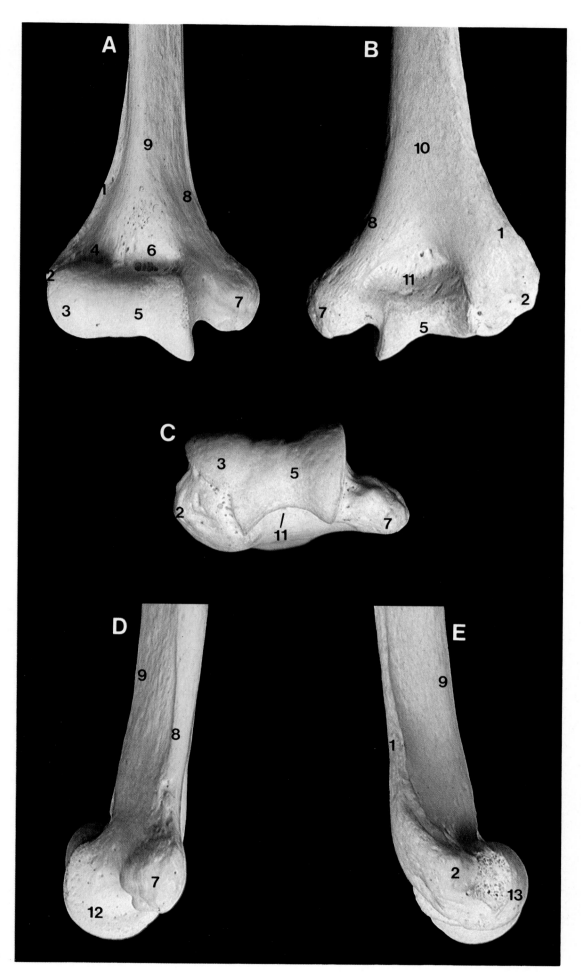

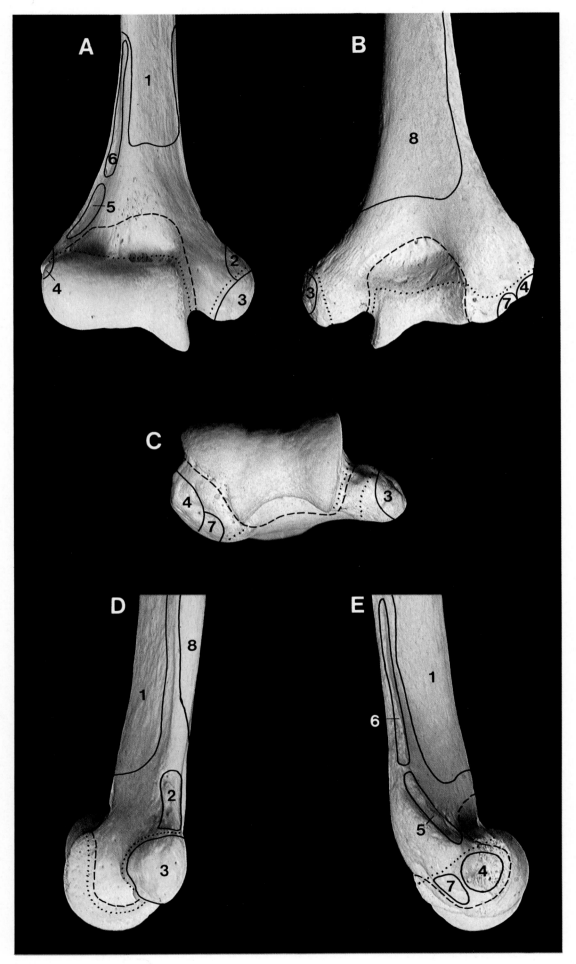

Right humerus, lower end, A from the front, B from behind, C from below, D from the medial side, E from the lateral side. Attachments

(Epiphysial line, dotted; capsule attachment, interrupted line)

1 Brachialis
2 Pronator teres
3 Common flexor origin
4 Common extensor origin
5 Extensor carpi radialis longus
6 Brachioradialis
7 Anconeus
8 Medial head of triceps

● The ulnar and radial collateral ligaments of the elbow joint are attached to the medial and lateral epicondyles respectively (beneath the common flexor and extensor origins).

Right radius, upper end, A from the front, B from behind, C from the medial side, D from the lateral side

1 Head
2 Neck
3 Tuberosity
4 Anterior oblique line
5 Interosseous border
6 Anterior surface
7 Anterior border
8 Lateral surface
9 Posterior border
10 Posterior surface
11 Rough area for pronator teres

● The head of the radius is at its upper end; the head of the ulna is at its lower end (page 100).

● The tuberosity is rough posteriorly for the attachment of the biceps tendon, and smooth anteriorly where it is covered by the intervening bursa.

● The shaft is triangular in cross section, and its surfaces are anterior, posterior and lateral; its borders are interosseous, anterior and posterior (compare with the ulna, page 100).

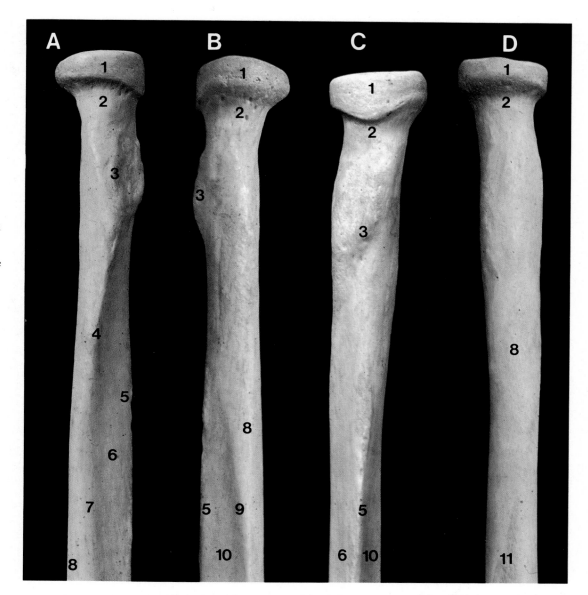

Right radius, lower end, E from the front, F from behind, G from the medial side, H from the lateral side

1 Anterior surface
2 Interosseous border
3 Ulnar notch
4 Styloid process
5 Lateral surface
6 Posterior surface
7 Groove for extensor digitorum and extensor indicis
8 Groove for extensor pollicis longus
9 Dorsal tubercle
10 Groove for extensor carpi radialis brevis
11 Groove for extensor carpi radialis longus
12 Groove for extensor pollicis brevis
13 Groove for abductor pollicis longus

● The lower end of the radius is concave anteriorly, with the ulnar notch medially and the dorsal tubercle on the posterior surface.

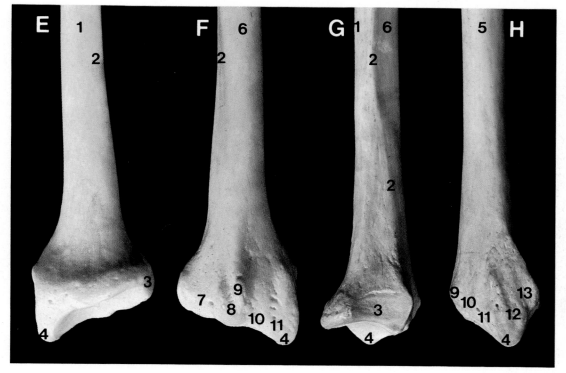

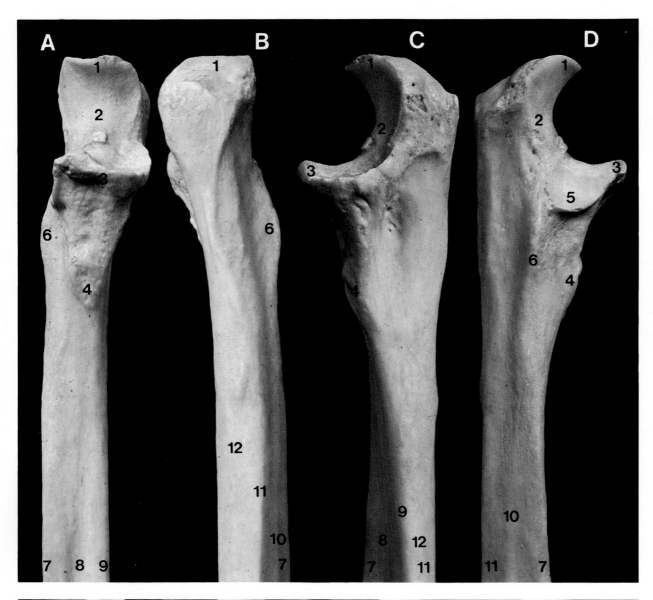

Right ulna, upper end, A from the front, B from behind, C from the medial side, D from the lateral side

1 Olecranon
2 Trochlear notch
3 Coronoid process
4 Tuberosity
5 Radial notch
6 Supinator crest
7 Interosseous border
8 Anterior surface
9 Anterior border
10 Posterior surface
11 Posterior border
12 Medial surface

● The trochlear notch faces forwards, with the radial notch on the lateral side.
● The upper part of the shaft is triangular in cross section but the lower quarter is almost cylindrical. The surfaces of the shaft are anterior, posterior and medial; the borders are interosseous, anterior and posterior (compare with the radius, page 99).

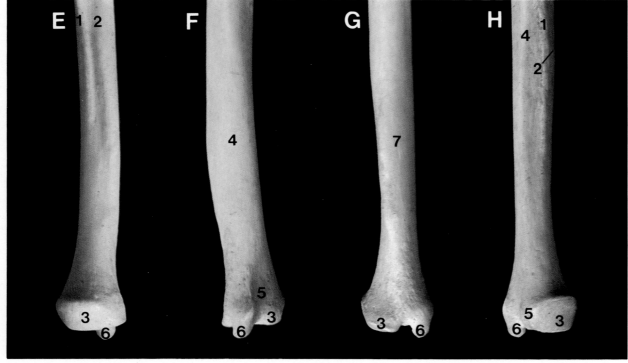

Right ulna, lower end, E from the front, F from behind, G from the medial side, H from the lateral side

1 Interosseous border
2 Anterior surface
3 Head
4 Posterior surface
5 Groove for extensor carpi ulnaris
6 Styloid process
7 Medial surface

● The head of the ulna is at its lower end, with the styloid process situated posteromedially.

A Right radius and ulna, upper ends, from above and in front

1 Olecranon
2 Trochlear notch
3 Coronoid process
4 Tuberosity of ulna
5 Tuberosity of radius
6 Neck
7 Head

B Right radius and ulna, lower ends, from below

1 Styloid process of radius
2 Surface for scaphoid
3 Surface for lunate
4 Attachment of articular disc
5 Surface for disc
6 Styloid process of ulna
7 Groove for extensor carpi ulnaris
8 Groove for extensor digitorum and extensor indicis
9 Groove for extensor pollicis longus
10 Dorsal tubercle
11 Groove for extensor carpi radialis brevis
12 Groove for extensor carpi radialis longus

Articulation of right humerus, radius and ulna, C from the front, D from behind

1 Lateral epicondyle ⎫
2 Capitulum   ⎬ of humerus
3 Trochlea   ⎪
4 Medial epicondyle ⎭
5 Coronoid process of ulna
6 Head of radius
7 Olecranon

● The elbow joint is the articulation of the humerus with the radius and ulna – the capitulum of the humerus with the head of the radius, and the trochlea of the humerus with the trochlear notch of the ulna.

● The head of the radius also articulates with the radial notch of the ulna, forming the proximal radio-ulnar joint.

● The elbow joint and the proximal radio-ulnar joint are both synovial, and the joint cavities are in continuity with one another.

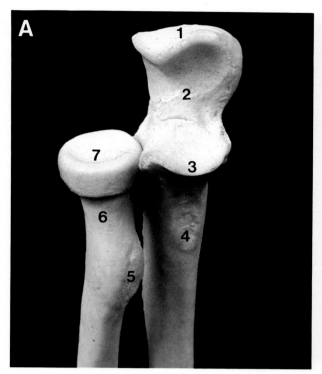

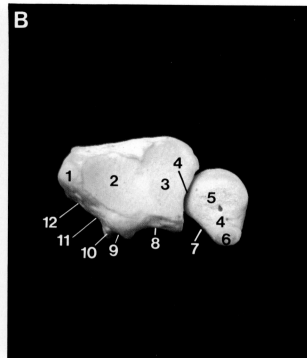

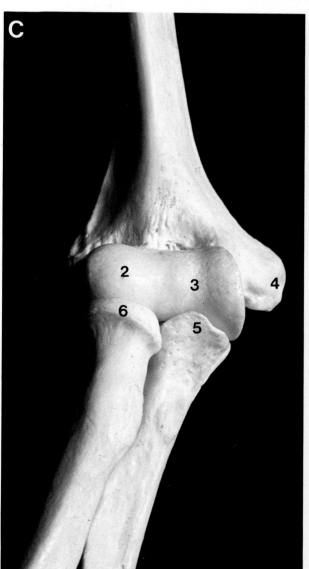

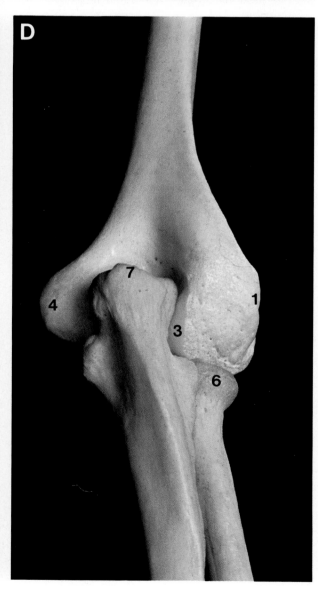

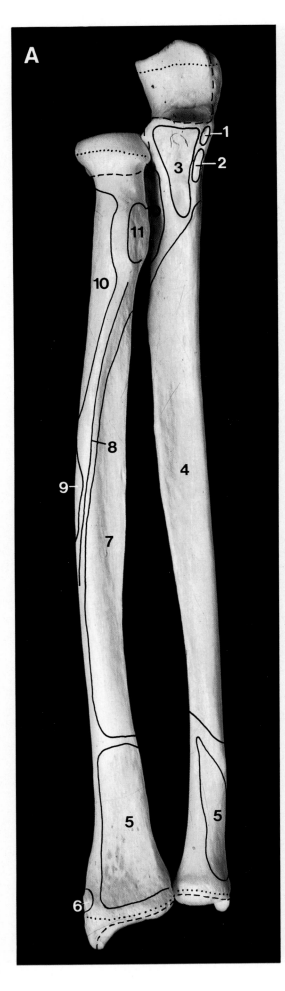

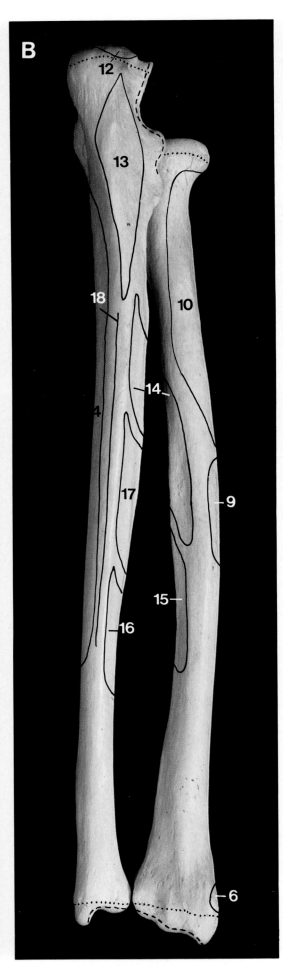

Right radius and ulna, A from the front, B from behind. Attachments
(Epiphysial line, dotted; capsule attachment, interrupted line)

  1 Flexor digitorum superficialis, ulnar head
  2 Pronator teres
  3 Brachialis
  4 Flexor digitorum profundus
  5 Pronator quadratus
  6 Brachioradialis
  7 Flexor pollicis longus
  8 Flexor digitorum superficialis, radial head
  9 Pronator teres
 10 Supinator
 11 Biceps
 12 Triceps
 13 Anconeus
 14 Abductor pollicis longus
 15 Extensor pollicis brevis
 16 Extensor indicis
 17 Extensor pollicis longus
 18 Aponeurotic attachment of flexor digitorum profundus, flexor carpi ulnaris and extensor carpi ulnaris

● Flexor pollicis longus has an occasional small additional origin from the lateral (or rarely the medial) side of the coronoid process of the ulna (beside the lower part of the brachialis attachment).

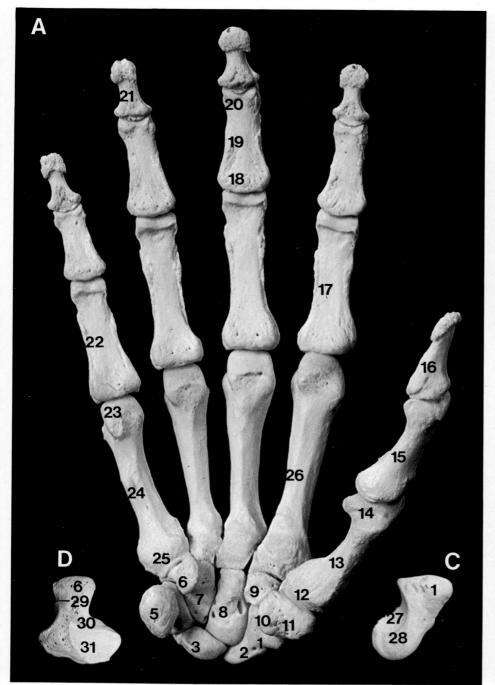

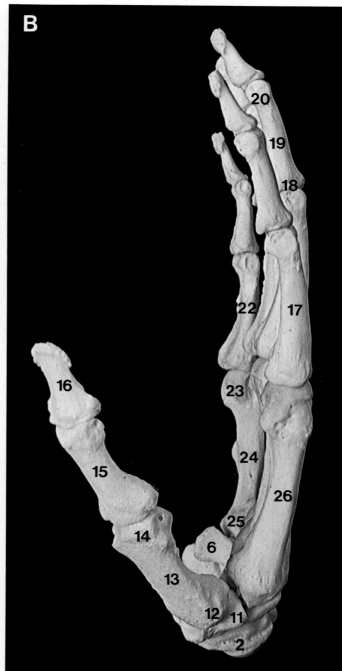

**Bones of the right hand, A palmar surface,
B from the lateral side, C scaphoid, palmar
surface, D hamate from the medial side**

 1 Tubercle of scaphoid
 2 Scaphoid
 3 Lunate
 4 Triquetral
 5 Pisiform
 6 Hook of hamate
 7 Hamate
 8 Capitate
 9 Trapezoid
10 Tubercle of trapezium
11 Trapezium
12 Base ⎤
13 Shaft ⎬ of first metacarpal
14 Head ⎦

15 Proximal ⎤
16 Distal ⎬ phalanx of thumb
17 Proximal phalanx of index finger
18 Base ⎤ of middle
19 Shaft ⎬ phalanx of
20 Head ⎦ middle finger
21 Distal phalanx of ring finger
22 Proximal phalanx of little finger
23 Head ⎤
24 Shaft ⎬ of fifth metacarpal
25 Base ⎦
26 Second metacarpal
27 Surface for capitate
28 Surface for lunate
29 Groove for deep branch of ulnar nerve
30 Palmar surface
31 Surface for triquetral

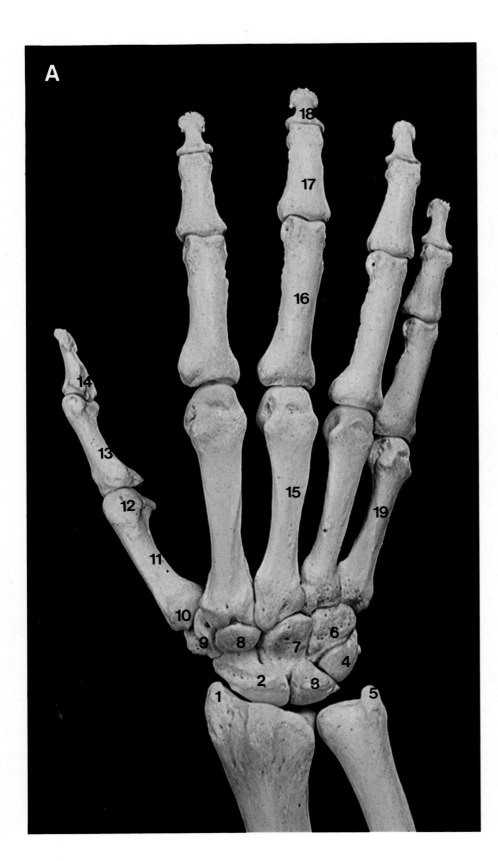

Bones of the right hand, A dorsal surface

1 Styloid process of radius
2 Scaphoid
3 Lunate
4 Triquetral
5 Styloid process of ulna
6 Hamate
7 Capitate
8 Trapezoid
9 Trapezium
10 Base ⎫
11 Shaft ⎬ of first metacarpal
12 Head ⎭
13 Proximal ⎫
14 Distal ⎬ phalanx of thumb
15 Third metacarpal
16 Proximal ⎫
17 Middle ⎬ phalanx of middle finger
18 Distal ⎭
19 Fifth metacarpal

Bones of the right hand, B palmar surface, C dorsal surface. Attachments

1 Flexor carpi ulnaris
2 Abductor digiti minimi
3 Pisohamate ligament
4 Pisometacarpal ligament
5 Flexor digiti minimi brevis
6 Opponens digiti minimi
7 Fourth ⎫
8 Third ⎬ palmar interosseous
9 Second ⎪
10 First ⎭
11 First ⎫
12 Second ⎬ dorsal interosseous
13 Third ⎪
14 Fourth ⎭
15 Transverse ⎫ head of adductor pollicis
16 Oblique ⎬
17 Flexor carpi radialis
18 Flexor pollicis brevis
19 Opponens pollicis
20 Abductor pollicis brevis
21 Abductor pollicis longus
22 Extensor pollicis brevis
23 Extensor pollicis longus
24 Flexor digitorum superficialis
25 Flexor digitorum profundus
26 Flexor pollicis longus
27 Dorsal digital expansion
28 Extensor carpi ulnaris
29 Extensor carpi radialis brevis
30 Extensor carpi radialis longus

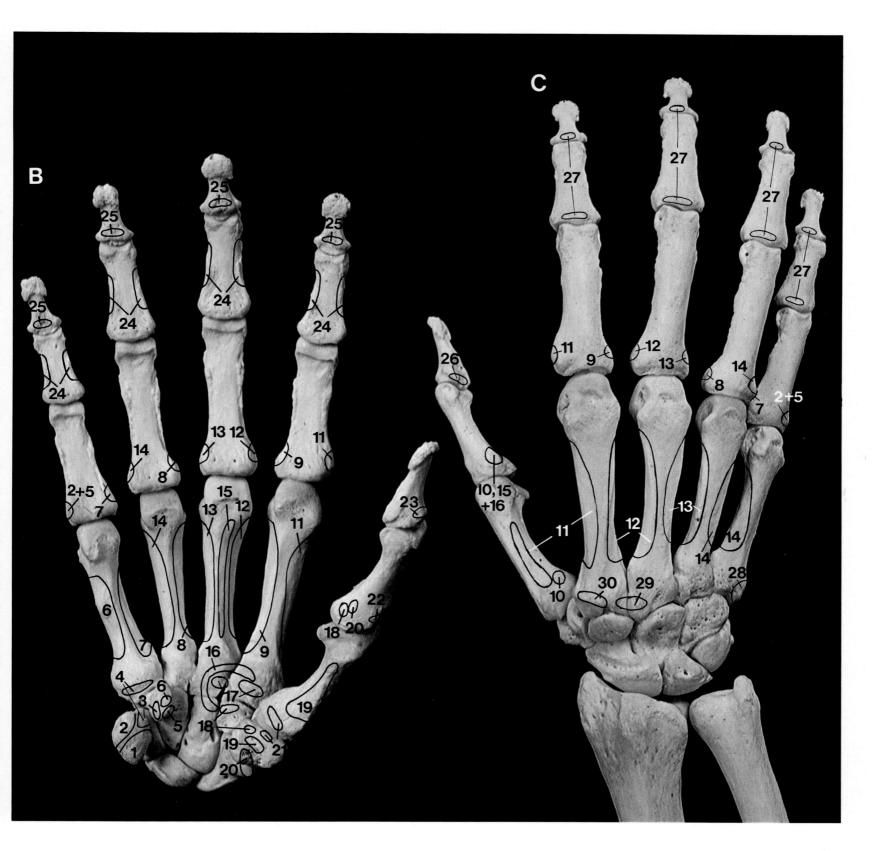

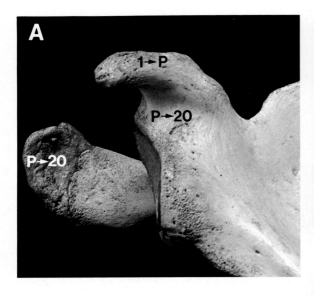

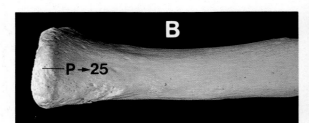

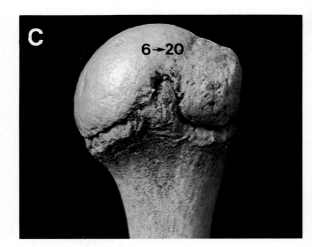

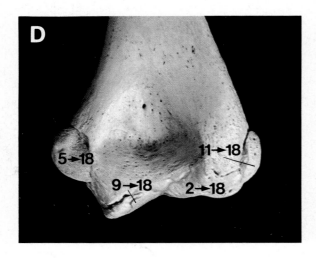

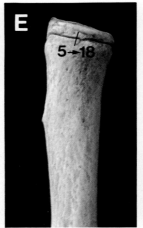

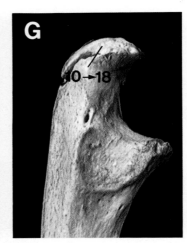

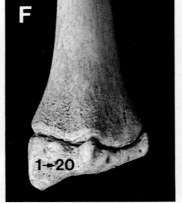

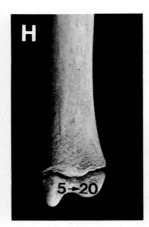

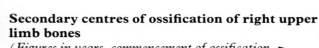

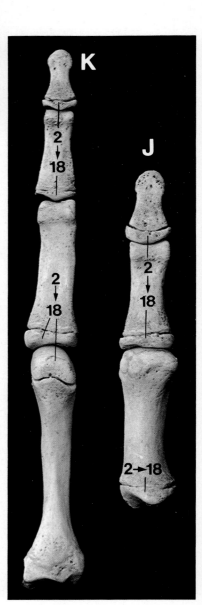

Secondary centres of ossification of right upper limb bones

(Figures in years, commencement of ossification → fusion; P: puberty)

A Upper lateral part of scapula, **B** sternal end of clavicle, **C** upper and **D** lower end of humerus, **E** upper and **F** lower end of radius, **G** upper and **H** lower end of ulna, **J** first metacarpal and phalanges of thumb, **K** second metacarpal and phalanges of index finger

● For simplicity single average dates have been given here (and for lower limb bone centres on pages 290 and 291) but there may be considerable individual variations.

● Apart from the acromial, coracoid and subcoracoid centres illustrated, the scapula usually has other centres for the inferior angle, medial border, and the lower part of the rim of the glenoid cavity (all P ► 20).

● The centre illustrated at the upper end of the humerus is the result of the union at 6 years of centres for the head (1 year), greater tubercle (3 years) and lesser tubercle (5 years).

● At the lower end of the humerus the centres for the capitulum, trochlea and lateral epicondyle fuse together before uniting with the shaft.

● All the carpal bones are cartilaginous at birth and none has a secondary centre.

● All the phalanges, and the first metacarpal, have a secondary centre at their proximal ends; the other metacarpals have one at their distal ends.

Right shoulder, from the front (with the arm slightly abducted)

1 Tip of shoulder (deltoid overlying head of humerus)
2 Acromioclavicular joint
3 Anterior margin of deltoid
4 Infraclavicular fossa
5 Clavicular part of pectoralis major
6 Clavicle
7 Supraclavicular fossa
8 Anterior border of trapezius
9 Lateral (clavicular) ⎱
10 Medial (sternal)   ⎰ head of sternocleidomastoid
11 Sternal part of pectoralis major
12 Areola
13 Nipple
14 Serratus anterior
15 Lower border of pectoralis major
16 Deltopectoral groove and cephalic vein
17 Biceps

● The nipple in the male normally lies at the level of the fourth intercostal space.
● The lower part of pectoralis major forms the anterior axillary fold.

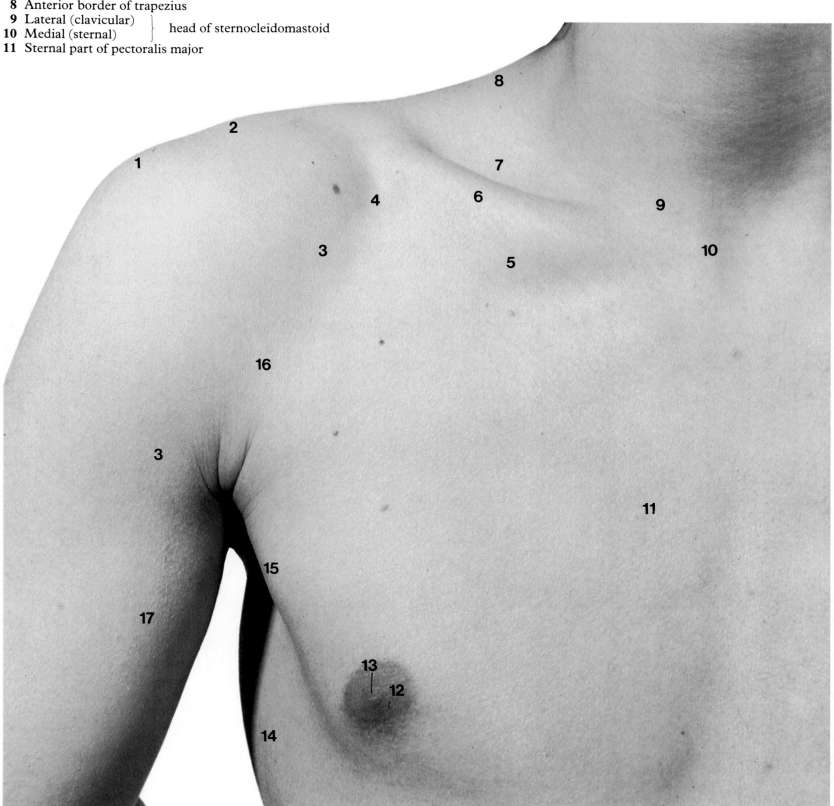

Right shoulder and neck, from the front. Superficial dissection

1 Deltoid
2 Supraclavicular nerves
3 Trapezius
4 Cervical nerve to trapezius
5 Spinal part of accessory nerve
6 Lesser occipital nerve
7 Great auricular nerve
8 Sternocleidomastoid
9 Transverse cutaneous nerve of neck
10 Superior belly of omohyoid
11 Thyrohyoid
12 Sternohyoid
13 Sternothyroid
14 Pectoralis major
15 Cephalic vein overlying thoraco-acromial vessels
16 Clavipectoral fascia in infraclavicular fossa
17 Venous plexus overlying inferior belly of omohyoid

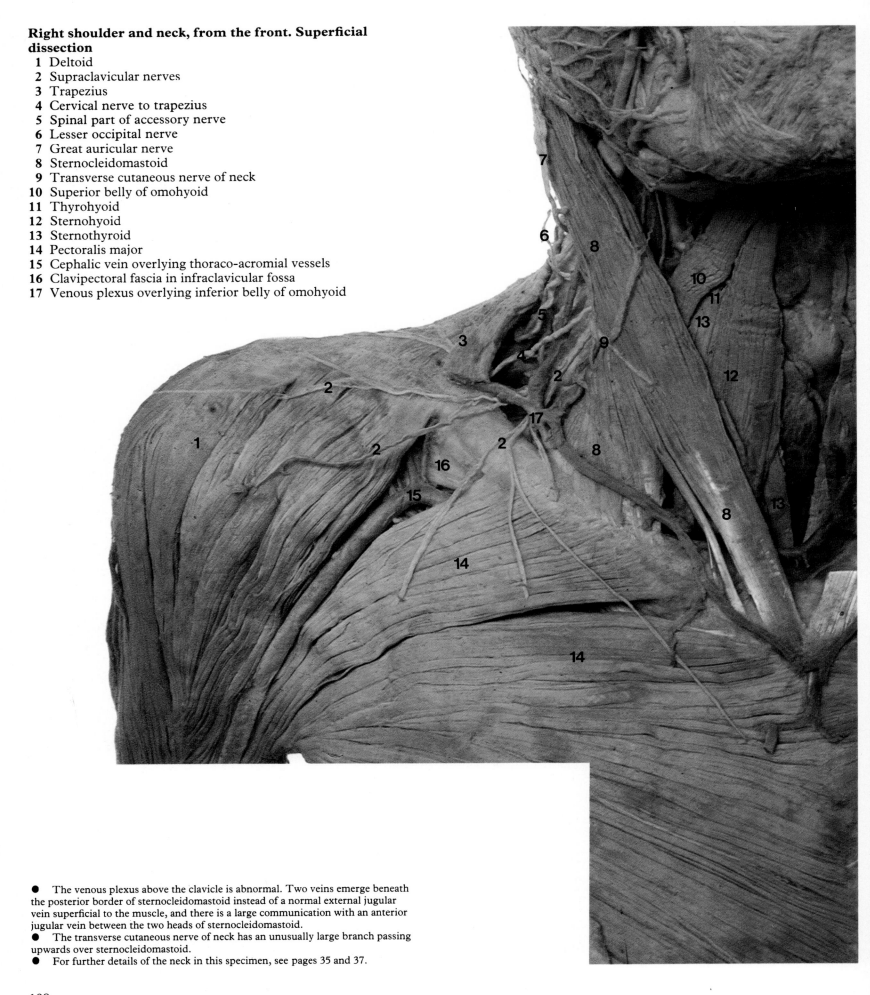

● The venous plexus above the clavicle is abnormal. Two veins emerge beneath the posterior border of sternocleidomastoid instead of a normal external jugular vein superficial to the muscle, and there is a large communication with an anterior jugular vein between the two heads of sternocleidomastoid.
● The transverse cutaneous nerve of neck has an unusually large branch passing upwards over sternocleidomastoid.
● For further details of the neck in this specimen, see pages 35 and 37.

Left shoulder and neck, from the front, with most of deltoid and pectoralis major and the clavipectoral fascia removed

1 Sternohyoid
2 Sternothyroid
3 Internal jugular vein
4 Phrenic nerve overlying scalenus anterior
5 Nerve to subclavius
6 Trunks of brachial plexus
7 Suprascapular nerve
8 Scalenus medius
9 Long thoracic nerve (to serratus anterior)
10 Inferior belly of omohyoid (displaced upwards)
11 Trapezius
12 Deltoid
13 Coracoid process and acromial branch of thoraco-acromial artery
14 Coracobrachialis
15 Short head of biceps
16 Subscapularis
17 Tendon of long head of biceps
18 Pectoralis major
19 Cephalic vein
20 Intercostobrachial nerve
21 Median nerve
22 Axillary lymph nodes
23 Lateral thoracic artery
24 Branch of medial pectoral nerve
25 Pectoralis minor
26 Anterior circumflex humeral artery and musculocutaneous nerve
27 Branches of lateral pectoral nerve
28 Pectoral branch of thoraco-acromial artery
29 Axillary vein
30 Subclavian vein
31 First rib
32 Subclavius
● For further details of the neck in this specimen see pages 35 and 37.

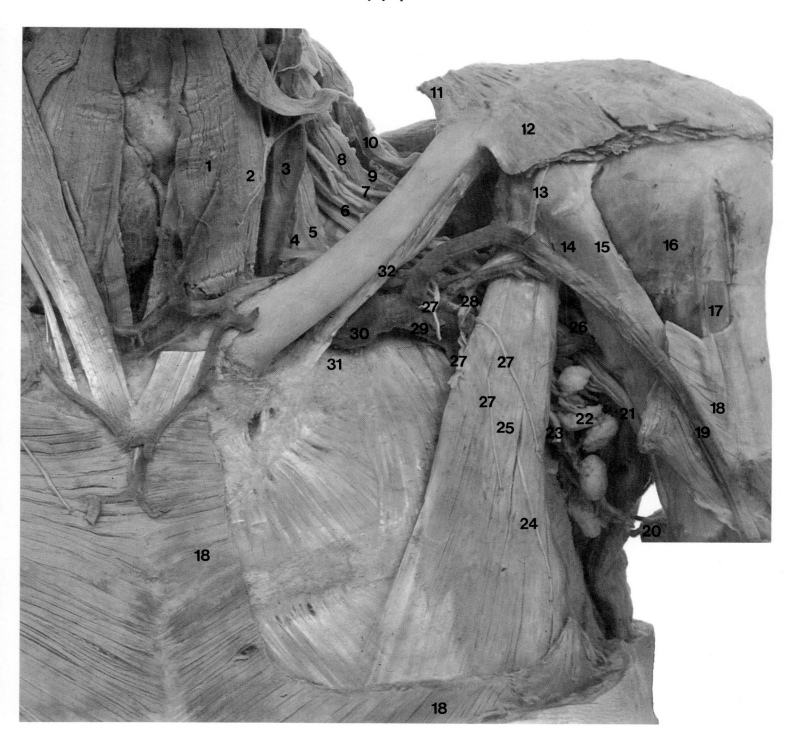

109

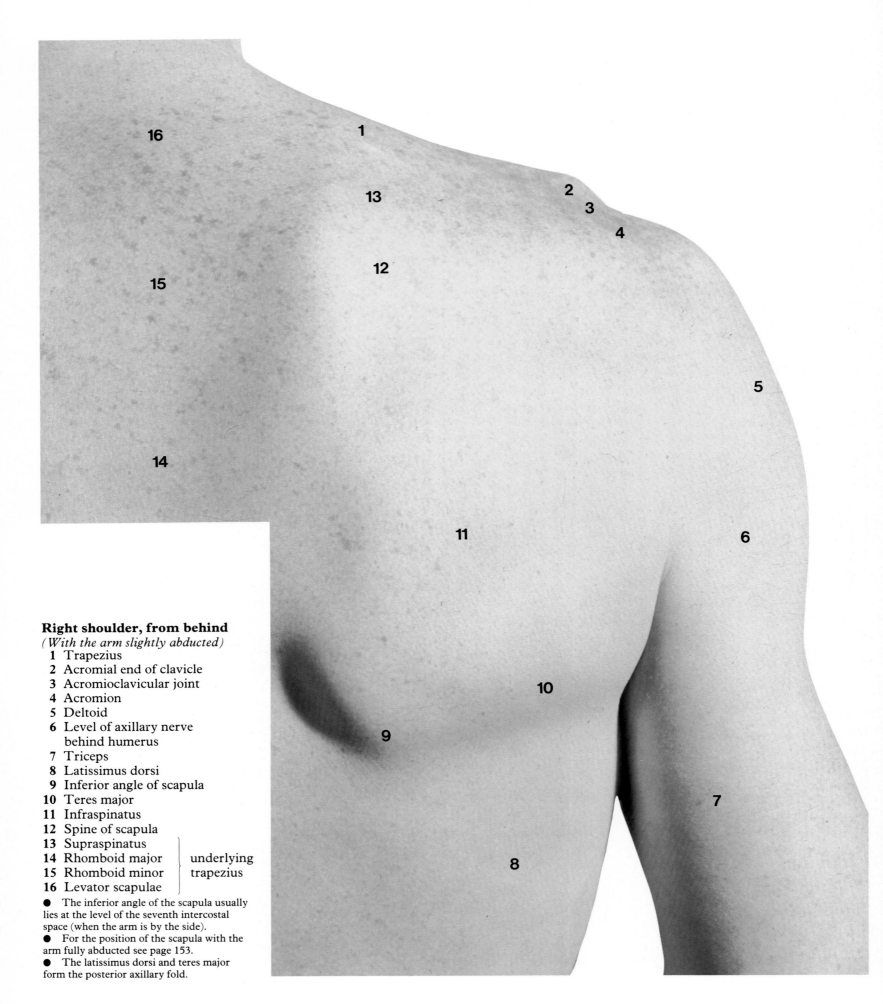

Right shoulder, from behind
(With the arm slightly abducted)
 1 Trapezius
 2 Acromial end of clavicle
 3 Acromioclavicular joint
 4 Acromion
 5 Deltoid
 6 Level of axillary nerve
    behind humerus
 7 Triceps
 8 Latissimus dorsi
 9 Inferior angle of scapula
10 Teres major
11 Infraspinatus
12 Spine of scapula
13 Supraspinatus
14 Rhomboid major ⎤ underlying
15 Rhomboid minor ⎟ trapezius
16 Levator scapulae ⎦

● The inferior angle of the scapula usually
lies at the level of the seventh intercostal
space (when the arm is by the side).
● For the position of the scapula with the
arm fully abducted see page 153.
● The latissimus dorsi and teres major
form the posterior axillary fold.

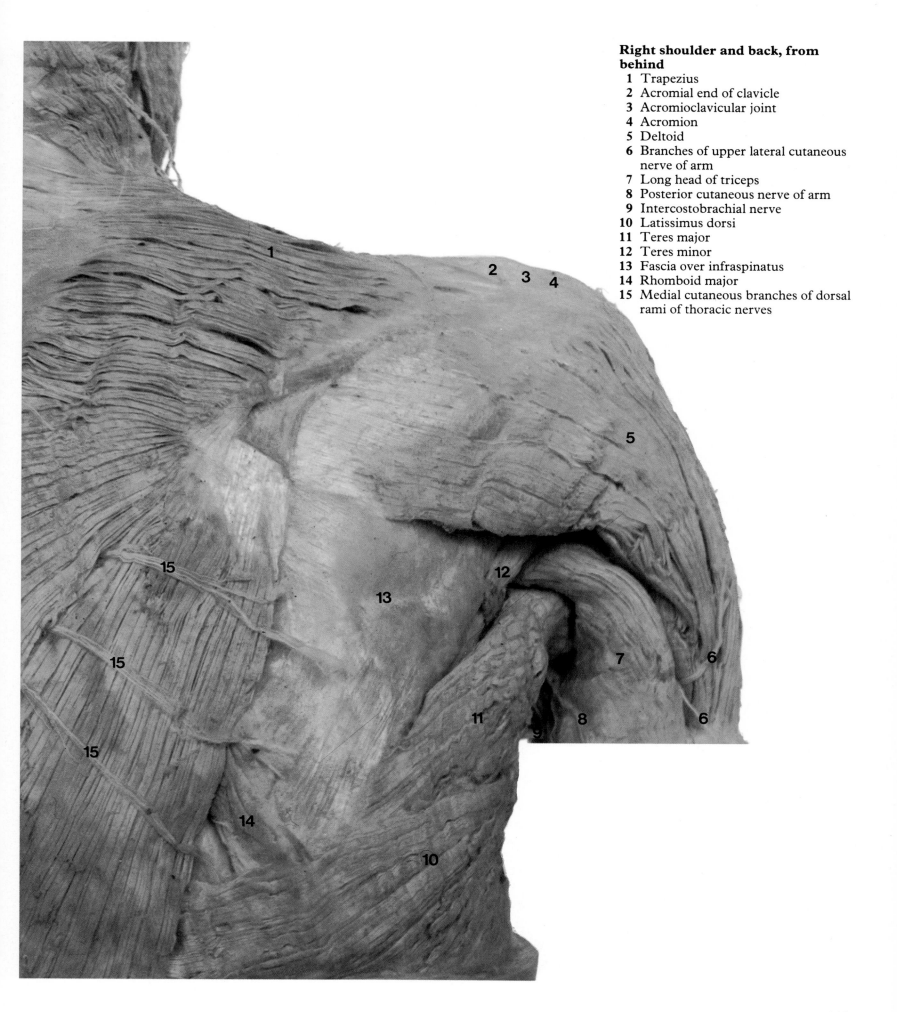

1 Trapezius
2 Acromial end of clavicle
3 Acromioclavicular joint
4 Acromion
5 Deltoid
6 Branches of upper lateral cutaneous nerve of arm
7 Long head of triceps
8 Posterior cutaneous nerve of arm
9 Intercostobrachial nerve
10 Latissimus dorsi
11 Teres major
12 Teres minor
13 Fascia over infraspinatus
14 Rhomboid major
15 Medial cutaneous branches of dorsal rami of thoracic nerves

Left shoulder, from behind, with most of trapezius and deltoid removed

1 Deltoid
2 Acromion
3 Acromioclavicular joint
4 Acromial end of clavicle
5 Trapezius
6 Supraspinatus
7 Levator scapulae
8 Rhomboid minor
9 Rhomboid major
10 Branch of dorsal ramus of a thoracic nerve
11 Erector spinae
12 Thoracolumbar fascia
13 Latissimus dorsi
14 Teres major
15 Long head of triceps
16 Posterior circumflex humeral vessels and axillary nerve
17 Teres minor
18 Infraspinatus
19 Spine of scapula

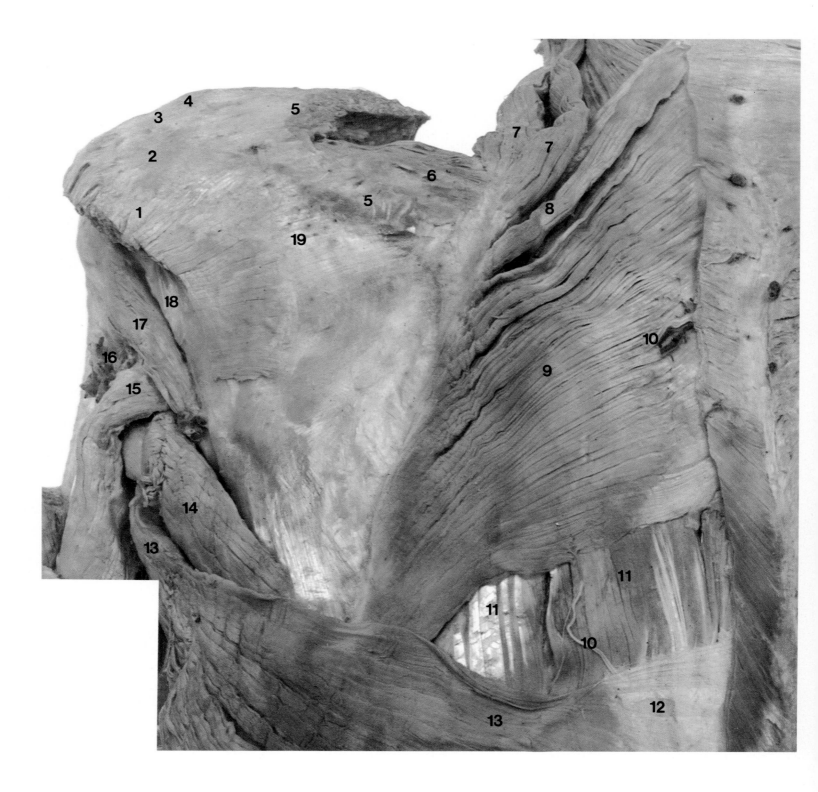

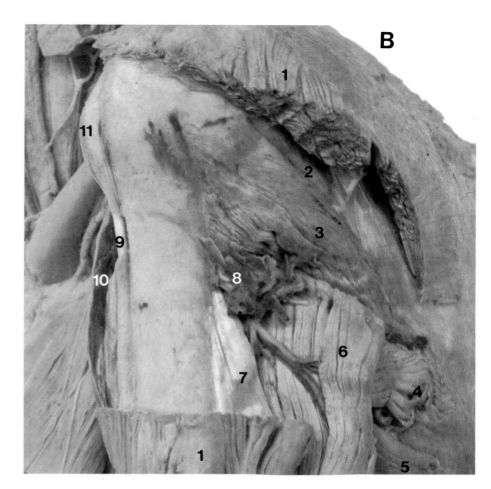

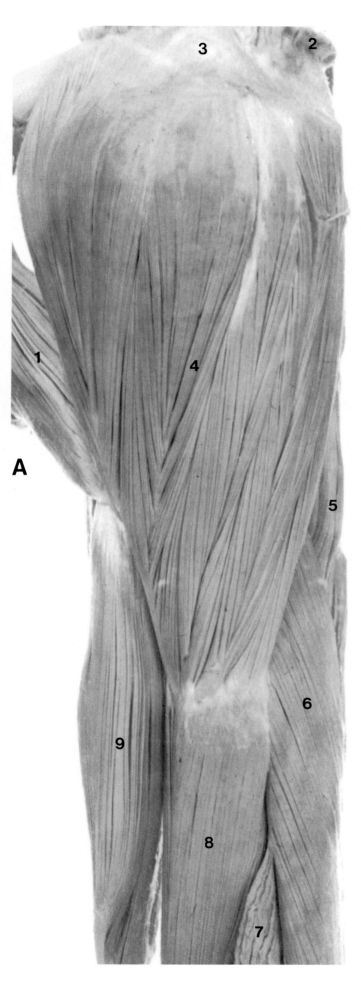

B Left shoulder, from the lateral side, with deltoid removed

1 Deltoid
2 Infraspinatus
3 Teres minor
4 Teres major
5 Latissimus dorsi
6 Long head of triceps
7 Lateral head of triceps
8 Posterior circumflex humeral vessels and axillary nerve
9 Tendon of long head of biceps
10 Cephalic vein
11 Lesser tubercle

● The deltoid covers the shoulder region at the front and back and laterally. The most lateral part, overlying the greater tubercle of the humerus, forms the tip of the shoulder.

A Left shoulder, from the lateral side

1 Pectoralis major
2 Trapezius
3 Acromion
4 Deltoid
5 Long head of triceps
6 Lateral head of triceps
7 Brachioradialis
8 Brachialis
9 Biceps

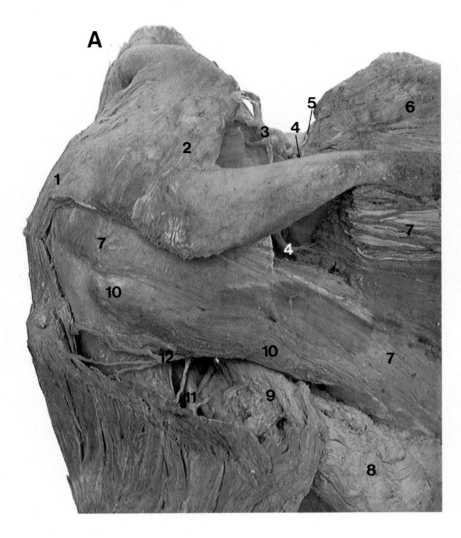

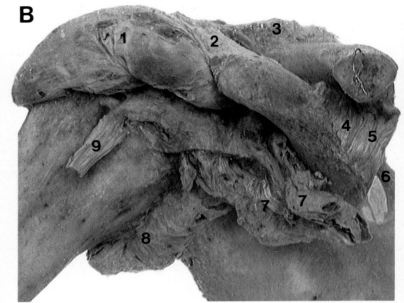

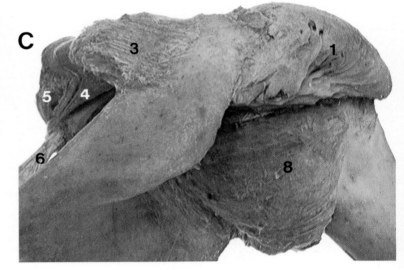

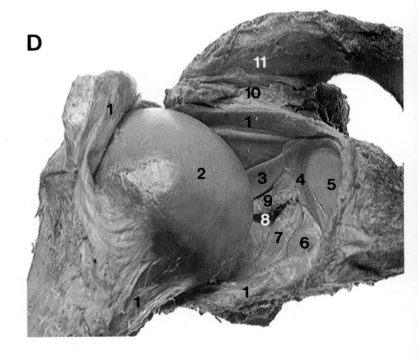

A Left shoulder, from the left and behind. Suprascapular and axillary nerves

(Part of supraspinatus and infraspinatus removed)

 1 Deltoid
 2 Acromioclavicular joint
 3 Suprascapular artery
 4 Suprascapular nerve
 5 Superior transverse scapular (suprascapular) ligament
 6 Supraspinatus
 7 Infraspinatus
 8 Teres major
 9 Long head of triceps
10 Teres minor
11 Posterior circumflex humeral artery
12 Axillary nerve

● The suprascapular artery passes into the supraspinous fossa superficial to the superior transverse scapular ligament; the suprascapular nerve passes deep to the ligament.

● The axillary nerve and posterior circumflex humeral vessels pass backwards through the quadrilateral space which (viewed from behind) is bounded above by teres minor, below by teres major, medially by the long head of triceps and laterally by the humerus. (Viewed from the front, the upper boundary of the space is subscapularis – see page 118.)

● As it lies just beneath the capsule of the shoulder joint, the axillary nerve may be injured by dislocation of the joint.

Right shoulder joint, B from the front, C from behind, with resin injection of the synovial cavity and of the subacromial bursa

1 Subacromial bursa
2 Coraco-acromial ligament
3 Acromioclavicular joint
4 Trapezoid ligament
5 Conoid ligament
6 Superior transverse scapular (suprascapular) ligament
7 Subscapularis bursa
8 Capsule of shoulder joint
9 Tendon of long head of biceps

● The subscapularis bursa normally communicates with the synovial cavity of the shoulder joint.

● The subacromial bursa does *not* normally communicate with the shoulder joint; it is separated from the joint by the supraspinatus tendon. Only if the tendon is ruptured can the two cavities become continuous with one another.

D Left shoulder joint, opened from below and behind, with much of the capsule removed

1 Capsule
2 Head of humerus
3 Long head of biceps
4 Glenoid labrum
5 Glenoid cavity
6 Inferior glenohumeral ligament
7 Middle glenohumeral ligament
8 Opening into subscapularis bursa
9 Superior glenohumeral ligament
10 Supraspinatus
11 Acromion

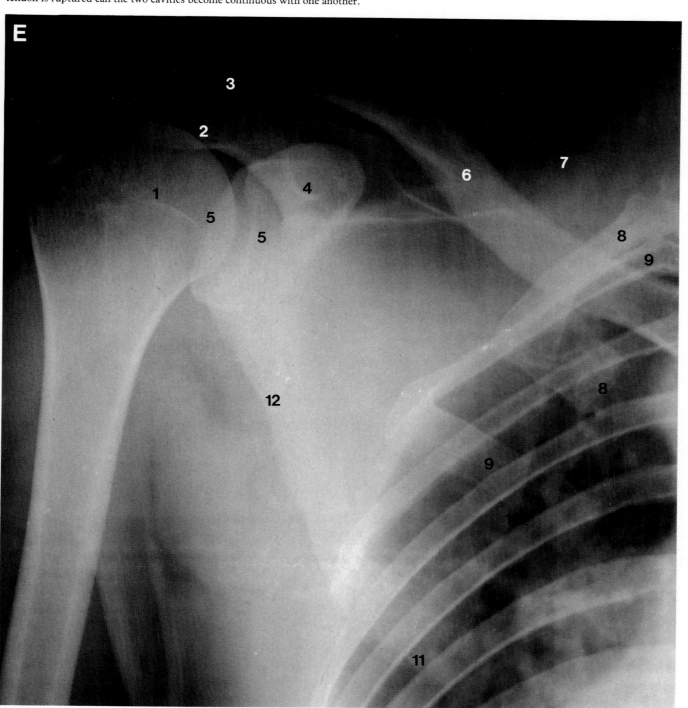

E Radiograph of the left shoulder, from behind

1 Head of humerus
2 Acromion
3 Acromioclavicular joint
4 Coracoid process
5 Rim of glenoid cavity
6 Clavicle
7 Superior angle of scapula
8 First rib
9 Second rib
10 Medial border of scapula
11 Inferior angle of scapula
12 Lateral border of scapula

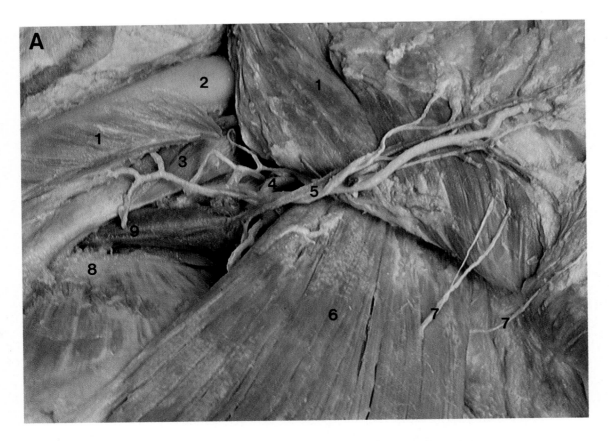

Left axilla, anterior wall *(with pectoralis major reflected)*
1 Pectoralis major
2 Clavicle
3 Subclavius
4 Cephalic vein
5 Thoraco-acromial vessels and lateral pectoral nerve
6 Pectoralis minor
7 Branches of medial pectoral nerve
8 First rib
9 Subclavian vein

● The *lateral* pectoral nerve is related to the *medial* (upper) border of pectoralis minor. The *medial* pectoral nerve is related to the *lateral* (lower) border of pectoralis minor.

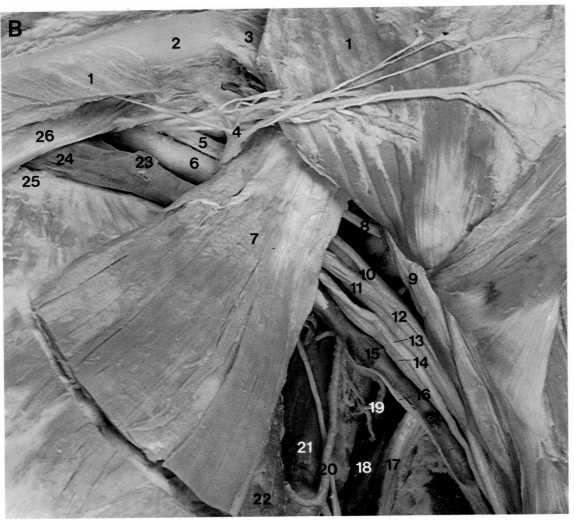

Left axilla and brachial plexus *(with pectoralis major reflected)*
1 Pectoralis major
2 Clavicle
3 Deltoid
4 Thoraco-acromial vessels and lateral pectoral nerve
5 Lateral cord of brachial plexus
6 Axillary artery
7 Pectoralis minor
8 Musculocutaneous nerve
9 Coracobrachialis
10 Lateral root ⎱ of median nerve
11 Medial root ⎰
12 Median nerve
13 Ulnar nerve
14 Medial cutaneous nerve of forearm
15 Axillary vein
16 Medial cutaneous nerve of arm
17 Latissimus dorsi
18 Teres major
19 Circumflex scapular artery
20 Thoracodorsal artery and nerve
21 Subscapularis
22 Serratus anterior
23 Entry of cephalic vein
24 Subclavian vein
25 First rib
26 Subclavius

Left brachial plexus *(with the arm partially abducted, pectoralis major and minor reflected and the axillary vein and its tributaries removed)*

1 Clavicle
2 Pectoralis major
3 Subclavius
4 Lateral pectoral nerve
5 Lateral cord
6 Axillary artery
7 Thoraco-acromial artery
8 Loop between medial and lateral pectoral nerves
9 Pectoralis minor
10 Musculocutaneous nerve
11 Lateral root ⎫
12 Medial root ⎬ of median nerve
13 Median nerve ⎭
14 Radial nerve
15 Axillary nerve
16 Anterior circumflex humeral artery
17 Coracobrachialis and short head of biceps
18 Long head of biceps
19 Deltoid
20 Ulnar nerve
21 Medial cutaneous nerve of forearm
22 Medial cutaneous nerve of arm
23 Latissimus dorsi
24 Teres major
25 Lower subscapular nerve
26 Circumflex scapular artery
27 Thoracodorsal artery
28 Thoracodorsal nerve
29 Subscapularis
30 Serratus anterior
31 Long thoracic nerve
32 Intercostobrachial nerve (cut end)
33 Communication between 22 and 32
34 Branch from first thoracic nerve to intercostobrachial nerve
35 Lateral thoracic artery
36 Axillary vein
37 Entry of cephalic vein
38 Subclavian vein
39 First rib

● The thoracodorsal artery is the name given to the continuation of the subscapular artery distal to the origin of the circumflex scapular branch.

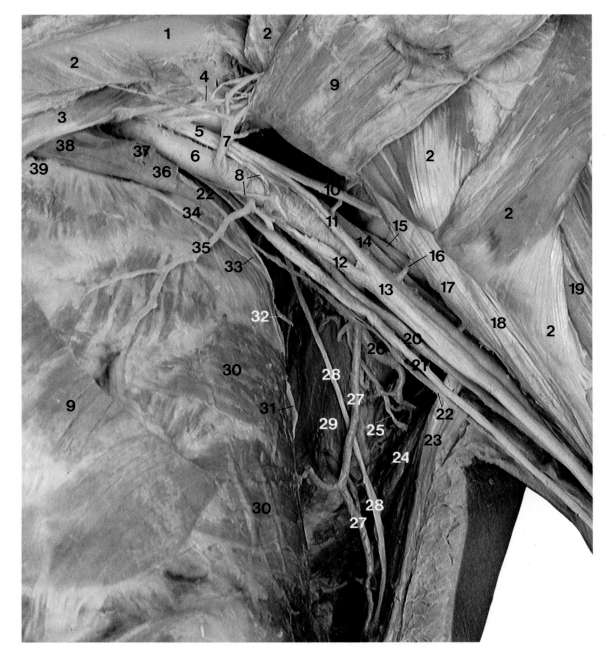

● The cords of the brachial plexus are arranged round the axillary artery according to their names – medial, lateral and posterior.
● To sort out the major branches of the medial and lateral cords, note that the largest branches form the shape of a capital M. Identify the median nerve (the middle stem of the M) in front of the axillary artery. Follow its lateral root upwards to the lateral cord, from which the musculocutaneous nerve arises (as the lateral stem of the M) to run into the coracobrachialis muscle. Follow the medial root of the median nerve upwards to the medial cord, whose largest branch is the ulnar nerve (the medial stem of the M).
● The radial nerve (one of the two terminal branches of the posterior cord and the largest of all the branches of the plexus) is most easily identified as it lies behind the axillary artery and in front of the latissimus dorsi tendon. Follow the nerve upwards to find the axillary nerve (the other terminal branch of the posterior cord) passing laterally and backwards through the quadrilateral space.

Right brachial plexus and branches, from the front and medial side, with all vessels removed and some displacement of the cords of the plexus to reveal the branches more clearly

1 Lateral cord
2 Posterior cord
3 Medial cord
4 Pectoralis minor and lateral pectoral nerve
5 Musculocutaneous nerve
6 Axillary nerve
7 Lateral root of median nerve
8 Radial nerve
9 Medial root of median nerve
10 Upper subscapular nerves
11 Thoracodorsal nerve
12 Lower subscapular nerve
13 Medial cutaneous nerve of arm
14 Ulnar nerve
15 Medial cutaneous nerve of forearm
16 Intercostobrachial nerve
17 Subscapularis
18 Teres major
19 Latissimus dorsi
20 Long head of triceps
21 Lateral head of triceps
22 Medial head of triceps
23 Radial nerve branches to triceps
24 Median nerve
25 Coracobrachialis
26 Biceps
27 Deltoid

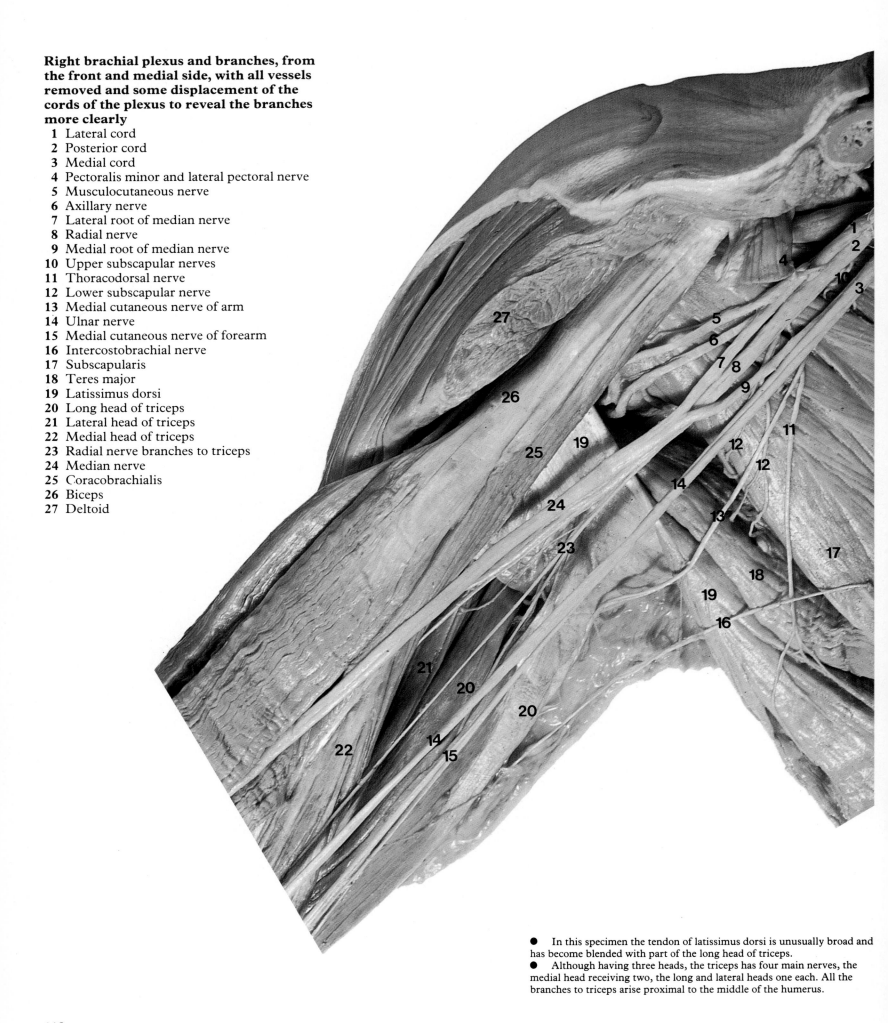

● In this specimen the tendon of latissimus dorsi is unusually broad and has become blended with part of the long head of triceps.
● Although having three heads, the triceps has four main nerves, the medial head receiving two, the long and lateral heads one each. All the branches to triceps arise proximal to the middle of the humerus.

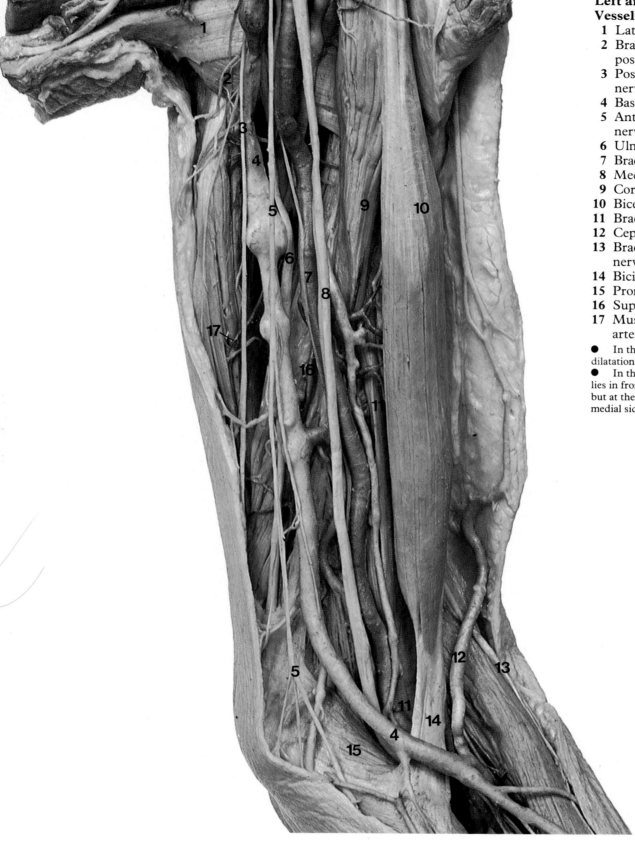

**Left arm, from the medial side.
Vessels and nerves**

1 Latissimus dorsi
2 Branches of medial cutaneous and posterior cutaneous nerves of arm
3 Posterior branch of medial cutaneous nerve of forearm
4 Basilic vein
5 Anterior branch of medial cutaneous nerve of forearm
6 Ulnar nerve
7 Brachial artery and venae comitantes
8 Median nerve
9 Coracobrachialis
10 Biceps
11 Brachialis
12 Cephalic vein
13 Brachioradialis and lateral cutaneous nerve of forearm
14 Bicipital aponeurosis
15 Pronator teres
16 Superior ulnar collateral artery
17 Muscular branch of profunda brachii artery

● In this specimen the basilic vein shows several dilatations.
● In the upper part of the arm the median nerve lies in front of the lateral side of the brachial artery, but at the elbow (cubital fossa) the nerve lies on the medial side of the artery.

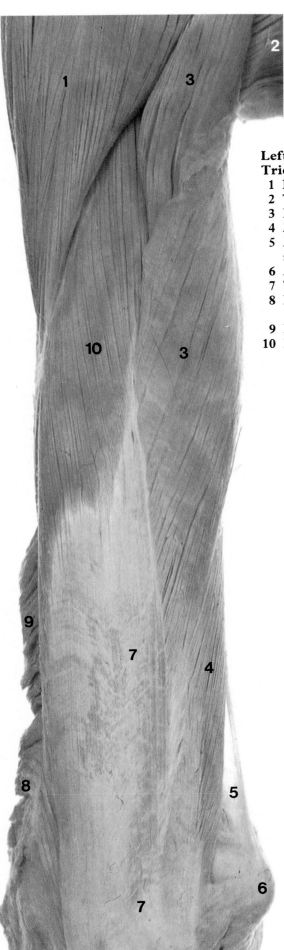

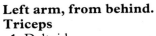

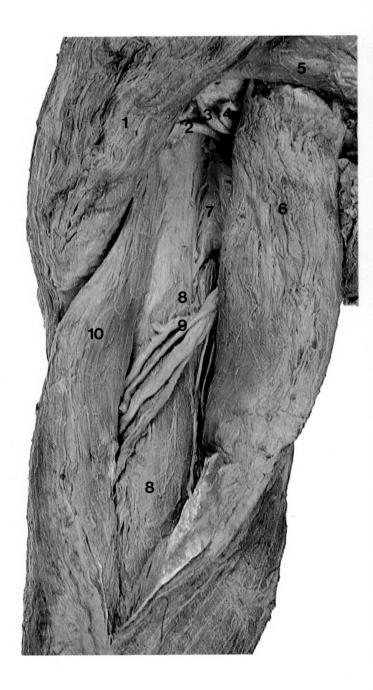

**Left arm, from behind.
Triceps**
1 Deltoid
2 Teres major
3 Long head of triceps
4 Medial head of triceps
5 Medial intermuscular
  septum
6 Medial epicondyle
7 Tendon of triceps
8 Extensor carpi radialis
  longus
9 Brachioradialis
10 Lateral head of triceps

**Left upper arm, from behind. Triceps and the
radial nerve**
1 Deltoid
2 Posterior circumflex humeral artery
3 Axillary nerve
4 Nerve to teres minor
5 Teres minor
6 Long head of triceps
7 Teres major
8 Medial head of triceps
9 Profunda brachii artery and radial nerve with
  branches to triceps
10 Lateral head of triceps
● The long and lateral heads of triceps have been separated to reveal
the upper part of the medial (deep) head.
● The radial nerve and accompanying vessels cross the uppermost
part of the attachment of the medial head of triceps before coming into
contact with the radial groove of the humerus.
● The radial nerve is most commonly injured by fractures of the shaft
of the humerus in the region of the radial groove.

Left elbow, from behind

1 Triceps
2 Medial epicondyle
3 Ulnar nerve
4 Olecranon
5 Posterior border of ulna
6 Flexor carpi ulnaris
7 Extensor muscles
8 Proximal radio-ulnar joint and head of radius
9 Lateral epicondyle

● The ulnar nerve can be palpated easily (and injured) as it lies behind the medial epicondyle before passing into the forearm between the two heads of flexor carpi ulnaris.
● The head of the radius can be palpated easily in the depression beside the lateral epicondyle.

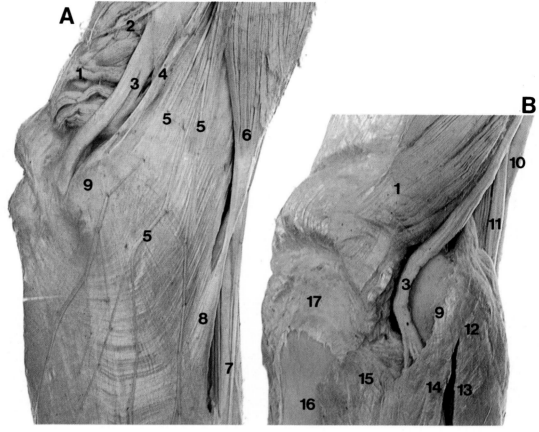

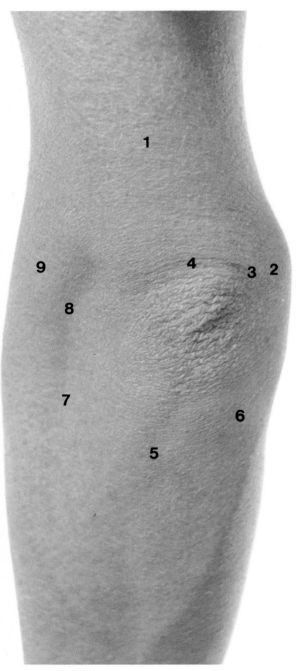

Left elbow region, A from the medial side, B from the medial side and behind

1 Triceps
2 Medial cutaneous nerve of arm
3 Ulnar nerve
4 Medial intermuscular septum
5 Branches of medial cutaneous nerve of forearm
6 Biceps
7 Brachioradialis and lateral cutaneous nerve of forearm
8 Bicipital aponeurosis and deep fascia overlying pronator teres
9 Medial epicondyle
10 Brachial artery
11 Median nerve
12 Common flexor origin
13 Palmaris longus
14 Humeral ⎱ head of flexor
15 Ulnar ⎰ carpi ulnaris
16 Posterior border of ulna
17 Olecranon

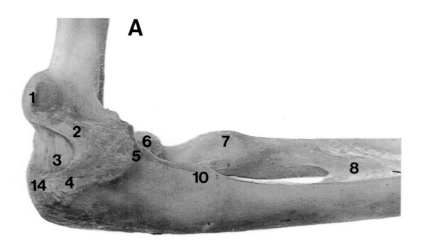

A

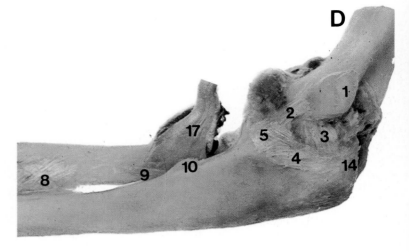

D

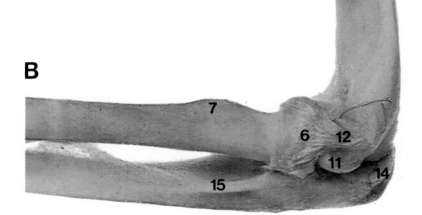

B

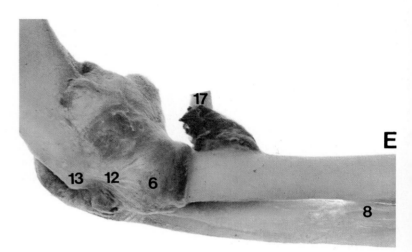

E

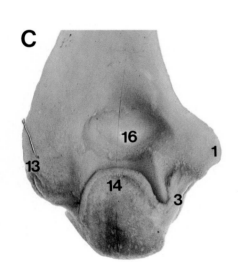

C

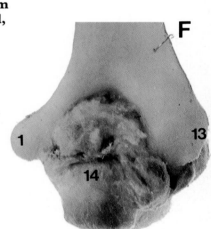

F

Left elbow joint and proximal radio-ulnar joint, A from the medial side, B from the lateral side, C from behind, with the forearm flexed to a right angle

 1 Medial epicondyle
 2 Upper band ⎫
 3 Posterior band ⎬ of ulnar collateral ligament
 4 Oblique band ⎭
 5 Coronoid process of ulna
 6 Head of radius covered by annular ligament
 7 Tuberosity of radius
 8 Interosseous membrane
 9 Oblique cord
 10 Tuberosity of ulna
 11 Capitulum
 12 Radial collateral ligament
 13 Lateral epicondyle
 14 Olecranon of ulna
 15 Supinator crest of ulna
 16 Olecranon fossa
 17 Biceps tendon and underlying bursa

Right elbow joint and proximal radio-ulnar joint, D from the medial side, E from the lateral side, F from behind, with the forearm partially flexed and resin injection of the synovial cavity
Identifying figures as above

● The synovial cavity of the proximal radio-ulnar joint is continuous with that of the elbow joint (the synovial cavity of the inferior radio-ulnar joint is *not* continuous with that of the wrist joint).

● Posteriorly and above, the capsule of the elbow joint is attached to the upper part of the *floor* of the olecranon fossa, not to the upper margin of the fossa.

A

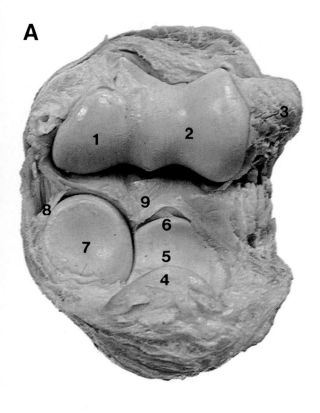

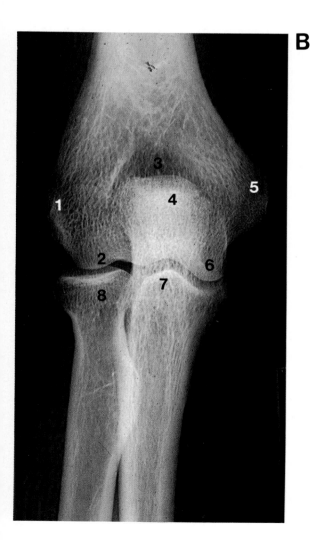

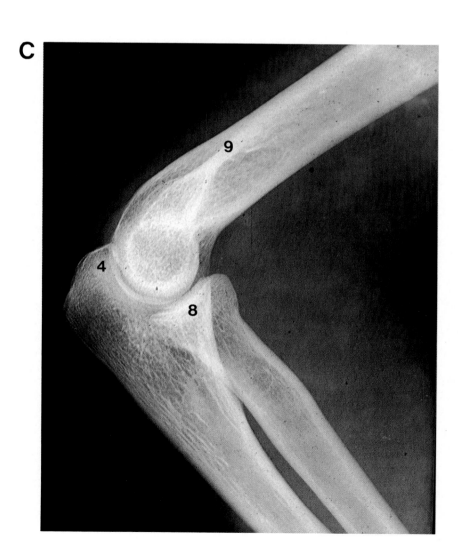

A Left elbow joint, opened from behind, with the humerus viewed from below and the forearm in forced flexion

1 Capitulum
2 Trochlea ⎫ of humerus
3 Medial epicondyle ⎭
4 Olecranon ⎫
5 Trochlear notch ⎬ of ulna
6 Coronoid process ⎭
7 Head of radius
8 Annular ligament
9 Anterior part of capsule

Radiograph of the left elbow, B from behind in extension, C from the medial side in semiflexion

1 Lateral epicondyle of humerus
2 Capitulum
3 Olecranon fossa
4 Olecranon of ulna
5 Medial epicondyle
6 Medial margin of trochlea
7 Coronoid process of ulna
8 Head of radius (in C superimposed on coronoid process)
9 Medial supracondylar ridge

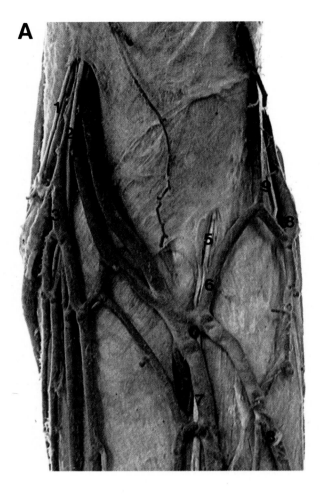

A

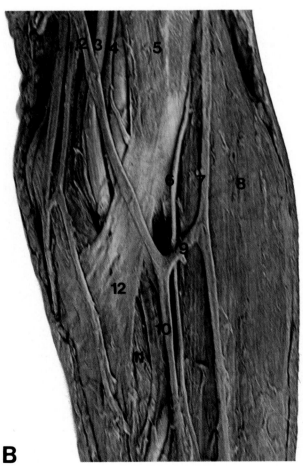

B

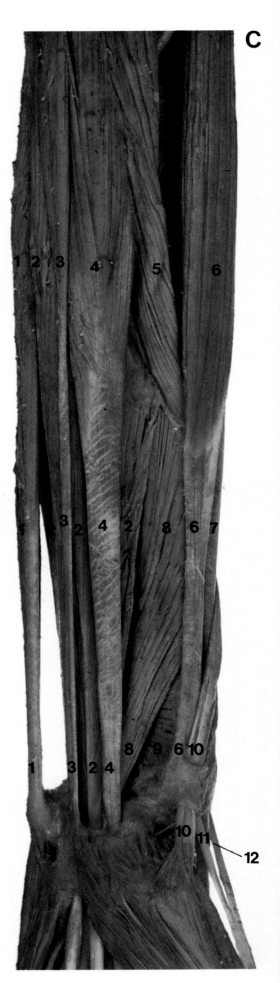

C

A Left cubital fossa.
Superficial veins and nerves
1 Posterior branch of medial cutaneous nerve of forearm
2 Anterior branch of medial cutaneous nerve of forearm
3 Basilic vein
4 Median basilic vein (double)
5 Anterior branch of lateral cutaneous nerve of forearm
6 Median cephalic vein
7 Median vein of forearm
8 Cephalic vein
9 Lateral cutaneous nerve of forearm

● The pattern of veins in the cubital region is very variable. The principal veins are the cephalic (laterally) and the basilic (medially), with one or more communications between them, and often a median vein in the centre of the forearm.
● The readily visible veins in the cubital region (and the dorsum of the hand) are commonly used as sites for intravenous injections and infusions.
● The anterior branch of the medial cutaneous nerve of the forearm usually passes deep to the median cubital vein, not superficial to it as in this specimen.
● The posterior branch of the medial cutaneous nerve of the forearm usually passes in front of the medial epicondyle, not behind it as in this specimen.

B Left cubital fossa. Superficial dissection
1 Basilic vein (double)
2 Median basilic vein
3 Median nerve
4 Brachial artery and vena comitans
5 Biceps
6 Lateral cutaneous nerve of forearm
7 Cephalic vein
8 Brachioradialis
9 Median cephalic vein
10 Median vein of forearm
11 Pronator teres
12 Bicipital aponeurosis

C Left forearm, from the front, in the midprone position. Superficial muscles
1 Flexor carpi ulnaris
2 Flexor digitorum superficialis
3 Palmaris longus
4 Flexor carpi radialis
5 Pronator teres
6 Brachioradialis
7 Extensor carpi radialis longus
8 Flexor pollicis longus
9 Pronator quadratus
10 Abductor pollicis longus (double tendon)
11 Extensor pollicis brevis
12 Extensor pollicis longus

B Right cubital fossa and forearm. Arteries and nerves (part of pronator teres and flexor carpi radialis removed)

  1 Lateral cutaneous nerve of forearm
  2 Brachialis
  3 Biceps
  4 Brachial artery
  5 Median nerve
  6 Humeral head of pronator teres
  7 Common flexor origin
  8 Humero-ulnar head of flexor digitorum superficialis
  9 Flexor carpi ulnaris (displaced medially)
10 Ulnar nerve and artery
11 Radial artery
12 Superficial terminal branch of radial nerve overlying extensor carpi radialis longus
13 Radial head of flexor digitorum superficialis
14 Anterior interosseous nerve
15 Ulnar head of pronator teres
16 Ulnar artery
17 Muscular branch of median nerve
18 Radial recurrent artery
19 Brachioradialis (displaced laterally)

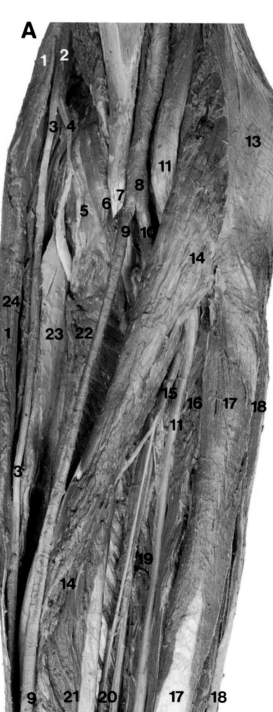

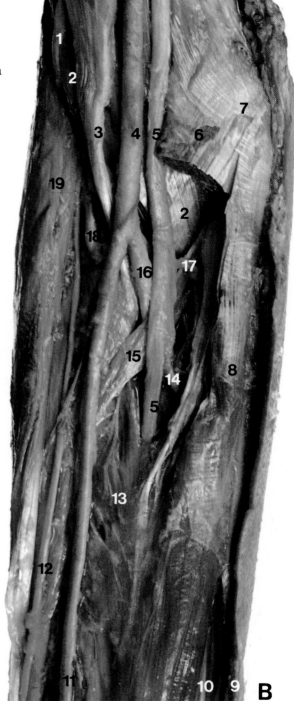

A Right cubital fossa and forearm. Arteries and nerves
(palmaris longus and radial head of flexor digitorum superficialis removed)

  1 Brachioradialis (displaced laterally)
  2 Radial nerve
  3 Superficial terminal branch of radial nerve
  4 Posterior interosseous nerve (deep terminal branch of radial nerve)
  5 Nerve to supinator
  6 Brachialis
  7 Biceps
  8 Brachial artery
  9 Radial artery
10 Ulnar artery
11 Median nerve
12 Medial epicondyle
13 Common flexor origin
14 Pronator teres
15 Anterior interosseous nerve
16 Humero-ulnar head of flexor digitorum superficialis
17 Flexor carpi radialis (displaced medially)
18 Flexor carpi ulnaris
19 Flexor digitorum profundus
20 Anterior interosseous nerve and artery overlying interosseous membrane
21 Flexor pollicis longus
22 Supinator
23 Extensor carpi radialis brevis
24 Extensor carpi radialis longus

● The median nerve passes between the humeral (superficial) and ulnar (deep) heads of pronator teres; the ulnar artery passes deep to the ulnar head. In specimen B the humeral head has been removed to show the ulnar head lying between the median nerve and the ulnar artery.
● In the lower part of B flexor carpi ulnaris has been displaced medially to show the underlying ulnar nerve and artery.
● At the level of the lateral epicondyle and under cover of brachioradialis the radial nerve divides into its superficial and deep terminal branches. The deep terminal branch is commonly called the posterior interosseous nerve.

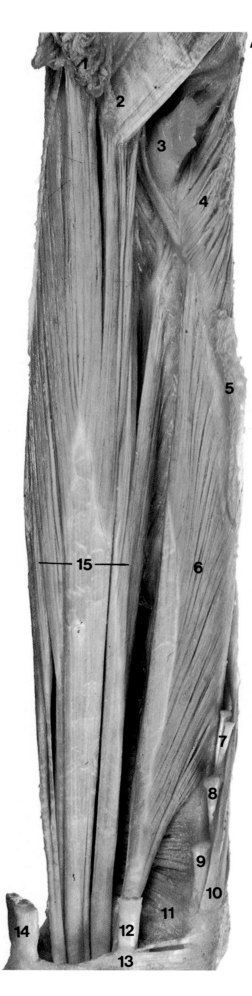

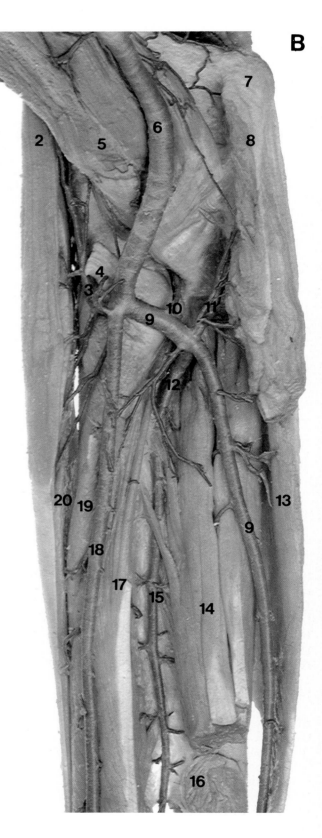

A Left forearm, from the front. Deep muscles
1 Common flexor origin
2 Brachialis
3 Biceps
4 Supinator
5 Pronator teres
6 Flexor pollicis longus
7 Extensor carpi radialis brevis
8 Extensor carpi radialis longus
9 Brachioradialis
10 Abductor pollicis longus
11 Pronator quadratus
12 Flexor carpi radialis
13 Flexor retinaculum
14 Flexor carpi ulnaris
15 Flexor digitorum profundus

B Right cubital fossa and forearm. Arteries
1 Brachioradialis
2 Extensor carpi radialis longus
3 Radial recurrent artery overlying supinator
4 Biceps tendon
5 Brachialis
6 Brachial artery
7 Medial epicondyle of humerus
8 Common flexor origin
9 Ulnar artery
10 Posterior ulnar recurrent artery
11 Anterior ulnar recurrent artery
12 Common interosseous artery
13 Flexor carpi ulnaris
14 Flexor digitorum profundus
15 Anterior interosseous artery overlying interosseous membrane
16 Pronator quadratus
17 Flexor pollicis longus
18 Radial artery
19 Pronator teres
20 Extensor carpi radialis brevis

● The radial artery usually appears to be the direct continuation of the brachial, with the ulnar artery leaving the main trunk almost at a right angle.
● The small unnamed vessels are muscular branches.

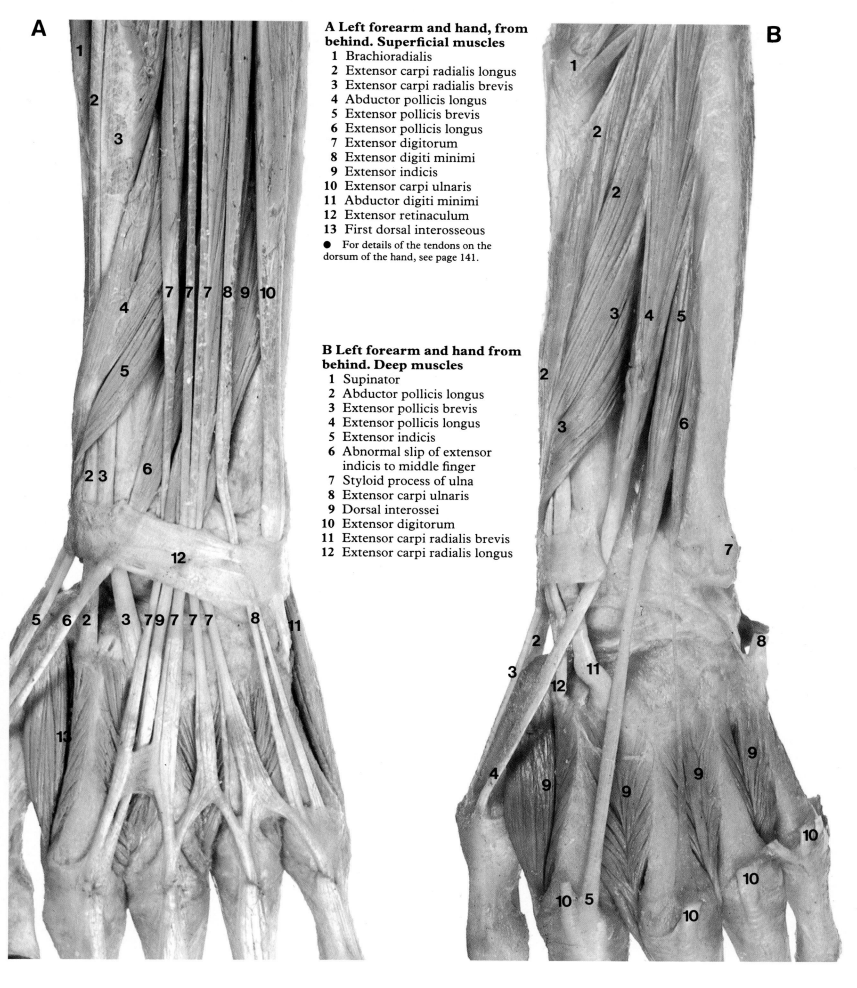

A Left forearm and hand, from behind. Superficial muscles

1 Brachioradialis
2 Extensor carpi radialis longus
3 Extensor carpi radialis brevis
4 Abductor pollicis longus
5 Extensor pollicis brevis
6 Extensor pollicis longus
7 Extensor digitorum
8 Extensor digiti minimi
9 Extensor indicis
10 Extensor carpi ulnaris
11 Abductor digiti minimi
12 Extensor retinaculum
13 First dorsal interosseous

● For details of the tendons on the dorsum of the hand, see page 141.

B Left forearm and hand from behind. Deep muscles

1 Supinator
2 Abductor pollicis longus
3 Extensor pollicis brevis
4 Extensor pollicis longus
5 Extensor indicis
6 Abnormal slip of extensor indicis to middle finger
7 Styloid process of ulna
8 Extensor carpi ulnaris
9 Dorsal interossei
10 Extensor digitorum
11 Extensor carpi radialis brevis
12 Extensor carpi radialis longus

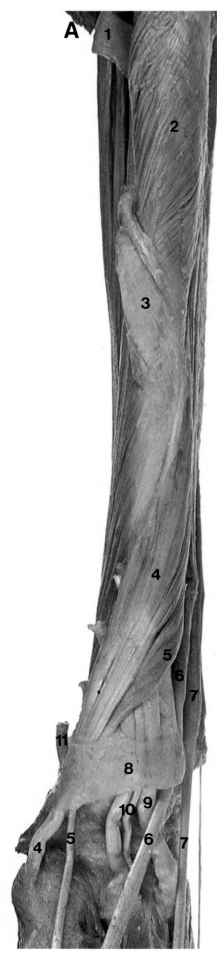

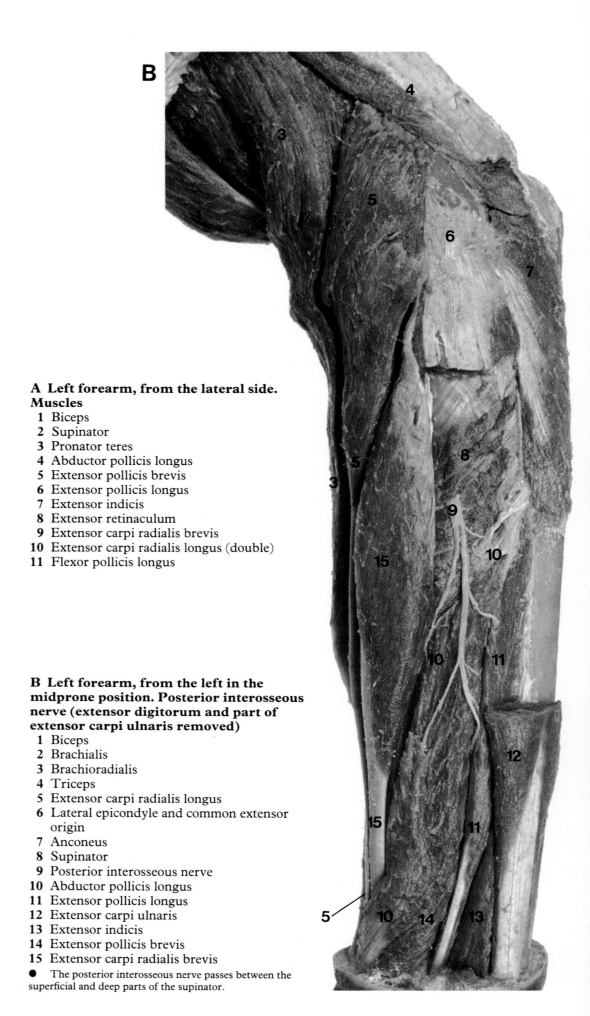

A Left forearm, from the lateral side. Muscles
1 Biceps
2 Supinator
3 Pronator teres
4 Abductor pollicis longus
5 Extensor pollicis brevis
6 Extensor pollicis longus
7 Extensor indicis
8 Extensor retinaculum
9 Extensor carpi radialis brevis
10 Extensor carpi radialis longus (double)
11 Flexor pollicis longus

B Left forearm, from the left in the midprone position. Posterior interosseous nerve (extensor digitorum and part of extensor carpi ulnaris removed)
1 Biceps
2 Brachialis
3 Brachioradialis
4 Triceps
5 Extensor carpi radialis longus
6 Lateral epicondyle and common extensor origin
7 Anconeus
8 Supinator
9 Posterior interosseous nerve
10 Abductor pollicis longus
11 Extensor pollicis longus
12 Extensor carpi ulnaris
13 Extensor indicis
14 Extensor pollicis brevis
15 Extensor carpi radialis brevis
● The posterior interosseous nerve passes between the superficial and deep parts of the supinator.

Left elbow and forearm, in the midprone position, A from the medial side, B from the front, C from the lateral side. Interosseous membrane and supinator muscle

1 Medial epicondyle of humerus
2 Trochlea
3 Upper band of ulnar collateral ligament
4 Coronoid process of ulna
5 Tuberosity of radius
6 Posterior interosseous nerve
7 Supinator
8 Interosseous membrane
9 Pronator quadratus
10 Capitulum
11 Lateral epicondyle
12 Radial collateral ligament
13 Annular ligament

● The posterior interosseous vessels pass backwards through the gap above the upper border of the interosseous membrane.

● The fibres of the interosseous membrane pass obliquely downwards and medially from the interosseous border of the radius to that of the ulna, so transmitting weight from the hand and radius to the ulna.

● The oblique cord (see page 122) is an unimportant inconstant fibrous band, whose fibres pass (at right angles to those of the interosseous membrane) from the tuberosity of the ulna to the radius just below its tuberosity.

● The supinator muscle arises from the lateral epicondyle of the humerus, the radial collateral ligament of the elbow joint, the annular ligament of the proximal radio-ulnar joint, the supinator crest of the ulna and the area of bone in front of the crest, and from an aponeurosis overlying the muscle. From these origins the fibres wrap round the upper end of the radius (the fibres from the ulna passing behind the radius), and are attached to the lateral surface of the radius above the pronator teres attachment, extending anteriorly and posteriorly as far as the radial tuberosity.

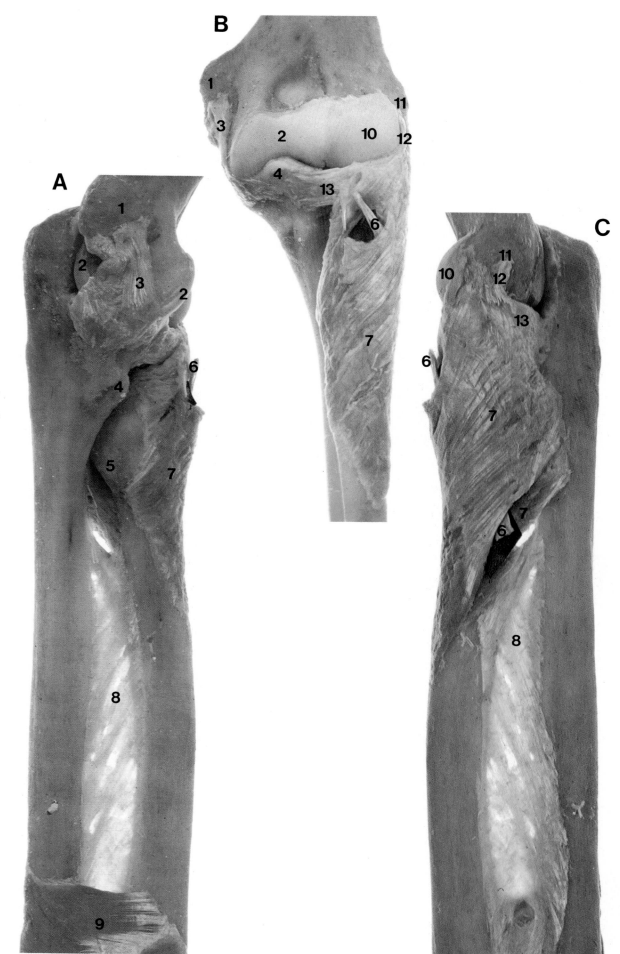

129

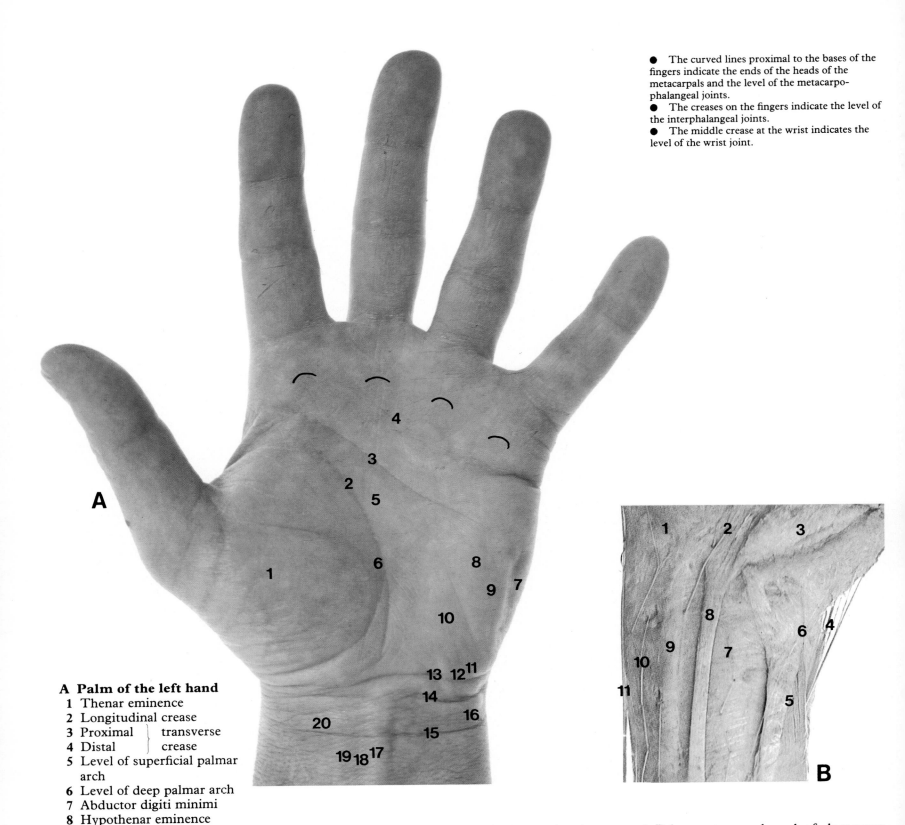

● The curved lines proximal to the bases of the fingers indicate the ends of the heads of the metacarpals and the level of the metacarpophalangeal joints.
● The creases on the fingers indicate the level of the interphalangeal joints.
● The middle crease at the wrist indicates the level of the wrist joint.

A Palm of the left hand
1 Thenar eminence
2 Longitudinal crease
3 Proximal ⎱ transverse
4 Distal ⎰ crease
5 Level of superficial palmar arch
6 Level of deep palmar arch
7 Abductor digiti minimi
8 Hypothenar eminence
9 Palmaris brevis
10 Hook of hamate
11 Pisiform
12 Ulnar artery and nerve
13 Distal ⎱
14 Middle ⎰ wrist crease
15 Proximal ⎰
16 Flexor carpi ulnaris
17 Palmaris longus
18 Median nerve
19 Flexor carpi radialis
20 Radial artery

B Left wrist, from the front, in ulnar deviation (adduction). Cutaneous nerves
1 Lateral part of palmar aponeurosis overlying thenar muscles
2 Palmar cutaneous branch of median nerve overlying palmaris longus attachment to flexor retinaculum
3 Medial part of palmar aponeurosis overlying hypothenar muscles
4 Branches of dorsal branch of ulnar nerve
5 Flexor carpi ulnaris
6 Palmar cutaneous branch of ulnar nerve
7 Medial cutaneous nerve of forearm and fascia overlying flexor digitorum superficialis
8 Palmaris longus
9 Flexor carpi radialis
10 Lateral cutaneous nerve of forearm
11 Superficial terminal branch of radial nerve

● The palmar cutaneous branch of the ulnar nerve normally pierces the deep fascia lateral to flexor carpi ulnaris, not medial to it as in this specimen.

130

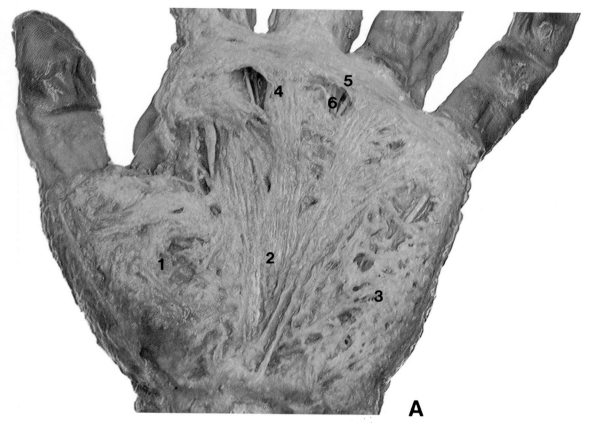

A Palm of the left hand. Palmar aponeurosis

1 Lateral part of aponeurosis overlying thenar muscles
2 Central part of aponeurosis
3 Medial part of aponeurosis overlying hypothenar muscles
4 Digital slip of aponeurosis
5 Superficial transverse metacarpal ligament
6 Palmar digital vessels and nerves in interval between slips

● The palmar aponeurosis is continuous with the distal edge of the flexor retinaculum; the palmaris longus tendon is attached to the aponeurosis and the distal part of the retinaculum.

B Palm of the left hand. Superficial dissection

1 Flexor retinaculum and palmar branch of median nerve
2 Abductor pollicis brevis
3 Flexor pollicis brevis
4 Adductor pollicis and digital branches of median nerve
5 First lumbrical
6 Central part of palmar aponeurosis and filaments of palmar branch of median nerve
7 Palmar digital vessels and nerves
8 Fibrous sheath (partly removed)
9 Flexor digitorum profundus tendon overlying superficialis tendon
10 Flexor digiti minimi brevis
11 Abductor digiti minimi
12 Palmaris brevis and filament of palmar branch of ulnar nerve
13 Flexor carpi ulnaris
14 Ulnar nerve and artery passing beneath superficial part of flexor retinaculum
15 Flexor digitorum superficialis
16 Median nerve and overlying palmar branch
17 Flexor carpi radialis
18 Radial artery

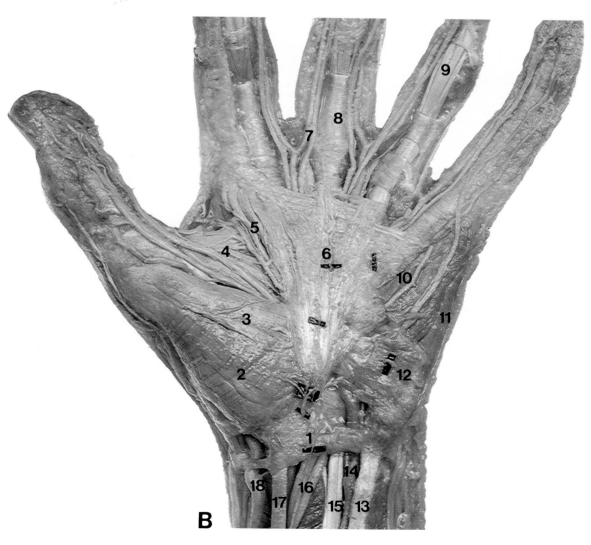

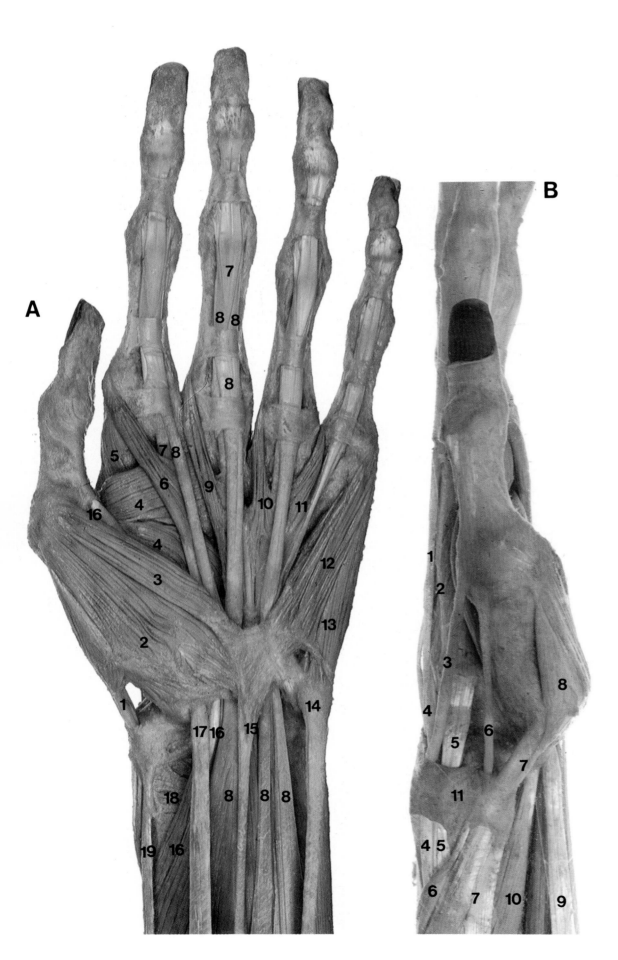

A Left wrist and palm. Muscles and tendons (digital fibrous sheaths partly removed)

1 Abductor pollicis longus overlying extensor pollicis brevis
2 Abductor pollicis brevis
3 Flexor pollicis brevis
4 Adductor pollicis
5 First dorsal interosseous
6 First lumbrical
7 Flexor digitorum profundus
8 Flexor digitorum superficialis
9 Second lumbrical
10 Third lumbrical
11 Fourth lumbrical
12 Flexor digiti minimi brevis
13 Abductor digiti minimi
14 Flexor carpi ulnaris and pisiform
15 Palmaris longus
16 Flexor pollicis longus
17 Flexor carpi radialis
18 Pronator quadratus
19 Brachioradialis

● The lumbrical muscles arise from the tendons of flexor digitorum profundus – the first and second lumbricals from the tendons of the index and middle fingers respectively, and the third and fourth from adjacent sides of the middle and ring, and ring and little, fingers respectively.

B Left wrist and hand, from the lateral side

1 Extensor digitorum
2 First dorsal interosseous
3 Extensor pollicis longus
4 Extensor carpi radialis brevis
5 Extensor carpi radialis longus
6 Extensor pollicis brevis
7 Abductor pollicis longus (giving slip to brevis)
8 Abductor pollicis brevis
9 Flexor carpi radialis
10 Flexor pollicis longus
11 Extensor retinaculum

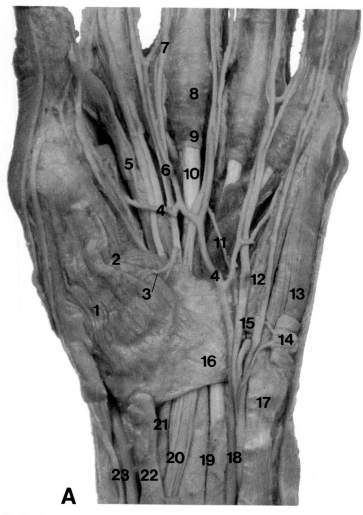

A

A Palm of the left hand, with resin injection of digital synovial sheaths

1 Abductor pollicis brevis
2 Flexor pollicis brevis
3 Muscular (recurrent) branch of median nerve
4 Superficial palmar arch
5 First lumbrical
6 Common palmar digital artery and nerve
7 Palmar digital artery and nerve
8 Fibrous sheath
9 Synovial sheath
10 Flexor digitorum superficialis tendon overlying profundus tendon
11 Communication between median and ulnar nerves
12 Flexor digiti minimi brevis
13 Abductor digiti minimi
14 Palmaris brevis
15 Deep branch of ulnar nerve and artery
16 Flexor retinaculum
17 Pisiform and flexor carpi ulnaris
18 Ulnar artery and nerve
19 Flexor digitorum superficialis
20 Median nerve
21 Flexor pollicis longus
22 Flexor carpi radialis
23 Radial artery and superficial terminal branch of radial nerve

● Communications between digital branches of the median and ulnar nerves (as at 11) are common.
● The median nerve at the wrist is usually flat and ribbon-like rather than rounded, and is most commonly injured at this site.
● For a note on the synovial sheaths see page 135.

B Palm of the right hand. Superficial palmar arch

(thenar muscles, flexor tendons and part of the deep palmar arch removed)

1 Flexor retinaculum
2 Deep branches of ulnar artery and nerve
3 Abductor digiti minimi
4 Opponens digiti minimi and digital branches of ulnar nerve
5 Common palmar digital branch of superficial arch
6 Palmar digital artery
7 Common palmar digital branch of median nerve
8 Palmar digital nerve
9 Radialis indicis artery
10 Princeps pollicis artery
11 Common stem of radialis indicis and princeps pollicis arteries
12 Extensor pollicis brevis
13 Abductor pollicis longus
14 Radial artery
15 Superficial palmar branch of radial artery
16 Flexor carpi radialis
17 Flexor pollicis longus
18 Median nerve
19 Flexor digitorum superficialis
20 Ulnar artery and nerve
21 Flexor carpi ulnaris

● In the palm the superficial arterial arch and its branches lie superficial to the digital nerves, but on the fingers the palmar digital nerves are superficial (anterior) to their corresponding arteries.
● The common palmar digital arteries and nerves divide distally to form the palmar digital arteries and nerves that run along the sides of adjacent fingers.
● In this specimen the radial side of the superficial arch anastomoses with the vessels of the thumb and index fingers.

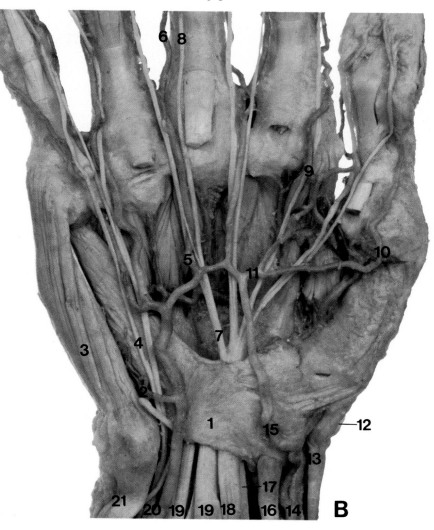

B

● In one third of hands the superficial palmar arch as in this specimen is not a complete arch. In another third it is completed by the superficial palmar branch of the radial artery which passes superficial to or through the muscles of the thenar eminence (see page 133) and in the remainder by the princeps pollicis or radialis indicis artery.

● On the palmar surface of the hand the ulnar nerve supplies the skin of the ulnar side of the palm and of the medial one-and-a-half fingers; the rest of the palm and palmar surfaces of the remaining fingers and thumb are supplied by the median nerve.

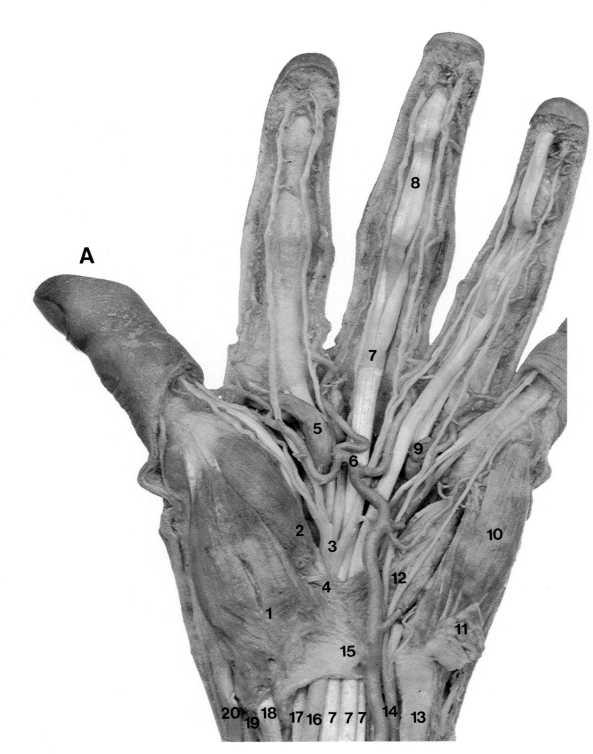

B Palm of the left hand, with resin injection of synovial sheaths

1 Abductor pollicis brevis
2 Flexor pollicis brevis
3 Adductor pollicis
4 First dorsal interosseous
5 First lumbrical arising from flexor digitorum profundus tendon and lying anterior to superficialis tendon
6 Second lumbrical
7 Flexor digitorum superficialis
8 Synovial sheath
9 Fibrous sheath
10 Third lumbrical (with abnormal part going to middle finger)
11 Fourth lumbrical
12 Opponens digiti minimi
13 Flexor digiti minimi brevis
14 Abductor digiti minimi
15 Deep branch of ulnar nerve
16 Flexor digitorum profundus
17 Flexor carpi ulnaris
18 Median nerve
19 Flexor pollicis longus
20 Flexor carpi radialis

● The deep branch of the ulnar nerve passes between flexor digiti minimi brevis and abductor digiti minimi, and then through opponens digiti minimi.

A Palm of the left hand. Incomplete superficial palmar arch

1 Abductor pollicis brevis
2 Flexor pollicis brevis
3 Median nerve dividing into common palmar digital nerves
4 Muscular (recurrent) branch of median nerve
5 First lumbrical
6 Ulnar artery forming superficial palmar arch giving off common palmar digital branches
7 Flexor digitorum superficialis
8 Flexor digitorum profundus
9 Fourth lumbrical
10 Abductor digiti minimi
11 Palmaris brevis
12 Opponens digiti minimi and common palmar digital branches of ulnar nerve
13 Flexor carpi ulnaris
14 Ulnar nerve and artery
15 Flexor retinaculum
16 Median nerve
17 Flexor pollicis longus
18 Flexor carpi radialis
19 Radial artery
20 Abductor pollicis longus

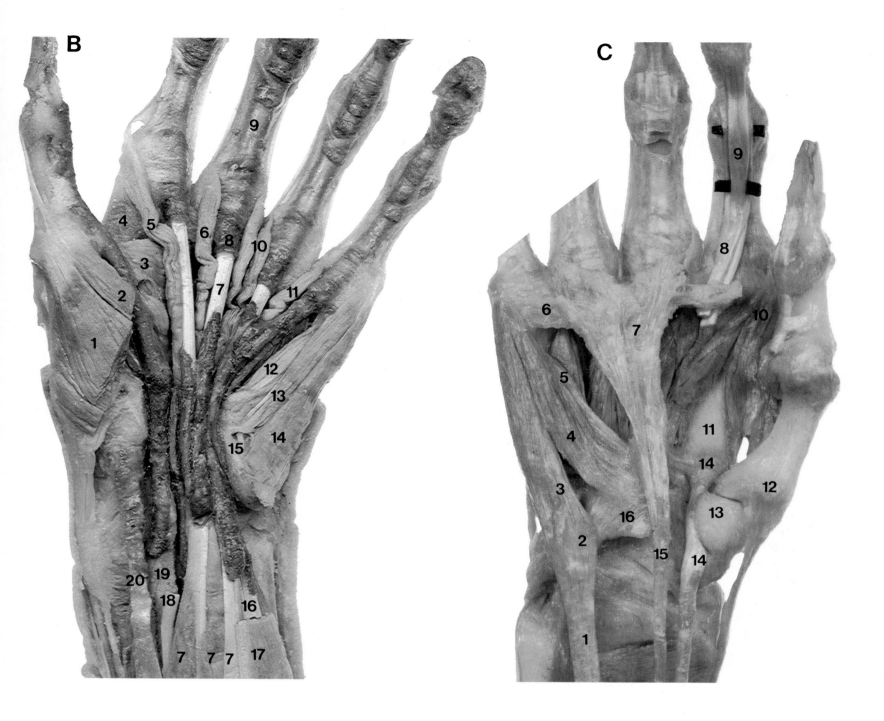

C Palm of the right hand. Flexor muscles

1 Flexor carpi ulnaris
2 Pisiform
3 Abductor digiti minimi
4 Flexor digiti minimi brevis
5 Opponens digiti minimi
6 Superficial transverse metacarpal ligament
7 Palmar aponeurosis
8 Flexor digitorum superficialis
9 Flexor digitorum profundus
10 First dorsal interosseous (with abnormal slip from ulnar side of second metacarpal)

11 Base of second metacarpal
12 Abductor pollicis longus and base of first metacarpal
13 Tubercle of trapezium
14 Flexor carpi radialis
15 Palmaris longus
16 Flexor retinaculum

● Near the bases of the proximal phalanges the flexor digitorum superficialis tendons divide to allow the profundus tendons to pass through to their insertions to the bases of the distal phalanges. The divided superficialis slips reunite and partially decussate before becoming attached to the sides of the shafts of the middle phalanges.

● In the carpal tunnel (beneath the flexor retinaculum), one synovial sheath envelops the eight tendons of flexor digitorum superficialis and profundus, another envelops the flexor pollicis longus tendon, and the flexor carpi radialis (in its own compartment of the flexor retinaculum) has its own sheath also. The synovial sheaths for flexor carpi radialis and flexor pollicis longus extend as far as the tendon insertions.

● The sheath of the long finger flexors is continuous with the digital synovial sheath of the little finger, but is *not* continuous with the digital synovial sheaths of the ring, middle or index fingers; these fingers have their own synovial sheaths whose proximal ends project slightly beyond the *fibrous* sheaths within which the digital *synovial* sheaths lie.

Palm of the right hand. Deep branch of the ulnar nerve

1 Pisiform
2 Abductor digiti minimi and palmar digital branch of ulnar nerve
3 Opponens digiti minimi
4 Fourth palmar interosseous
5 Fourth dorsal interosseous and common palmar digital branch of ulnar nerve
6 Third palmar interosseous
7 Third dorsal interosseous and common palmar digital branch of median nerve
8 Deep branch of ulnar nerve
9 Adductor pollicis (partly removed)
10 Second dorsal interosseous
11 Second palmar interosseous
12 First dorsal interosseous
13 Flexor pollicis longus
14 Flexor pollicis brevis
15 Abductor pollicis brevis
16 Flexor retinaculum
17 Flexor carpi radialis
18 Median nerve
19 Flexor digitorum superficialis
20 Ulnar artery and nerve
21 Flexor carpi ulnaris
22 Dorsal branch of ulnar nerve

● The deep branch of the ulnar nerve supplies all the small muscles of the hand, except abductor pollicis brevis, flexor pollicis brevis, opponens pollicis and the two lateral lumbricals (supplied by the median nerve).

● Anomalies in the innervation of the small muscles of the hand are frequent, especially in the case of flexor pollicis brevis, which in approximately one third of hands is supplied by the ulnar nerve, in one third by the median nerve, and in the remainder by both nerves.

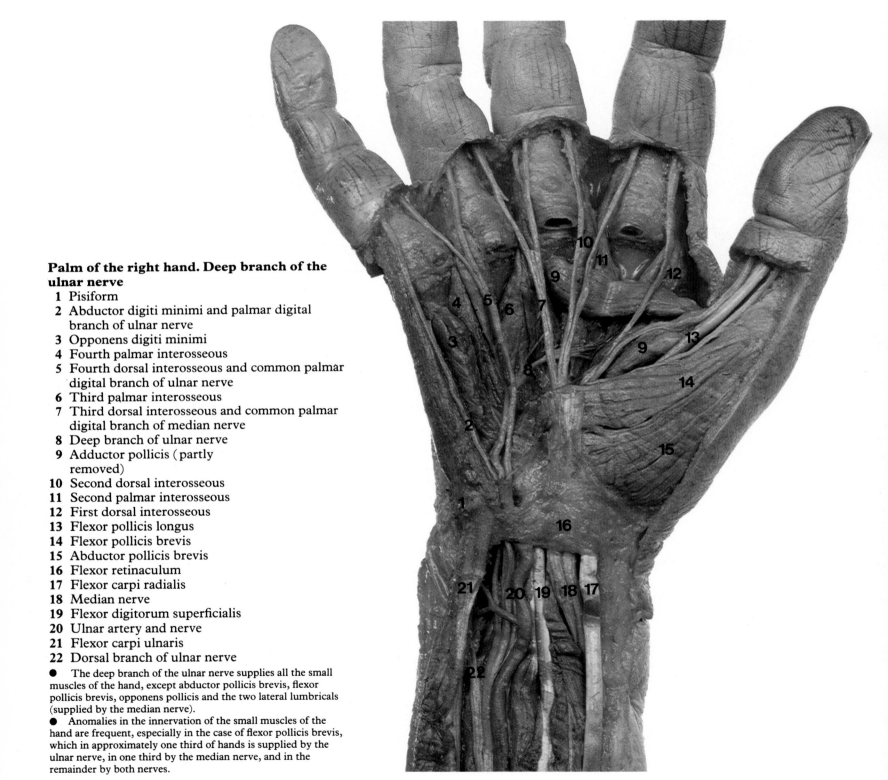

136

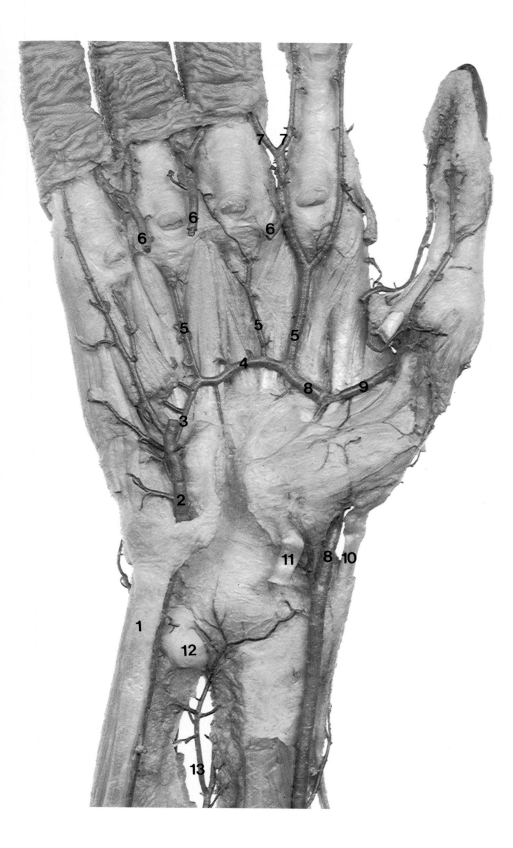

Palm of the right hand. Deep palmar arch

1 Flexor carpi ulnaris
2 Ulnar artery
3 Deep branch of ulnar artery
4 Deep palmar arch
5 Palmar metacarpal artery
6 Common palmar digital artery (from superficial arch)
7 Palmar digital artery
8 Radial artery
9 Princeps pollicis artery
10 Abductor pollicis longus
11 Flexor carpi radialis
12 Head of ulna
13 Branch of anterior interosseous artery to anterior carpal arch

● Unlike the superficial arch (see page 134), the deep arch is usually complete, being formed by the terminal part of the radial artery uniting with the deep branch of the ulnar.

● The most distal point of the deep arch lies about 1 cm proximal to the superficial arch.

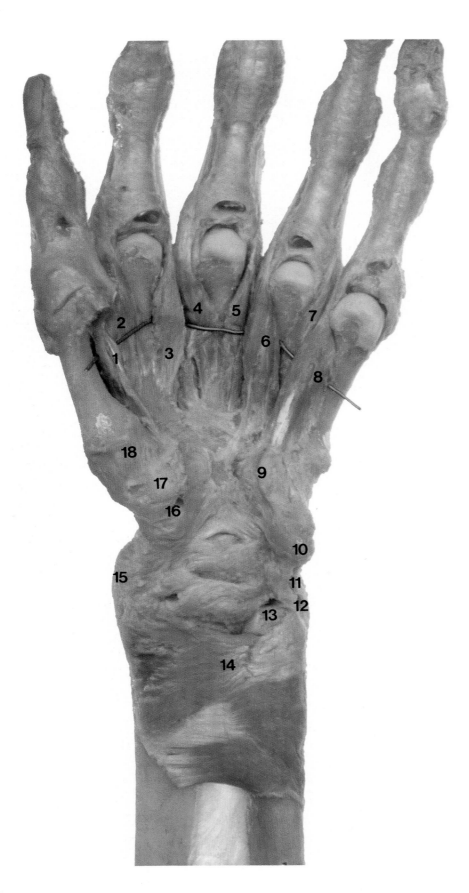

Left wrist and palm. Palmar interossei (superficial to the blue marker) and dorsal interossei (deep to the marker)

 1 First palmar
 2 First dorsal
 3 Second palmar
 4 Second dorsal
 5 Third dorsal
 6 Third palmar
 7 Fourth dorsal
 8 Fourth palmar
 9 Hook of hamate
10 Pisiform
11 Ulnar collateral ligament
12 Styloid process of ulna
13 Head of ulna
14 Pronator quadratus
15 Styloid process of radius
16 Scaphoid
17 Trapezium
18 Capsule of carpometacarpal joint of thumb

● The interossei are inserted partly into the extensor expansions of the extensor digitorum tendons, and partly into the sides of proximal phalanges (see page 145).

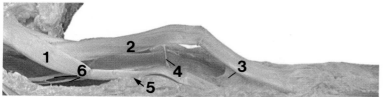

Long flexor tendons of the right middle finger, from the front and right. Long and short vincula

1 Flexor digitorum superficialis
2 Flexor digitorum profundus
3 Short vinculum of profundus tendon
4 Long vinculum of profundus tendon
5 Position of short vinculum of superficialis tendon
6 Long vincula of superficialis tendon

● The fibrous and synovial sheaths have been removed and the long tendons pulled anteriorly to reveal the vincula, which represent the remains of mesotendons and carry small blood vessels to the tendons.

Palm of the right hand. Ligaments and joints

 1 Ulnar collateral ligament of wrist joint
 2 Pisiform
 3 Pisometacarpal ligament
 4 Pisohamate ligament
 5 Hook of hamate
 6 Interosseous metacarpal ligament
 7 Deep transverse metacarpal ligament
 8 Palmar ligament of metacarpophalangeal joint with groove for flexor tendon
 9 Collateral ligament of interphalangeal joint (capsule removed)
10 Sesamoid bones of flexor pollicis brevis and adductor pollicis tendons
11 Palmar ligament of carpometacarpal joint of thumb
12 Lateral ligament of carpometacarpal joint
13 Tubercle of trapezium with marker in groove for flexor carpi radialis tendon
14 Head of capitate
15 Tubercle of scaphoid
16 Lunate
17 Palmar radiocarpal ligament
18 Articular disc of distal radio-ulnar joint
19 Sacciform recess of capsule of distal radio-ulnar joint

● The collateral ligaments of the metacarpophalangeal and interphalangeal joints pass obliquely forwards from the posterior part of the side of the head of the proximal bone to the anterior part of the side of the base of the distal bone. They become tightest in flexion.

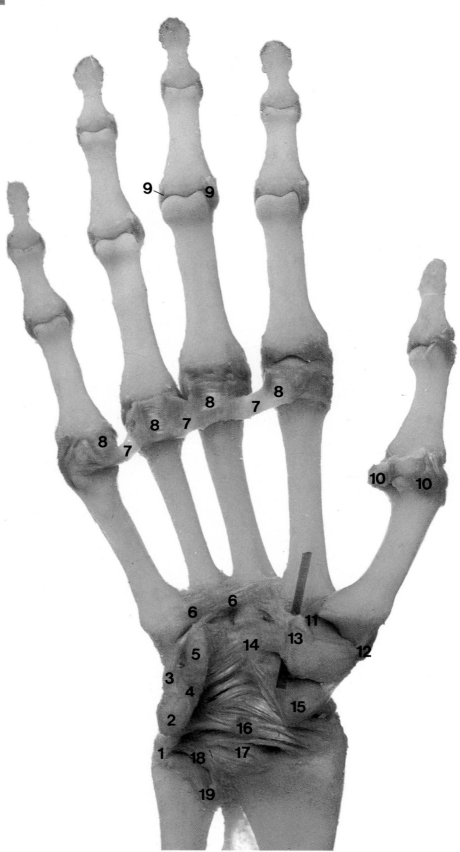

B Left wrist, from behind, in ulnar deviation (adduction). Cutaneous nerves
1 Branches of dorsal branch of ulnar nerve
2 Head of ulna
3 Extensor retinaculum
4 Lower end of radius
5 Superficial terminal branches of radial nerve
6 Branches of lateral cutaneous nerve of forearm

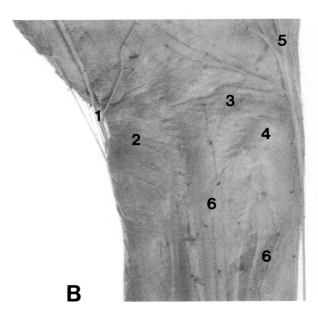

B

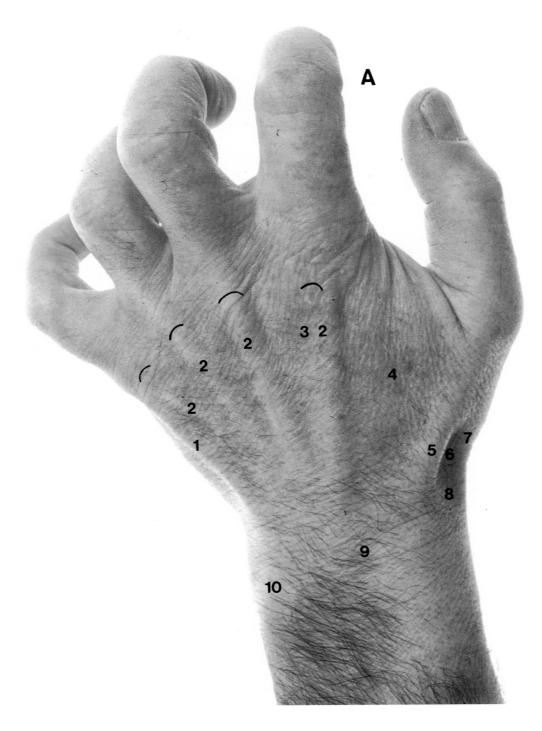

A

A Dorsum of the left hand
(The fingers are extended at the metacarpophalangeal joints and partially flexed at the interphalangeal joints. The thumb is extended at the carpometacarpal joint and partially flexed at the metacarpophalangeal and interphalangeal joints)
1 Extensor digiti minimi
2 Extensor digitorum
3 Extensor indicis
4 First dorsal interosseous
5 Extensor pollicis longus
6 Anatomical snuffbox
7 Extensor pollicis brevis and abductor pollicis longus
8 Styloid process of radius
9 Extensor retinaculum
10 Head of ulna
● The curved lines proximal to the bases of the fingers indicate the ends of the heads of the metacarpals and the level of the metacarpophalangeal joints. In a clenched fist the heads of the metacarpals form the knuckles.

Dorsum of the left hand

1 Abductor digiti minimi
2 Extensor digiti minimi
3 Slip from extensor digitorum to little finger
4 Extensor digitorum
5 Extensor indicis
6 First dorsal interosseous
7 Abductor pollicis longus
8 Extensor pollicis brevis
9 Extensor pollicis longus
10 Extensor carpi radialis longus
11 Extensor carpi radialis brevis
12 Extensor retinaculum
13 Extensor carpi ulnaris

● The tendon of extensor indicis lies on the ulnar side of the extensor digitorum tendon to the index finger.
● The tendon of extensor digiti minimi is normally double.
● The 'tendon' of extensor digitorum to the little finger consists of a slip from the digitorum tendon to the ring finger, joining the digiti minimi tendon just proximal to the metacarpophalangeal joint. Similar slips join adjacent digitorum tendons to the other fingers.

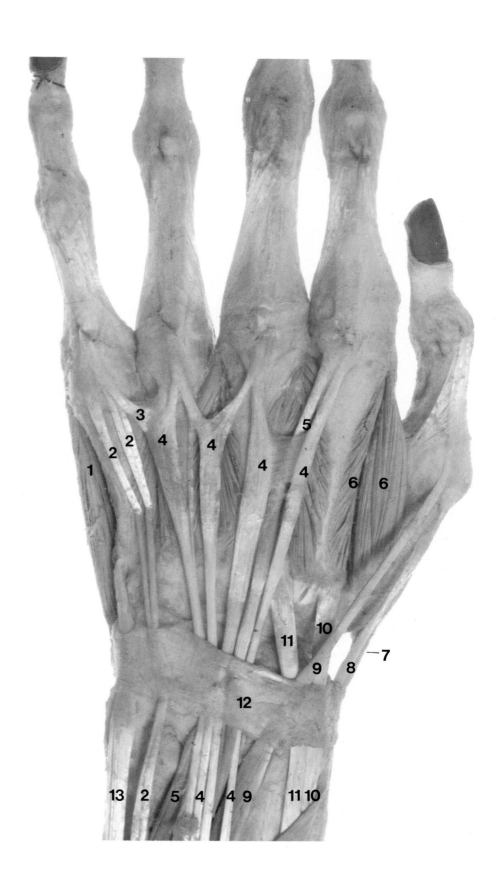

- In this specimen the extensor digitorum tendon to the ring finger is double, as well as giving a slip to the digiti minimi tendon, and to the extensor tendon of the middle finger. Some fascia distal to the extensor retinaculum is preserved.

- At the lateral side of the wrist the radial artery lies in the 'anatomical snuffbox' which is bounded laterally by the tendons of abductor pollicis longus and extensor pollicis brevis, and medially by the tendon of extensor pollicis longus.
- In this specimen the princeps pollicis artery has a more proximal origin than usual; it normally arises from the radial artery after that artery has passed through the first dorsal interosseous muscle.

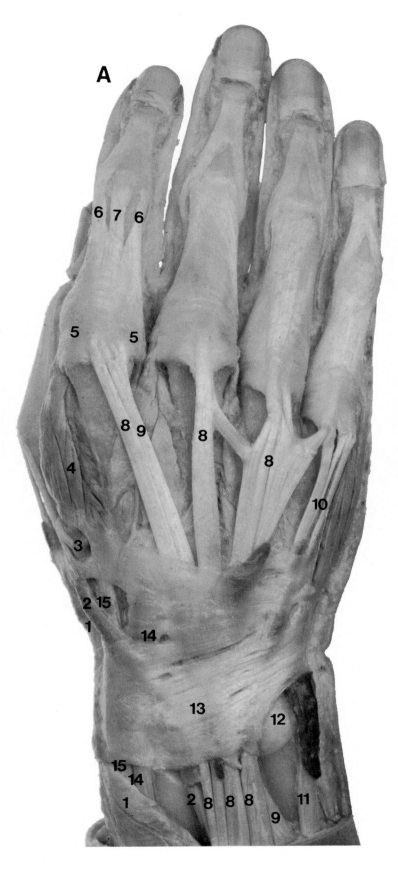

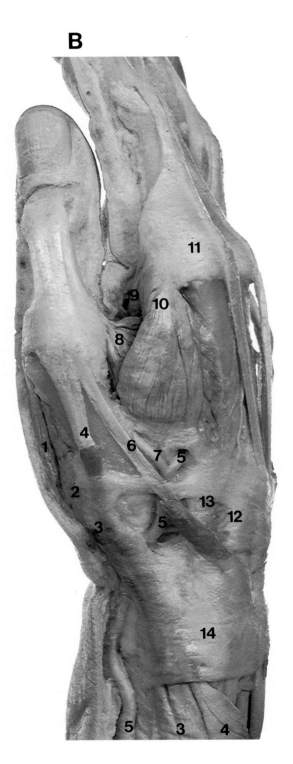

A Dorsum of the right hand, with resin injection of synovial sheaths

1 Extensor pollicis brevis
2 Extensor pollicis longus
3 Radial artery
4 First dorsal interosseous
5 Dorsal digital expansion of extensor digitorum tendon
6 Collateral slip of expansion to distal phalanx
7 Intermediate part of expansion to middle phalanx
8 Extensor digitorum
9 Extensor indicis
10 Extensor digiti minimi
11 Extensor carpi ulnaris
12 Head of ulna
13 Extensor retinaculum
14 Extensor carpi radialis brevis
15 Extensor carpi radialis longus

B Right wrist and hand, from the lateral side, with resin injection of synovial sheaths

1 Abductor pollicis brevis
2 Opponens pollicis
3 Abductor pollicis longus
4 Extensor pollicis brevis
5 Radial artery
6 Extensor pollicis longus
7 Princeps pollicis artery
8 Adductor pollicis
9 First lumbrical
10 First dorsal interosseous
11 Extensor expansion
12 Extensor carpi radialis brevis
13 Extensor carpi radialis longus
14 Extensor retinaculum

C Dorsum of the right hand. Arteries

1 Adductor pollicis and branch of princeps pollicis artery
2 First dorsal interosseous and first dorsal metacarpal artery
3 Second dorsal interosseous and second dorsal metacarpal artery
4 Abductor digiti minimi
5 Extensor carpi ulnaris
6 Dorsal carpal arch
7 Anterior interosseous artery
8 Posterior interosseous artery
9 Branch of anterior interosseous artery to anterior carpal arch
10 Extensor pollicis brevis
11 Abductor pollicis longus
12 Brachioradialis
13 Extensor carpi radialis brevis
14 Extensor carpi radialis longus
15 Radial artery
16 Extensor pollicis longus

● The *anterior* interosseous artery pierces the interosseous membrane above pronator quadratus (here removed) to anastomose with the *posterior* interosseous artery and join the *dorsal* carpal arch.

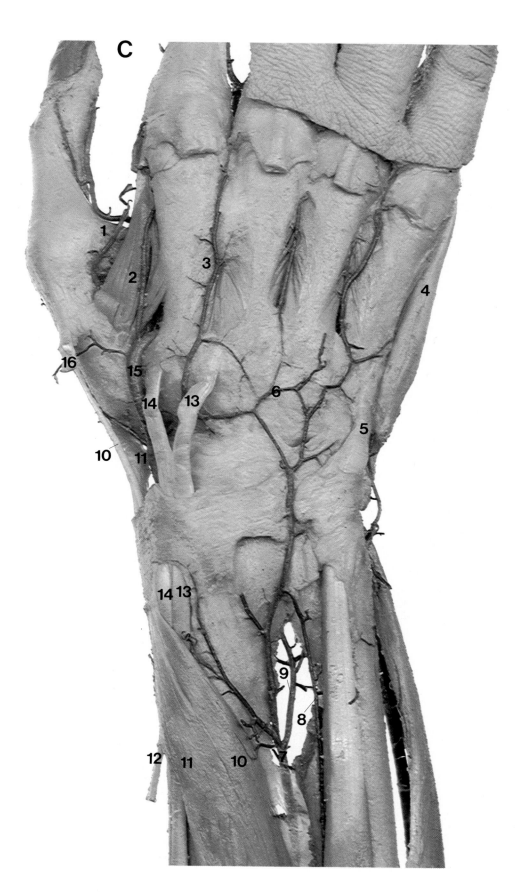

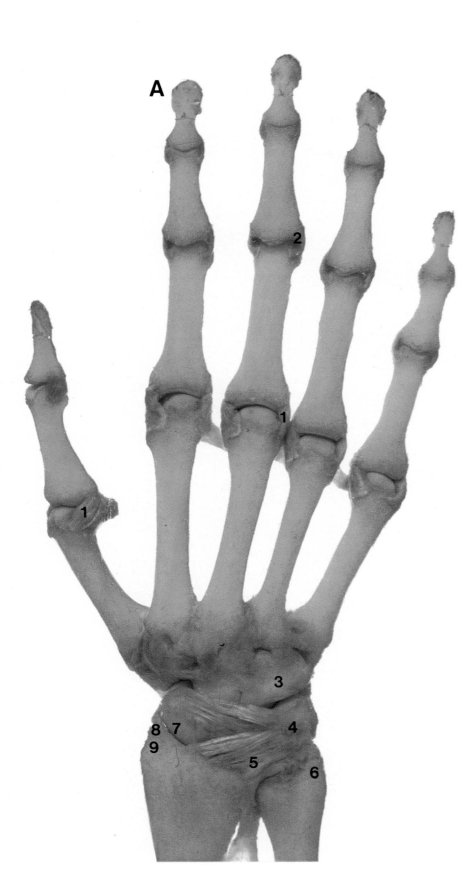

A Dorsum of the right hand. Ligaments and joints
1 Collateral ligament of metacarpophalangeal joint
2 Collateral ligament of interphalangeal joint
3 Hamate
4 Triquetral
5 Dorsal radiocarpal ligament
6 Styloid process of ulna
7 Scaphoid
8 Radial collateral ligament of wrist joint
9 Styloid process of radius
● The deep transverse metacarpal ligaments (of the palmar surface) are seen between the metacarpophalangeal joints (see page 139).

B Coronal section of the right wrist and hand, from behind
1 Lower end of radius
2 Sacciform recess of distal radio-ulnar joint
3 Head of ulna
4 Articular disc
5 Triquetral
6 Lunate
7 Scaphoid
8 Trapezium
9 Trapezoid
10 Capitate
11 Hamate
12 Head of fourth metacarpal
13 Head of third metacarpal
14 Head of second metacarpal

● The arrows indicate the line of the midcarpal joint.
● The section has passed through the carpus near the dorsal surface, and the first and fifth metacarpals have not been included in the sawcut.
● The cavity of the wrist joint does not communicate with that of the distal radio-ulnar, nor with the midcarpal, joint.

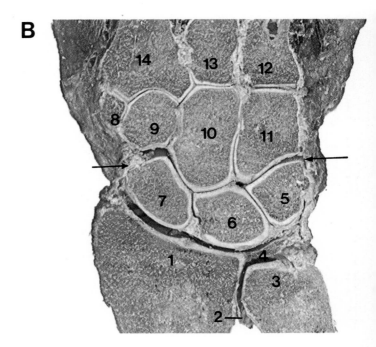

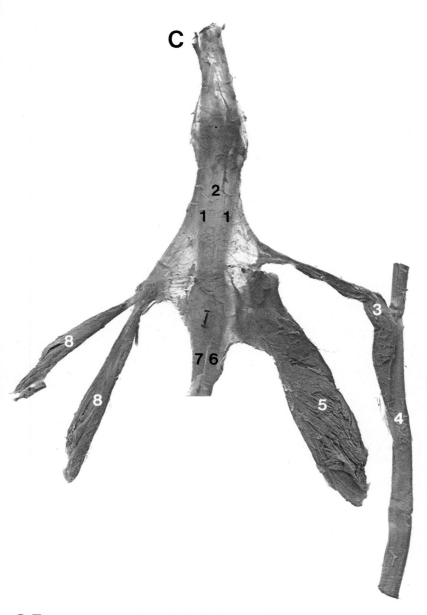

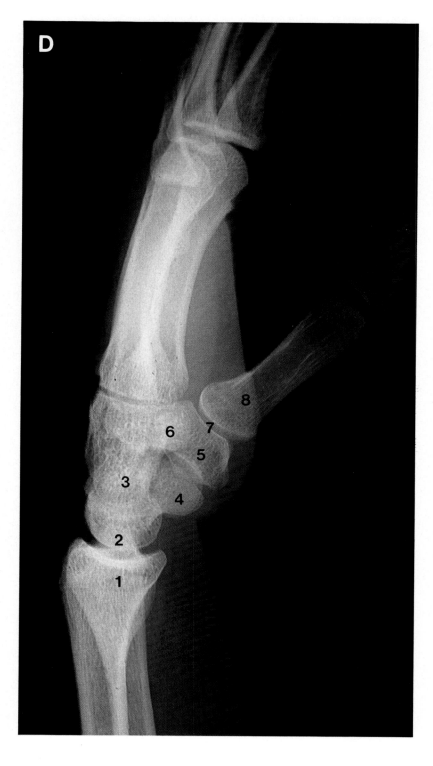

1 Lower end of radius
2 Lunate
3 Capitate
4 Pisiform
5 Trapezium
6 Hook of hamate
7 Carpometacarpal joint of thumb
8 First metacarpal

● Because of its rounded shape, the lunate is the carpal bone most frequently dislocated.

C Extensor expansion of the left index finger, dorsal surface

1 Collateral slip
2 Intermediate part
3 First lumbrical
4 Flexor digitorum profundus tendon
5 First dorsal interosseous
6 Extensor digitorum tendon
7 Extensor indicis tendon
8 First palmar interosseous (dissected out into two bellies)

● The lumbrical muscles are inserted entirely into the extensor expansions.
● The interossei are inserted partly into the extensor expansions and partly into the sides of proximal phalanges.

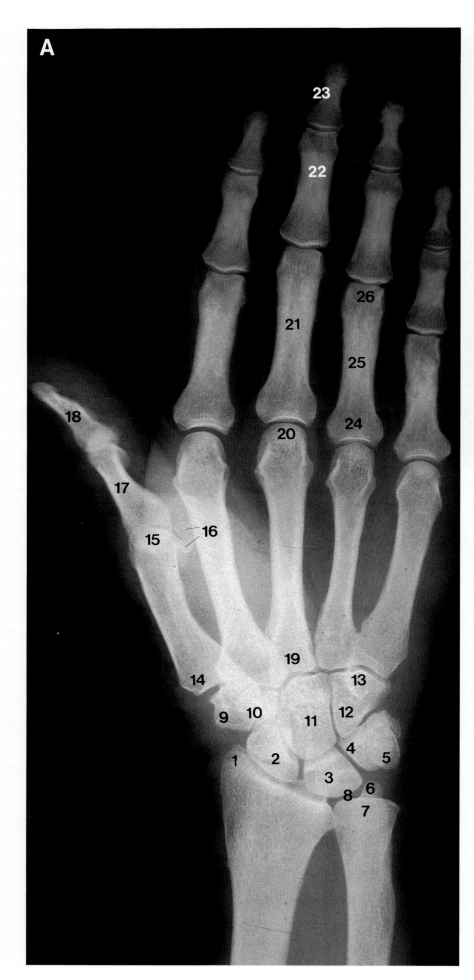

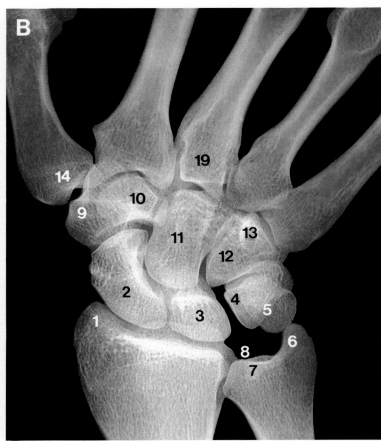

Radiograph of the left wrist and hand, A in the normal position, B in adduction (ulnar deviation)
  1 Styloid process of radius
  2 Scaphoid
  3 Lunate
  4 Triquetral
  5 Pisiform
  6 Styloid process of ulna
  7 Head of ulna
  8 Position of articular disc of distal radio-ulnar joint
  9 Trapezium
 10 Trapezoid
 11 Capitate
 12 Hamate
 13 Hook of hamate
 14 Base ⎫
 15 Head ⎬ of first metacarpal
 16 Sesamoid bones in flexor pollicis brevis and adductor pollicis tendons
 17 Proximal phalanx ⎫
 18 Distal phalanx ⎬ of thumb
 19 Base ⎫
 20 Head ⎬ of third metacarpal
 21 Proximal ⎫
 22 Middle ⎬ phalanx of middle finger
 23 Distal ⎭
 24 Base ⎫
 25 Shaft ⎬ of phalanx
 26 Head ⎭

● The wrist (radiocarpal) joint is the joint between the lower end of the radius and articular disc of the distal radio-ulnar joint proximally, and the scaphoid, lunate and triquetral distally.
● In the normal position the lunate articulates with the radius and the articular disc, but in adduction it moves completely on to the radius. In extreme adduction part of the triquetral may also make contact with the radius.

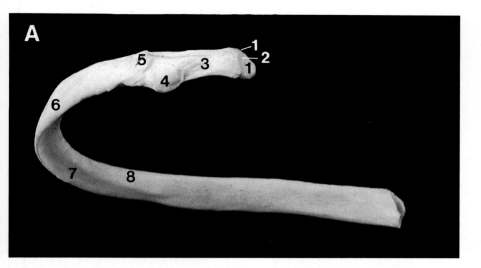

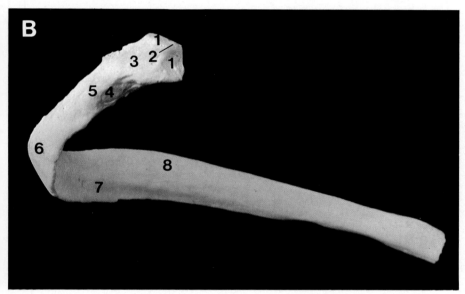

C Typical rib and vertebra articulated, from above

1 Non-articular ⎫
               ⎬ part of tubercle
2 Articular ⎭
3 Articular facet of transverse process
4 Neck of rib
5 Upper costal facet of head of rib
6 Upper costal facet of vertebral body

● The lower of the two facets on the head of a typical rib articulates with the upper costal facet on the vertebral body having the same number as the rib. The upper facet on the head of the rib articulates with the vertebral body above.

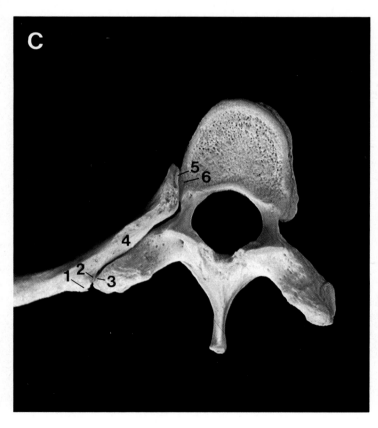

Typical ribs, from behind, A the left fifth rib (a typical upper rib), B the left seventh rib (a typical lower rib)

1 Articular facets of head
2 Crest of head
3 Neck
4 Articular facet of tubercle
5 Non-articular part of tubercle
6 Angle
7 Costal groove
8 Shaft

● Typical ribs (3–9) have a head with two facets, and a tubercle with articular and non-articular parts at the junction of the neck and shaft. The shaft has external and internal surfaces, an angle and a costal groove.

● In typical upper ribs (3–6) the articular facet of the tubercle is curved, but becomes increasingly flattened in lower ribs (7–9).

● The atypical ribs are the first, second, tenth, eleventh and twelfth.

● The first rib has a head with one facet, a prominent tubercle, no angle and no costal groove. The shaft has superior and inferior surfaces.

● The second rib has a head with two facets, an angle near the tubercle, a broad costal groove posteriorly, and an external surface facing upwards and outwards with the inner surface facing correspondingly downwards and inwards.

● The tenth rib has a head with one or two facets, a tubercle with or without an articular facet, and a costal groove.

● The eleventh rib has a head with one facet, no tubercle but there is an angle and a slight costal groove.

● The twelfth rib has a head with one facet but there is no tubercle, no angle and no costal groove. The shaft tapers at its end (the ends of all other ribs widen slightly).

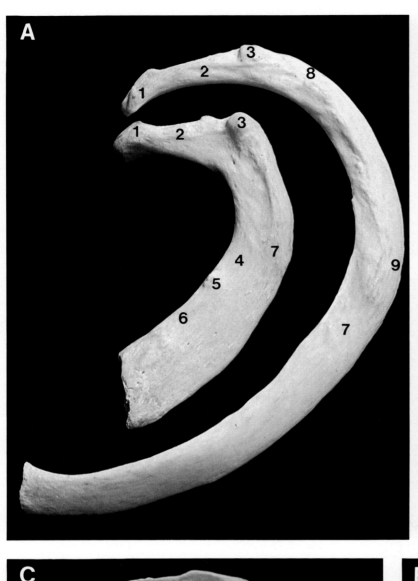

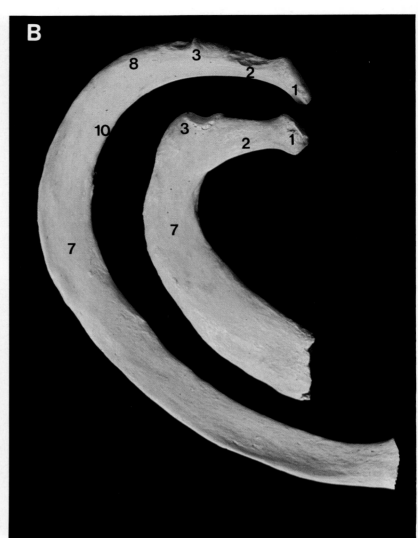

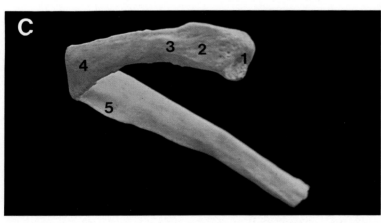

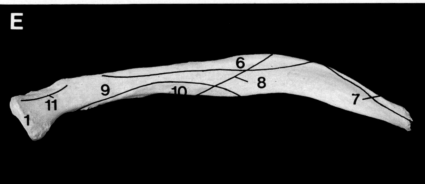

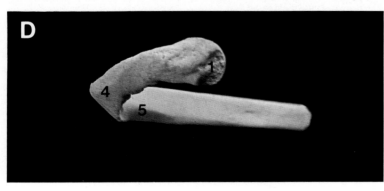

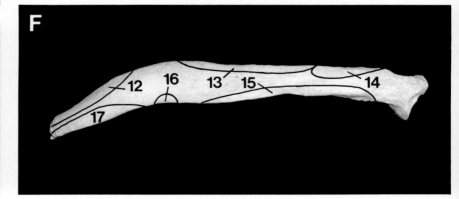

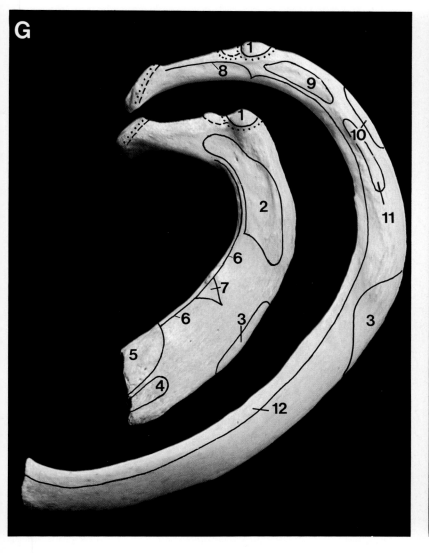

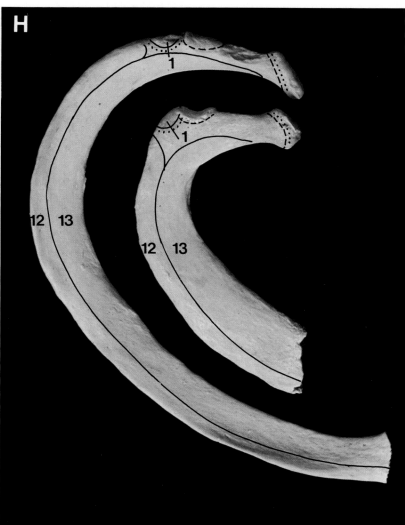

Left first rib (inner) and second rib (outer), A from above, B from below

1 Head
2 Neck
3 Tubercle
4 Groove for subclavian artery and first thoracic nerve
5 Scalene tubercle
6 Groove for subclavian vein
7 Shaft
8 Angle
9 Serratus anterior tuberosity
10 Costal groove

Atypical left lower ribs, C tenth rib from behind, D eleventh rib from behind, E twelfth rib from the front, with attachments, F twelfth rib from behind, with attachments

1 Head	10 Quadratus lumborum
2 Neck	11 Costotransverse ligament
3 Tubercle	12 Latissimus dorsi
4 Angle	13 External intercostal
5 Costal groove	14 Levator costae
6 Internal intercostal	15 Erector spinae
7 Diaphragm	16 Serratus posterior inferior
8 Line of pleural reflexion	17 External oblique
9 Area covered by pleura	

Left first rib (inner) and second rib (outer), G from above, H from below. Attachments

(Epiphysial line, dotted; capsule attachment, interrupted line)

1 Lateral costotransverse ligament
2 Scalenus medius
3 Serratus anterior
4 Subclavius
5 Costoclavicular ligament
6 Suprapleural membrane
7 Scalenus anterior
8 Superior costotransverse ligament
9 Levator costae
10 Serratus posterior superior
11 Scalenus posterior
12 Intercostal muscles and membranes
13 Area covered by pleura

● The second rib gives origin to part of the first, and the whole of the second, digitation of serratus anterior.

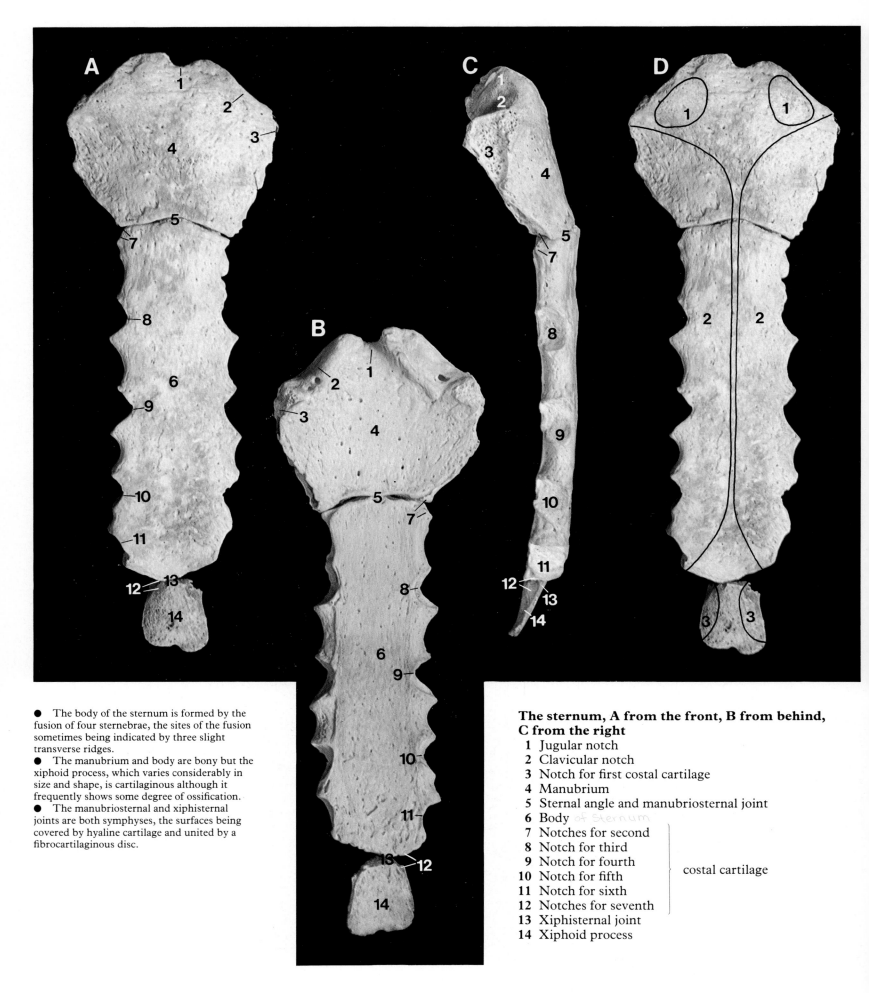

The body of the sternum is formed by the fusion of four sternebrae, the sites of the fusion sometimes being indicated by three slight transverse ridges.

The manubrium and body are bony but the xiphoid process, which varies considerably in size and shape, is cartilaginous although it frequently shows some degree of ossification.

The manubriosternal and xiphisternal joints are both symphyses, the surfaces being covered by hyaline cartilage and united by a fibrocartilaginous disc.

The sternum, A from the front, B from behind, C from the right

1 Jugular notch
2 Clavicular notch
3 Notch for first costal cartilage
4 Manubrium
5 Sternal angle and manubriosternal joint
6 Body of sternum
7 Notches for second
8 Notch for third
9 Notch for fourth
10 Notch for fifth   costal cartilage
11 Notch for sixth
12 Notches for seventh
13 Xiphisternal joint
14 Xiphoid process

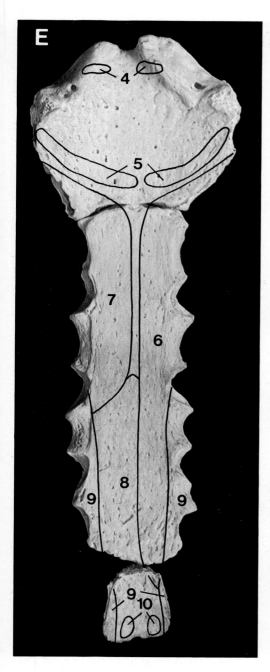

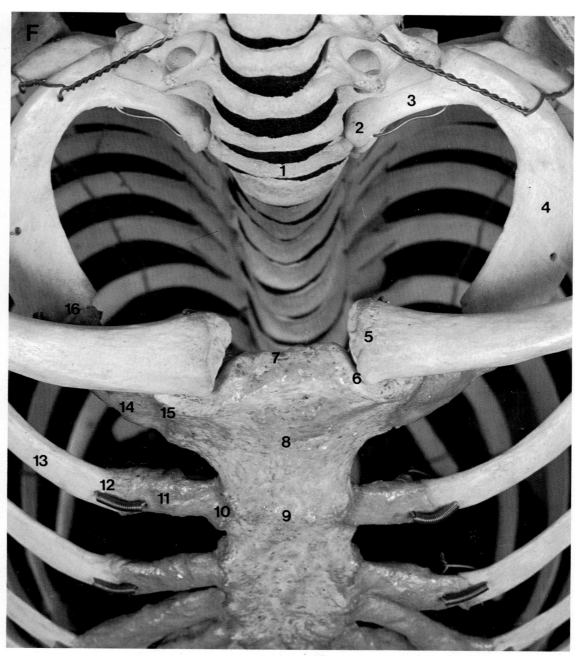

The sternum, D from the front, E from behind. Attachments

1 Sternocleidomastoid
2 Pectoralis major
3 Rectus abdominis
4 Sternohyoid
5 Sternothyroid
6 Area covered by right pleura
7 Area covered by left pleura
8 Area in contact with pericardium
9 Transverse thoracic
10 Diaphragm

● The two pleural sacs are in contact from the levels of the second to fourth costal cartilages.

F Thoracic inlet, from above and in front, in an articulated skeleton

1 First thoracic vertebra
2 Head ⎫
3 Neck ⎬ of first rib
4 Shaft ⎭
5 Sternal end of clavicle
6 Sternoclavicular joint
7 Jugular notch or Suprasternal Notch
8 Manubrium of sternum
9 Manubriosternal joint (angle of Louis)
10 Second sternocostal joint
11 Second costal cartilage
12 Costochondral joint
13 Second rib
14 First costal cartilage
15 First sternocostal joint
16 First costochondral joint

● The thoracic inlet (upper aperture of the thorax) is approximately the same size and shape as the outline of the kidney, and is bounded by the first thoracic vertebra, first ribs and costal cartilages, and the upper border of the manubrium of the sternum. It does not lie in a horizontal plane but slopes downwards and forwards.

Left hemithorax in the female, from the front. Surface markings of the heart and pleura

(Heart, interrupted line; pleura, dotted line)

1 Jugular notch
2 Sternocleidomastoid
3 Sternoclavicular joint
4 Midpoint of clavicle
5 Acromioclavicular joint
6 Axillary tail ⎫
7 Areola   ⎪
8 Nipple   ⎬ of breast
9 Areolar gland ⎪
10 Costal margin (at eighth costal cartilage)
11 Xiphisternal joint
12 Sixth ⎫
13 Fourth ⎪
14 Third ⎬ costal cartilage
15 Second ⎪
16 Manubriosternal joint
17 Pulmonary ⎫
18 Aortic   ⎪
19 Mitral   ⎬ valve
20 Tricuspid ⎪

● The manubriosternal joint is palpable and a guide to identifying the second costal cartilage which joins the sternum at this level.

● The pleura and lung extend into the neck for 2.5 cm above the medial third of the clavicle.

● In the midclavicular line the lower limit of the *pleura* reaches the eighth costal cartilage, in the midaxillary line it reaches the tenth rib, and at the lateral border of the erector spinae muscle it crosses the twelfth rib. The lower border of the *lung* is about two ribs higher than the pleural reflexion.

● Behind the sternum the pleural sacs are adjacent to one another in the midline from the level of the second to fourth costal cartilages, but then diverge due to the mass of the heart on the left.

● For a radiograph of the chest and heart see page 197.

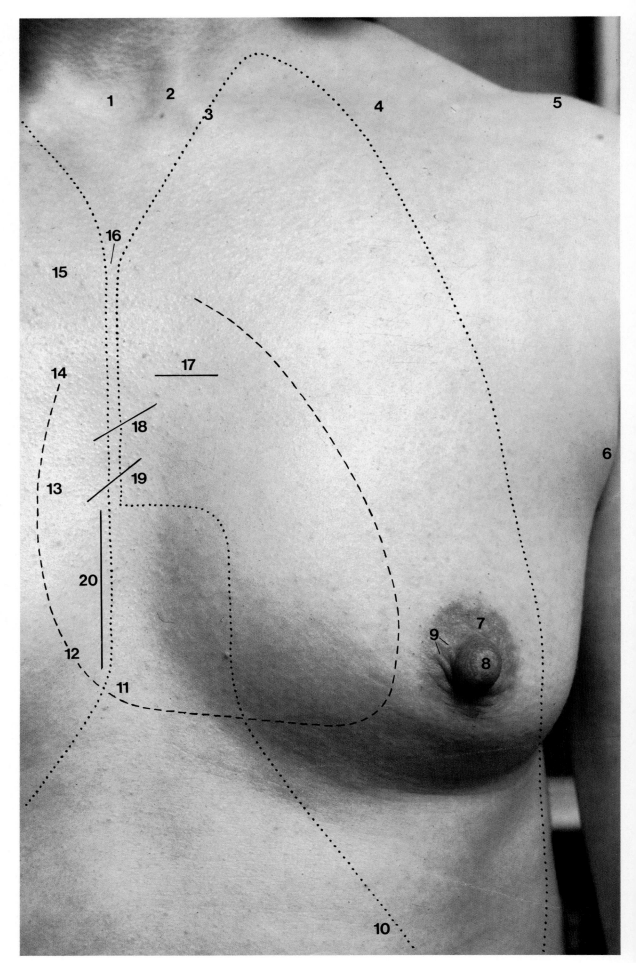

152

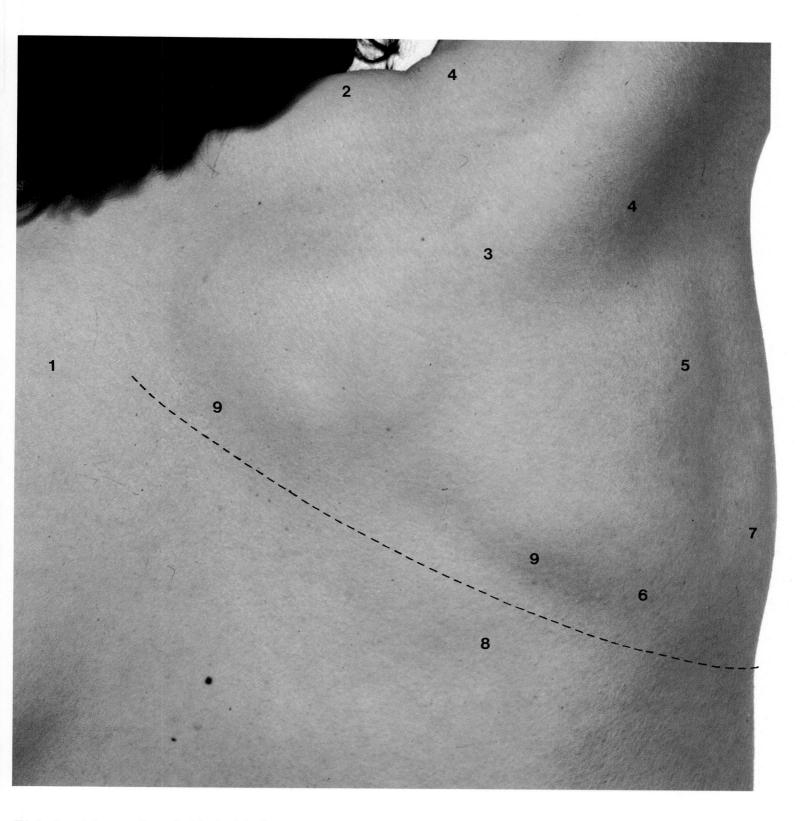

Right hemithorax, from behind with the arm abducted

Oblique fissure of the right lung (indicated by the interrupted line)

1 Spinous process of third thoracic vertebra
2 Trapezius
3 Spine of scapula
4 Deltoid
5 Teres major
6 Inferior angle of scapula
7 Latissimus dorsi

8 Fifth intercostal space
9 Medial border of scapula

● With the arm fully abducted the medial border of the scapula indicates approximately the line of the oblique fissure of the lung, which runs from the level of the spinous process of the third thoracic vertebra to the sixth costal cartilage at the lateral border of the sternum.

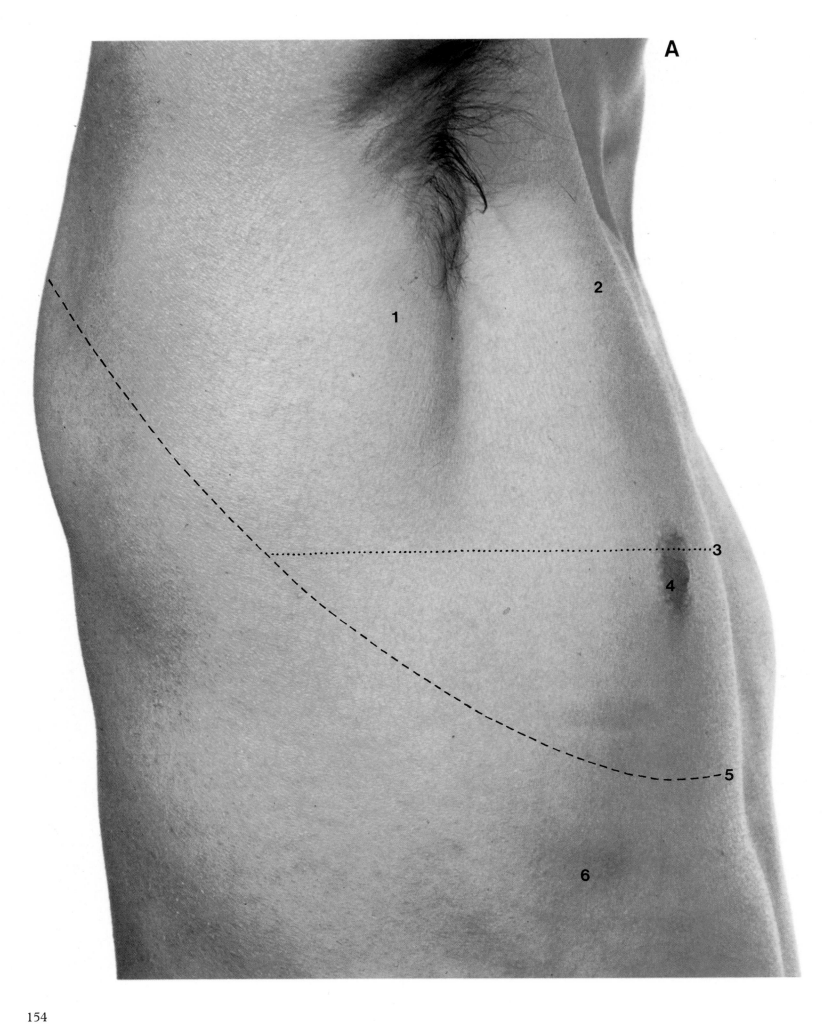

A Right hemithorax, from the right with the arm abducted
Oblique and transverse fissures of the right lung (indicated by the interrupted and dotted lines respectively)
1 Latissimus dorsi
2 Pectoralis major
3 Fourth costal cartilage
4 Nipple overlying fourth intercostal space
5 Sixth costal cartilage
6 Serratus anterior
● The transverse fissure of the right lung is represented by a line drawn horizontally backwards from the fourth costal cartilage until it meets the line of the oblique fissure. The triangle so outlined demarcates the middle lobe of the lung.

B Muscles of the thorax, left side, from the front. External and internal intercostal muscles
1 Sternal angle
2 Second costal cartilage
3 Second rib
4 External intercostal
5 Internal intercostal
6 Xiphoid process
7 Seventh ⎤
8 Eighth ⎥ costal cartilage
9 Ninth   ⎥
10 Tenth ⎦
● The external intercostal muscles are continuous anteriorly with the anterior intercostal membranes (here removed) which cover up the medial ends of the internal intercostal muscles.
● The seventh costal cartilage is the lowest to join the sternum, and together with the eighth, ninth and tenth costal cartilages forms the costal margin.

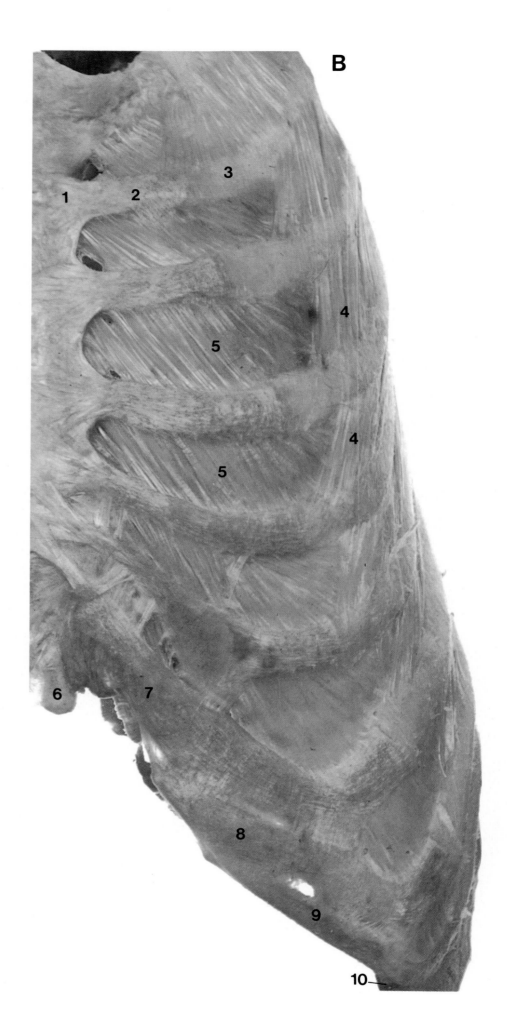

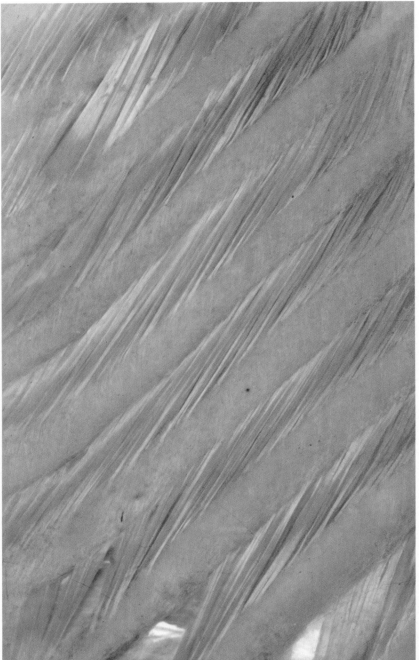

A

● The external intercostal muscles pass obliquely downwards and forwards from the rib above to the rib below.

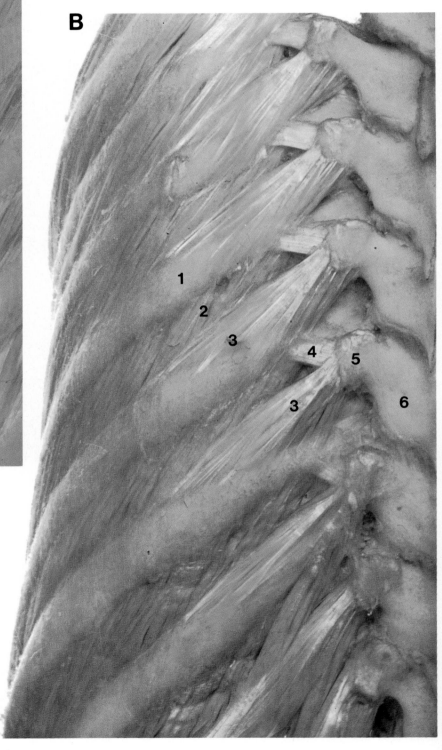

B

B Muscles of the thorax, left side, from behind. Levatores costarum muscles

1 Seventh rib
2 External intercostal
3 Levator costae
4 Lateral costotransverse ligament
5 Transverse process of eighth thoracic vertebra
6 Lamina of eighth thoracic vertebra

● The levatores costarum muscles pass from the tip of the transverse process of one vertebra to the rib below between the tubercle and angle.

● The internal intercostal muscles are continuous posteriorly with the posterior intercostal membranes which are covered up (as here) by the medial ends of the external intercostal muscles.

**Muscles of the thorax, lower
left side, from behind. Serratus
posterior inferior and related
muscles**

   1 Latissimus dorsi
   2 Tenth rib
   3 External intercostal
   4 Serratus posterior inferior
   5 Dorsal rami of lower thoracic
     and upper lumbar nerves
   6 Longissimus part of erector
     spinae
   7 Spinalis part of erector spinae
   8 Erector spinae
   9 Iliac crest
  10 Internal oblique
  11 Posterior (free) border of
     external oblique

● The medial part of the serratus
posterior *inferior* muscle (arising from the
last two thoracic and upper two lumbar
spinous processes and the supraspinous
ligament, and blending with the underlying
lumbar part of the thoracolumbar fascia) has
been removed, so displaying the medial and
intermediate parts of the erector spinae
muscle which belongs to the muscles of the
vertebral column (page 88). The lateral (iliocostalis) part of erector spinae is under cover
of the lateral part of the serratus muscle,
which becomes attached to the lower four
ribs lateral to their angles.

● The serratus posterior *superior* muscle
(not illustrated) passes to the second to fifth
ribs lateral to their angles, under cover of
the rhomboid muscles (page 112), having
arisen from the lower part of the
ligamentum nuchae and the spinous
processes of the seventh cervical and upper
two or three thoracic vertebrae and the
supraspinous ligament.

● On each side there is one serratus
anterior muscle (belonging to the group
connecting the upper limb to the trunk) and
two serratus *posterior* muscles (belonging to
the muscles of the thorax).

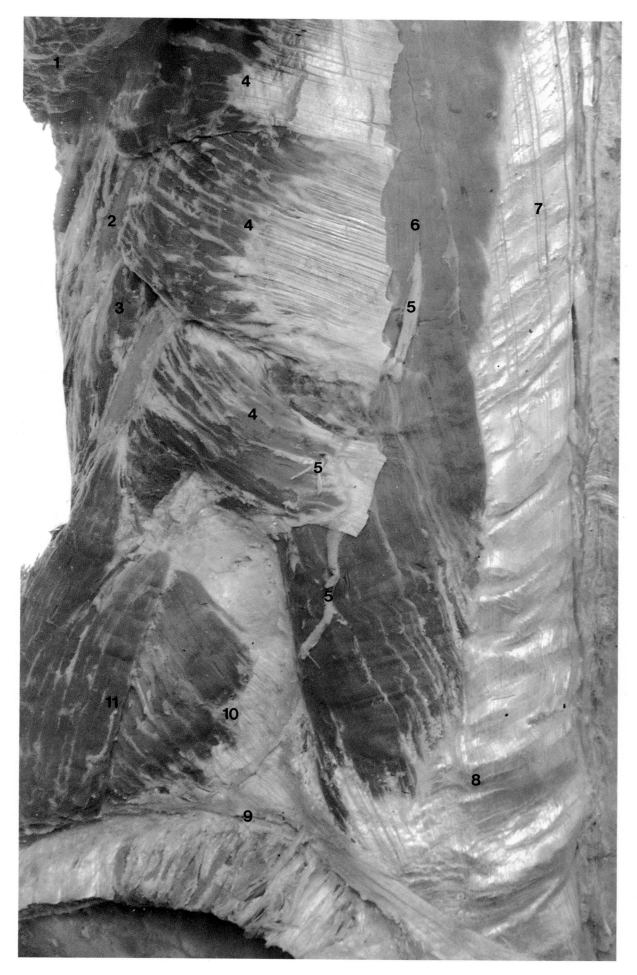

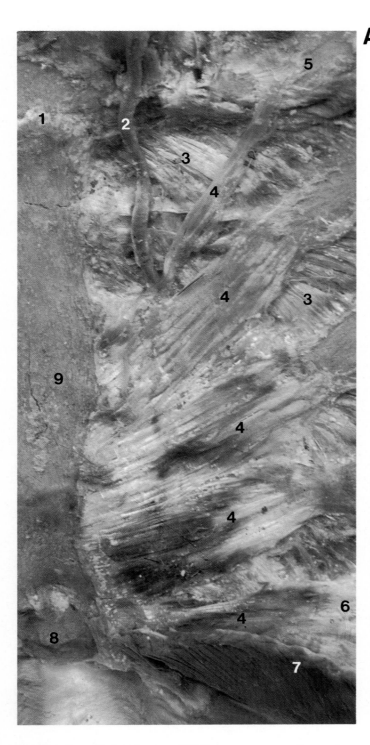

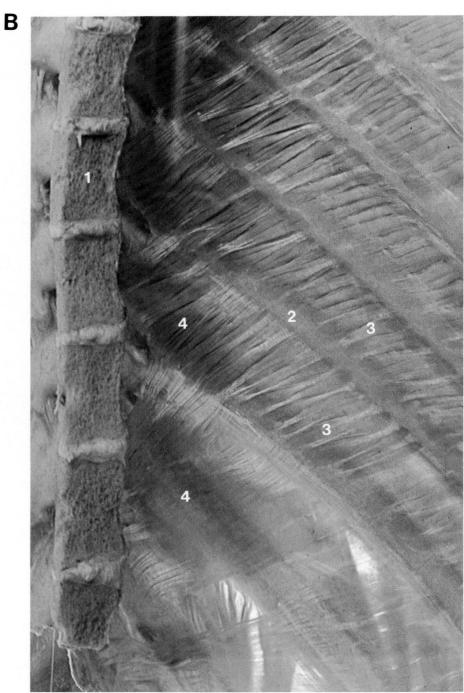

B Muscles of the thorax. Lower left subcostal and innermost intercostal muscles, from the right and the front

(Part of the vertebral column has been retained but the anterior parts of the vertebral bodies have been removed together with the pleura)

1 Eighth thoracic vertebra
2 Eighth rib
3 Innermost intercostal
4 Subcostal

● The subcostal and innermost intercostal muscles are often poorly developed especially in the upper part of the thorax. The subcostals (posteriorly) span more than one rib.

A Muscles of the thorax. Right transverse thoracic muscle (sternocostalis) on the internal surface of the anterior wall *(Pleura removed)*

1 Sternal angle
2 Internal thoracic artery
3 Internal intercostal
4 Slips of transverse thoracic muscle
5 Second rib
6 Sixth rib
7 Diaphragm
8 Xiphoid process
9 Body of sternum

● The transverse thoracic muscle is in the same plane as the innermost intercostals (laterally) and the subcostal muscles (posteriorly) and like them it separates the intercostal vessels and nerves from the pleura.

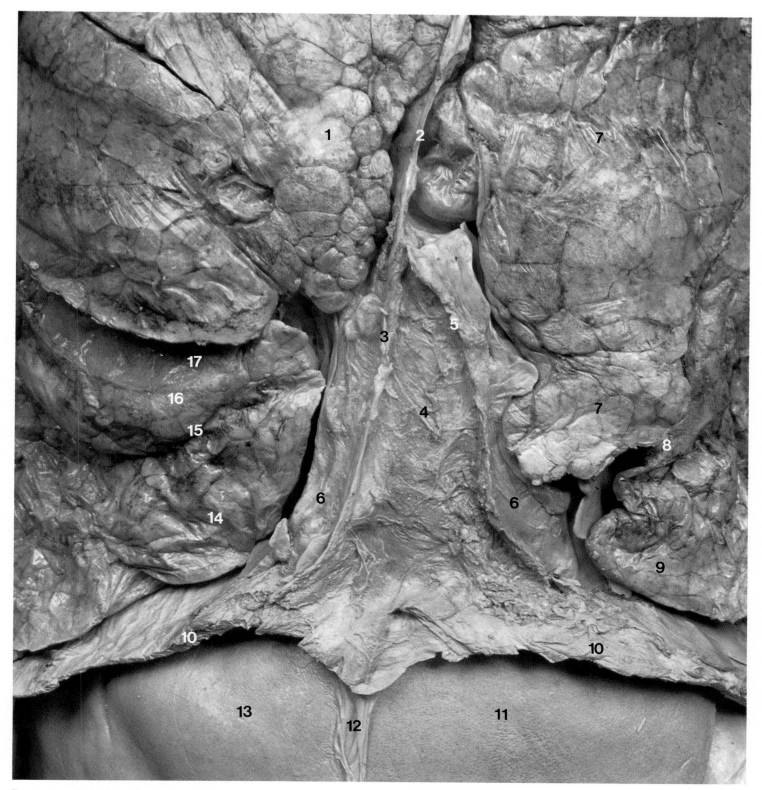

Lungs and pericardium, from the front with the anterior thoracic and abdominal walls removed

1 Superior lobe of right lung
2 Right and left parietal pleurae in contact
3 Line of reflexion of right pleura
4 Fibrous pericardium
5 Line of reflexion of left pleura
6 Pleura overlying pericardium
7 Superior lobe of left lung
8 Oblique fissure
9 Inferior lobe of left lung
10 Diaphragm
11 Left lobe of liver
12 Falciform ligament
13 Right lobe of liver
14 Inferior lobe ⎫
15 Oblique fissure ⎪
16 Middle lobe ⎬ of right lung
17 Transverse fissure ⎭

● The lungs show some degree of emphysema (balloon-like dilatation of the air sacs).
● The pleurae become separated at the level of the fourth costal cartilage due to the leftward bulge of the heart, and the central part of the fibrous pericardium is not covered by pleura.

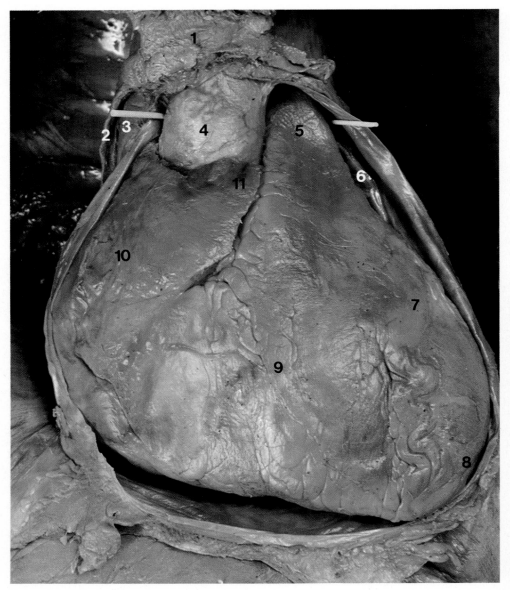

A

  1 Remains of thymus
  2 Pleura reflected from pericardium
  3 Superior vena cava
  4 Ascending aorta
  5 Pulmonary trunk
  6 Auricle of left atrium
  7 Left ventricle
  8 Apex
  9 Right ventricle
 10 Right atrium
 11 Auricle of right atrium

● The marker passes through the transverse sinus, behind the aorta and pulmonary trunk.

● The right border of the heart is formed by the right atrium, the left border by the auricle of the left atrium and the left ventricle, and the inferior border by the right ventricle with a small part of the left ventricle (at the apex).

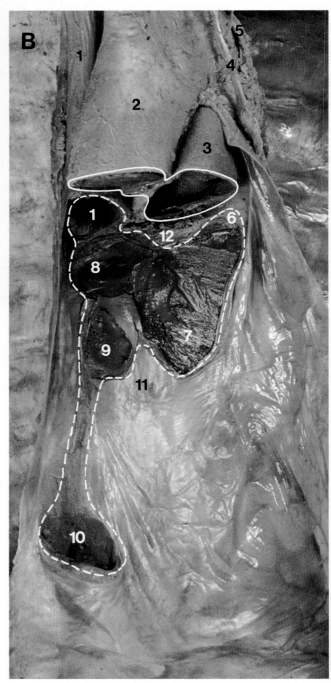

B Posterior part of the pericardium, with the heart removed

  1 Superior vena cava
  2 Arch of aorta
  3 Pulmonary trunk
  4 Left phrenic nerve
  5 Left vagus nerve
  6 Superior left ⎫
  7 Inferior left   ⎬ pulmonary veins
  8 Superior right ⎬ opening into
  9 Inferior right ⎭ left atrium
 10 Inferior vena cava
 11 Oblique sinus
 12 Transverse sinus

● The interrupted line indicates the line of reflexion between the parietal and serous pericardium that forms the upper and right boundaries of the oblique sinus.

● The continuous line indicates that the aorta and pulmonary trunk are enclosed within the same tube of serous pericardium. The space between these two great vessels (enclosed within their pericardial sleeve) and the pericardial reflexion round the pulmonary veins and superior vena cava is the transverse sinus.

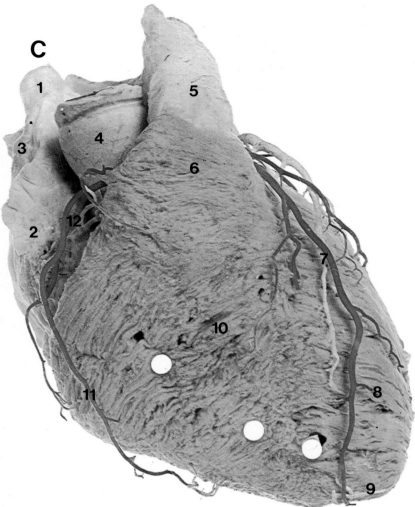

C

C The heart, sternocostal surface, with injection of major cardiac vessels

1 Superior vena cava
2 Right atrium
3 Auricle of right atrium (displaced laterally)
4 Ascending aorta
5 Pulmonary trunk
6 Infundibulum of right ventricle
7 Anterior interventricular branch of left coronary artery and great cardiac vein in interventricular groove
8 Left ventricle
9 Apex
10 Right ventricle
11 Marginal branch of right coronary artery
12 Right coronary artery in anterior atrioventricular groove

● The *sternocostal* surface is the *anterior* surface, formed mainly by the right ventricle, with parts of the left ventricle and right atrium.

● The *apex* of the heart is formed by the left ventricle.

● The infundibulum is the part of the right ventricle from which the pulmonary trunk arises.

● In this specimen the anterior atrioventricular groove has been opened up by displacing the auricle of the right atrium to show the right coronary artery more clearly. The marginal branch of this vessel has an unusually high origin.

● The *base* of the heart is the *posterior* surface, formed mainly by the left atrium with a small part of the right atrium.

● The *inferior* surface is the *diaphragmatic* surface, formed by the two ventricles (mainly the left).

● In this specimen there is a large ventricular branch of the left coronary artery passing superficial to the great cardiac vein.

D The heart from behind, with injection of major cardiac vessels

1 Left pulmonary artery
2 Superior left pulmonary vein
3 Auricle of left atrium
4 Inferior left pulmonary vein
5 Left atrium
6 Right pulmonary artery
7 Right atrium
8 Superior vena cava
9 Superior right pulmonary vein
10 Inferior right pulmonary vein
11 Inferior vena cava
12 Coronary sinus in posterior atrioventricular groove
13 Middle cardiac vein and posterior interventricular branch of right coronary artery in posterior interventricular groove
14 Right ventricle
15 Left ventricle
16 Posterior vein of left ventricle
17 Great cardiac vein and circumflex branch of left coronary artery
18 Great cardiac vein and anterior interventricular branch of left coronary artery

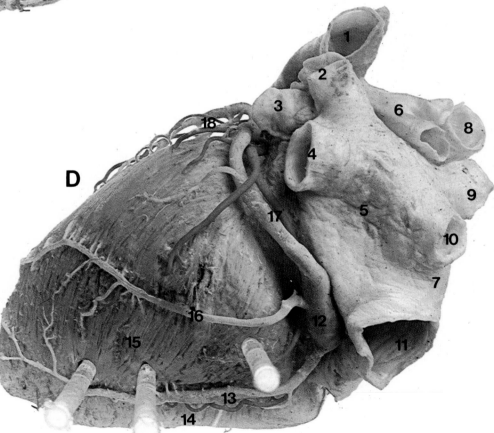

D

A

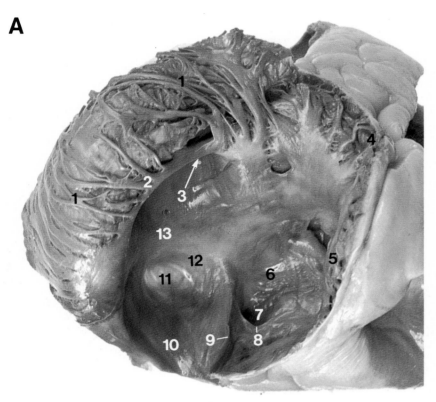

A The right atrium, from the right and the front, with the anterior wall opened and reflected to the right

1 Pectinate muscles
2 Crista terminalis
3 Superior vena cava
4 Auricle
5 Tricuspid valve
6 Position of atrioventricular node
7 Coronary sinus
8 Valve of coronary sinus
9 Valve of inferior vena cava
10 Inferior vena cava
11 Fossa ovalis
12 Limbus
13 Position of intervenous tubercle

● The fossa ovalis forms part of the interatrial septum, and the atrioventricular node is embedded within the myocardial fibres of the septum.

● The sinuatrial node (not illustrated) is horseshoe-shaped, beginning at the upper end of the crista terminalis in front of the opening of the superior vena cava, and embracing the left side of the opening. It extends through the full thickness of the myocardium, i.e. from epicardium to endocardium.

● The intervenous tubercle, which is rarely detectable in the human heart, may have served in the embryo to direct blood from the superior vena cava towards the tricuspid orifice.

B The right ventricle, from the front with most of the anterior wall removed

1 Right atrium
2 Auricle of right atrium
3 Anterior ⎤
4 Posterior ⎬ cusp of tricuspid valve
5 Septal ⎦
6 Supraventricular crest
7 Infundibulum
8 Anterior ⎤ papillary muscle
9 Posterior ⎦
10 Septomarginal trabecula
11 Chordae tendineae

● The septomarginal trabecula, which conducts the right limb of the atrioventricular bundle to the anterior papillary muscle, is sometimes called the moderator band.

● The chordae tendineae connect the valve cusps to the papillary muscles or ventricular wall. The anterior papillary muscle is large and connected with the anterior and posterior cusps; the posterior papillary muscle is small and often in two or three parts, and is connected with the posterior and septal cusps. Smaller septal papillary muscles may be present, connected with the septal and anterior cusps.

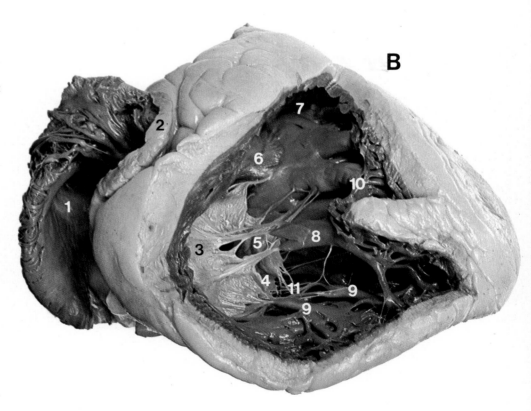

B

C The left ventricle and left atrium, opened from the left

1 Wall of left ventricle
2 Auricle of left atrium
3 Left atrium
4 Anterior cusp of mitral valve overlying posterior cusp
5 Chordae tendineae
6 Posterior ⎫
7 Anterior ⎬ papillary muscle
8 Aortic orifice

● This specimen shows a considerable amount of fat on the epicardial surface.

● The anterior and posterior papillary muscles are each connected by chordae tendineae to both cusps of the mitral valve.

● The aortic and mitral orifices are adjacent to one another, separated only by the anterior cusp of the mitral valve (see page 164).

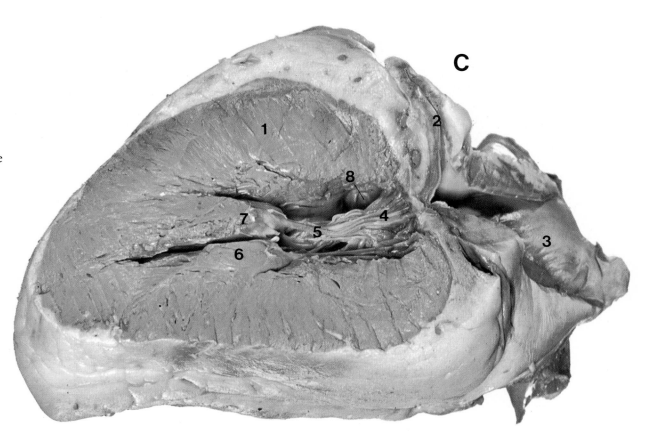

● The cusps of the aortic and pulmonary valves are here given their official names but some English texts use slightly different alternatives, as follows:

	Official	English
Aortic	Right	Anterior
	Left	Left posterior
	Posterior	Right posterior
Pulmonary	Left	Posterior
	Anterior	Left anterior
	Right	Right anterior

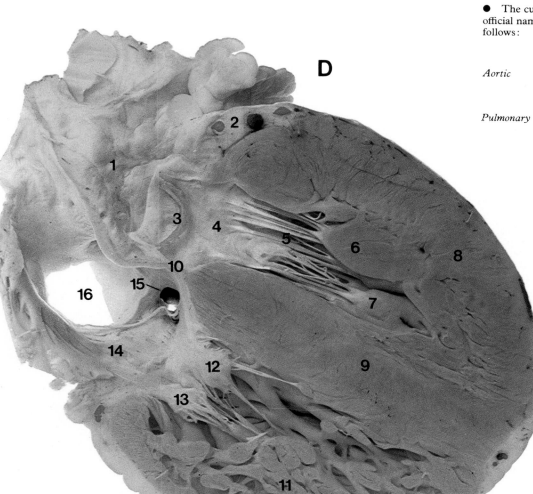

D The ventricles in section, from the front

1 Ascending aorta
2 Left coronary artery branches and great cardiac vein
3 Posterior cusp of aortic valve
4 Anterior cusp of mitral valve
5 Chordae tendineae
6 Anterior papillary muscle
7 Posterior papillary muscle
8 Left ventricular wall
9 Muscular ⎫ part of inter-
10 Membranous ⎬ ventricular septu
11 Right ventricular wall
12 Septal ⎫ cusp of
13 Posterior ⎬ tricuspid valve
14 Right atrium
15 Coronary sinus
16 Inferior vena cava

● The wall of the left ventricle is normally three times as thick as the wall of the right ventricle.

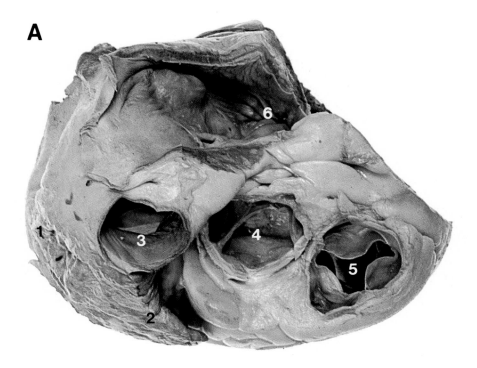

A

A The heart from above, with the great vessels and part of the left atrium and left ventricle removed
1 Right atrium
2 Auricle of right atrium
3 Superior vena cava
4 Cusps of aortic valve
5 Cusps of pulmonary valve
6 Cusps of mitral valve

B The atrioventricular orifices and fibrous rings, with the atria removed, from the right and behind

1 Left
2 Anterior } cusps of pulmonary valve
3 Right
4 Infundibulum of right ventricle
5 Right
6 Posterior } cusps of aortic valve
7 Left
8 Anterior
9 Posterior } cusps of tricuspid valve
10 Septal
11 Fibrous ring
12 Right fibrous trigone
13 Posterior
14 Anterior } cusps of mitral valve
15 Left fibrous trigone

● The fibrous rings form a figure-of-eight round the atrioventricular orifices, with extensions round the arterial orifices.
● The red marker is in the right fibrous trigone (between the aortic and the two atrio-ventricular orifices) and marks the position of the underlying atrioventricular bundle.

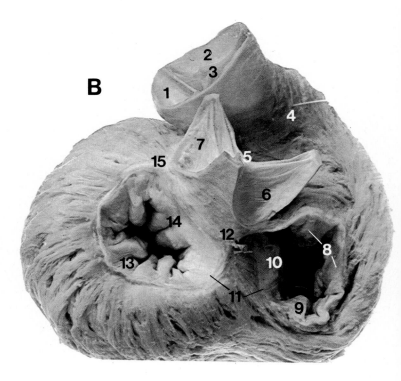

B

C Cast of the cardiac vessels, from the front
1 Ascending aorta
2 Pulmonary trunk and sinuses above pulmonary valve cusps
3 Anterior interventricular branch of left coronary artery and great cardiac vein
4 Vessels of interventricular septum
5 Middle cardiac vein and posterior interventricular branch of right coronary artery
6 Marginal branch of right coronary artery and small cardiac vein
7 Coronary sinus
8 Right coronary artery
9 Anterior cardiac vein

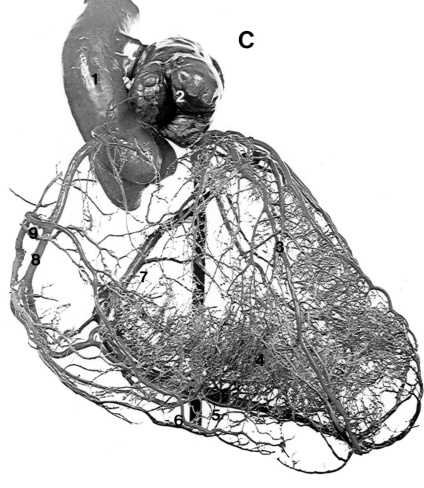

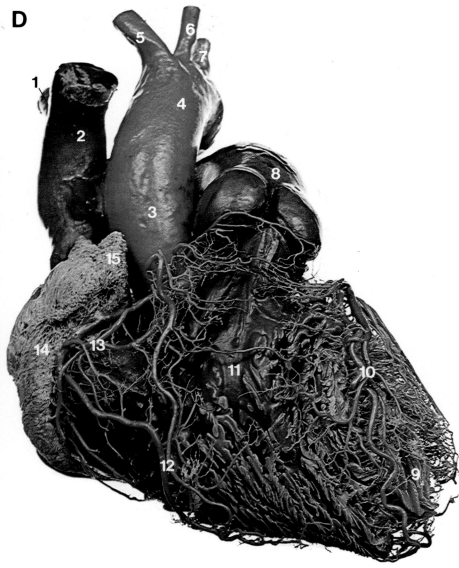

D Cast of the heart and great vessels, from the front
1 Azygos vein
2 Superior vena cava
3 Ascending aorta
4 Arch of aorta
5 Brachiocephalic trunk
6 Left common carotid artery
7 Left subclavian artery
8 Pulmonary trunk
9 Left ventricle
10 Anterior interventricular branch of left coronary artery and great cardiac vein
11 Right ventricle
12 Marginal branch of right coronary artery and small cardiac vein
13 Right coronary artery and anterior cardiac vein
14 Right atrium
15 Auricle of right atrium
● For a view of this specimen from behind see page 169.
● Like the veins of the brain, the veins of the heart do not have names that correspond to those of the arteries. The great cardiac vein accompanies the anterior interventricular and circumflex branches of the left coronary artery; the middle cardiac vein accompanies the posterior interventricular branch of the right coronary artery; and the small cardiac vein accompanies the marginal branch of the right coronary artery. These veins normally drain into the coronary sinus (see page 171). The anterior cardiac veins drain directly into the right atrium.

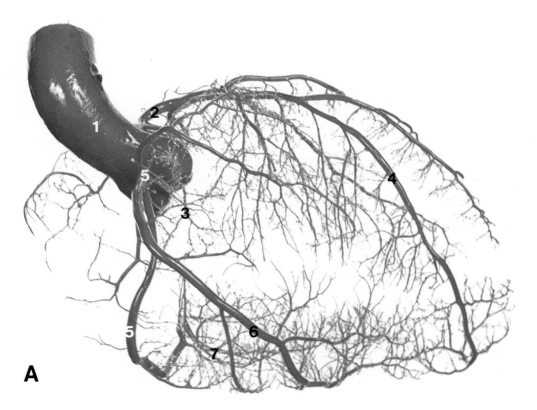

A Cast of the coronary arteries, from the front
1 Ascending aorta
2 Left coronary artery
3 Circumflex ⎤ branch of left
4 Anterior interventricular ⎦ coronary artery
5 Right coronary artery
6 Marginal ⎤ branch of right
7 Posterior interventricular ⎦ coronary artery
● Each coronary artery gives off two main branches – the circumflex and anterior interventricular from the left, the marginal and posterior interventricular from the right.

A

B Cast of the heart and vessels, from the front and above with the pulmonary trunk removed
1 Superior vena cava
2 Left atrium
3 Left pulmonary veins
4 Auricle of left atrium
5 Left coronary artery
6 Left (posterior) aortic sinus
7 Circumflex branch
8 Anterior interventricular branch
9 Great cardiac vein
10 Left ventricle
11 Right ventricle
12 Marginal branch of right coronary artery and small cardiac vein
13 Right coronary artery
14 Anterior aortic sinus
15 Ascending aorta
16 Auricle of right atrium
● The origin of the right coronary artery (from the anterior aortic sinus) is easily seen when dissecting the heart from the front, but the origin of the left coronary artery (from the left posterior aortic sinus) is hidden behind the pulmonary trunk (page 168).

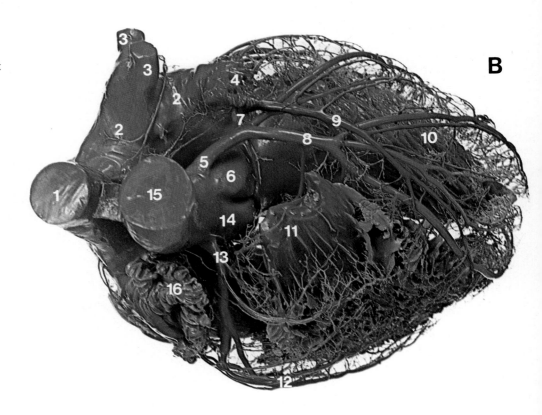

B

C Cast of the coronary arteries, from above. Origin of the sinuatrial nodal artery from the right coronary artery

1 Ascending aorta
2 Left coronary artery
3 Circumflex branch
4 Anterior interventricular branch
5 Right coronary artery
6 Sinuatrial nodal artery
7 Marginal branch
8 Posterior interventricular branch

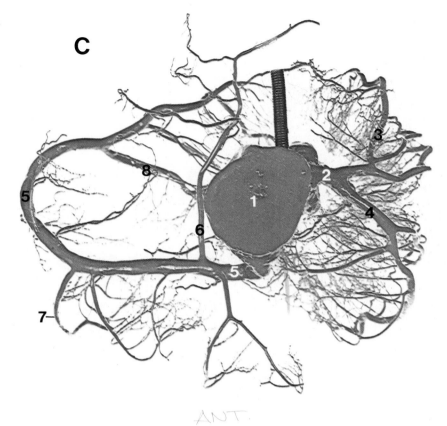

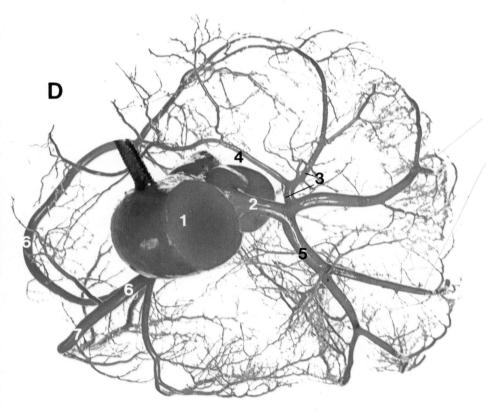

D Cast of the coronary arteries, from above. Origin of the sinuatrial nodal artery from the left coronary artery

1 Ascending aorta
2 Left coronary artery
3 Circumflex branch
4 Sinuatrial nodal artery
5 Anterior interventricular branch
6 Right coronary artery
7 Marginal branch

● In 55% of hearts the sinuatrial nodal artery arises from the right coronary artery. In 45% it arises from the circumflex branch of the left coronary artery.

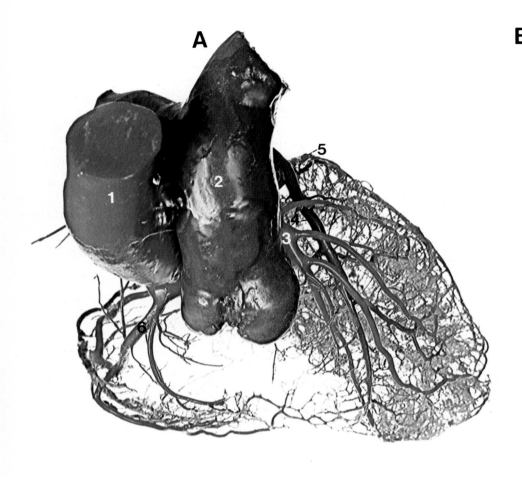

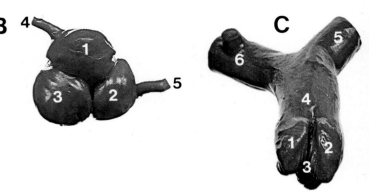

A Cast of the heart and vessels, from above
1 Ascending aorta
2 Pulmonary trunk
3 Anterior interventricular branch of left coronary artery
4 Great cardiac vein
5 Circumflex branch of left coronary artery
6 Right coronary artery

● The origin of the left coronary artery is obscured behind the pulmonary trunk (see page 166).

B Cast of the ascending aorta, from below
1 Right ⎫
2 Left ⎬ part of aortic sinus
3 Posterior ⎭
4 Right coronary artery
5 Left coronary artery

● The right coronary artery arises from the anterior aortic sinus, the left coronary from the left (posterior) sinus.

C Cast of the pulmonary trunk, from the front and above
1 Right ⎫
2 Anterior ⎬ part of pulmonary sinus
3 Left ⎭
4 Pulmonary trunk
5 Left pulmonary artery
6 Right pulmonary artery and branch to superior lobe of right lung

● There is no such thing as *the* pulmonary artery; the pulmonary *trunk* divides into *right* and *left* pulmonary arteries.

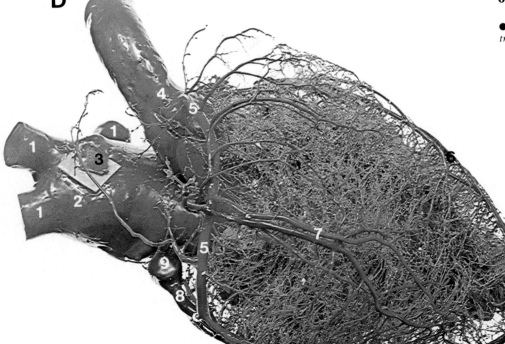

D Cast of the heart and vessels, from the front and the right, with the right atrium removed
1 Pulmonary veins
2 Left atrium
3 See note below
4 Ascending aorta
5 Right coronary artery
6 Anterior interventricular branch of left coronary artery and great cardiac vein
7 Marginal branch of right coronary artery and small cardiac vein
8 Middle cardiac vein
9 Opening of coronary sinus into right atrium

● The white marker lies behind resin that has passed from the left atrium into the right atrium through a patent foramen ovale.
● The small cardiac vein frequently drains directly into the right atrium (as in this specimen) and not into the coronary sinus.

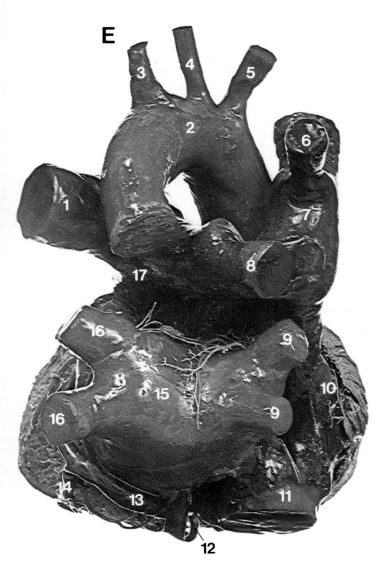

E

E Cast of the heart and great vessels, from behind
1 Left pulmonary artery
2 Arch of aorta
3 Left subclavian artery
4 Left common carotid artery
5 Brachiocephalic trunk
6 Azygos vein
7 Superior vena cava
8 Right pulmonary artery
9 Right pulmonary veins
10 Right atrium
11 Inferior vena cava
12 Middle cardiac vein
13 Coronary sinus
14 Posterior vein of left ventricle
15 Left atrium
16 Left pulmonary veins
17 Pulmonary trunk

● The *base* of the heart is its *posterior* surface, formed by the left atrium.
● For a view of this specimen from the front see page 165.

F Cast of the heart and vessels, from the left, below and behind
1 Pulmonary trunk
2 Left coronary artery
3 Ascending aorta
4 Superior vena cava
5 Right pulmonary veins
6 Right atrium
7 Inferior vena cava
8 Posterior interventricular branch of right coronary artery
9 Middle cardiac vein
10 Coronary sinus
11 Left ventricle
12 Posterior vein of left ventricle
13 Great cardiac vein
14 Circumflex branch of left coronary artery
15 Oblique vein of left atrium
16 Left atrium
17 Left pulmonary veins
18 Auricle of left atrium

● The coronary sinus which receives most of the venous blood from the heart (see page 171) lies in the posterior part of the atrioventricular groove between the left atrium and the left ventricle, and opens into the right atrium (page 162).

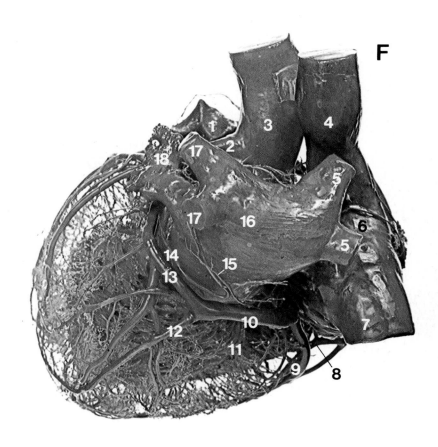

F

169

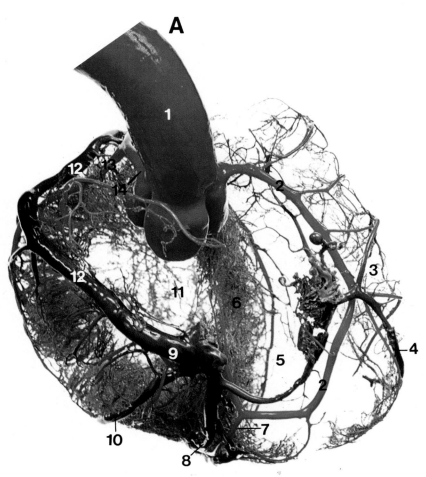

A Cast of cardiac vessels, from the right and behind. Interventricular septum

1 Ascending aorta
2 Right coronary artery
3 Anterior cardiac vein
4 Small cardiac vein entering right atrium
5 Right ventricle
6 Vessels of interventricular septum
7 Posterior interventricular branch of right coronary artery
8 Middle cardiac vein
9 Coronary sinus
10 Posterior vein of left ventricle
11 Left ventricle
12 Great cardiac vein
13 Circumflex branch of left coronary artery
14 Left coronary artery

● The position of the muscular interventricular septum is indicated by the deeply penetrating branches of the anterior and posterior interventricular arteries and their accompanying veins.

B Cast of the heart and vessels, from the right and behind. Interventricular septum

1 Pulmonary veins
2 Left atrium
3 Auricle of left atrium
4 Ascending aorta
5 Right coronary artery
6 Marginal branch and small cardiac vein
7 A large atrial branch
8 Vessels of interventricular septum
9 Posterior interventricular branch and middle cardiac vein
10 Coronary sinus
● For another view of this specimen see page 168.

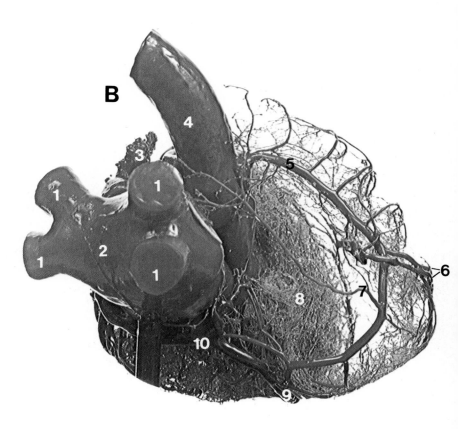

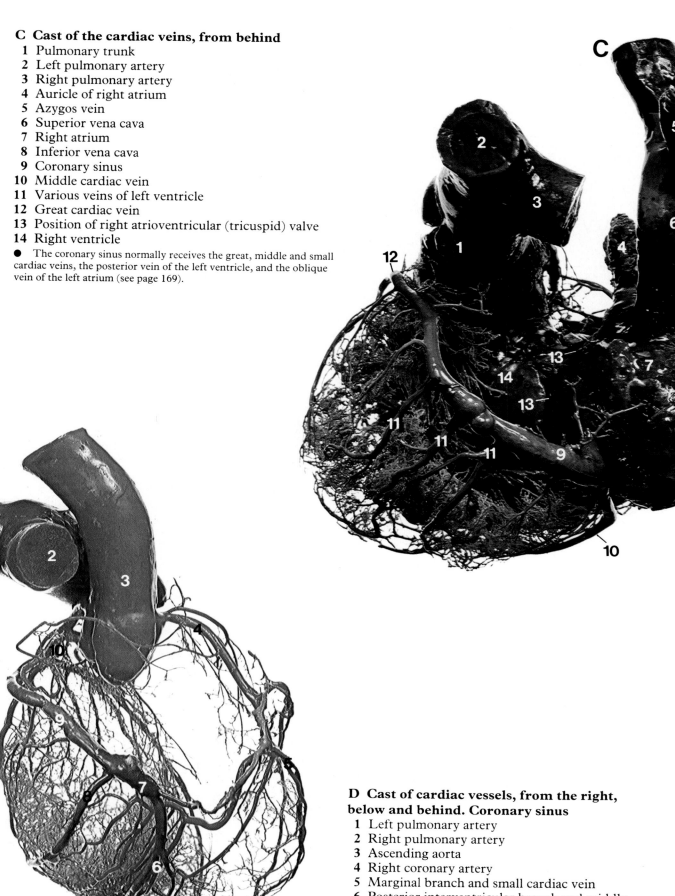

C Cast of the cardiac veins, from behind
1 Pulmonary trunk
2 Left pulmonary artery
3 Right pulmonary artery
4 Auricle of right atrium
5 Azygos vein
6 Superior vena cava
7 Right atrium
8 Inferior vena cava
9 Coronary sinus
10 Middle cardiac vein
11 Various veins of left ventricle
12 Great cardiac vein
13 Position of right atrioventricular (tricuspid) valve
14 Right ventricle
● The coronary sinus normally receives the great, middle and small cardiac veins, the posterior vein of the left ventricle, and the oblique vein of the left atrium (see page 169).

D Cast of cardiac vessels, from the right, below and behind. Coronary sinus
1 Left pulmonary artery
2 Right pulmonary artery
3 Ascending aorta
4 Right coronary artery
5 Marginal branch and small cardiac vein
6 Posterior interventricular branch and middle cardiac vein
7 Coronary sinus
8 Posterior vein of left ventricle
9 Great cardiac vein
10 Circumflex branch of left coronary artery

171

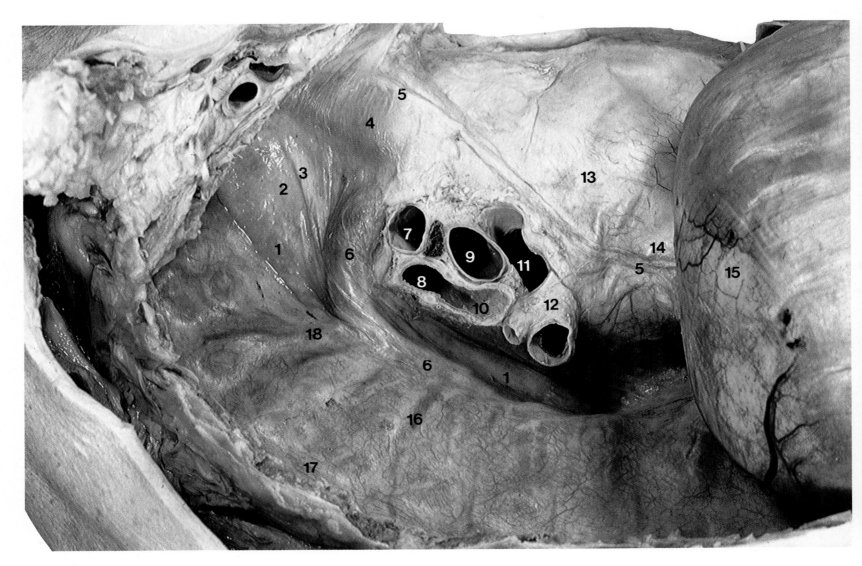

Right lung root and mediastinal pleura

1 Oesophagus
2 Trachea
3 Right vagus nerve
4 Superior vena cava
5 Right phrenic nerve and pericardiacophrenic vessels
6 Azygos vein
7 Branch of right pulmonary artery to superior lobe
8 Superior lobe bronchus
9 Right pulmonary artery
10 Right principal bronchus
11 Superior right pulmonary vein
12 Inferior right pulmonary vein
13 Mediastinal pleura and pericardium overlying right atrium
14 Inferior vena cava
15 Diaphragm
16 Posterior intercostal vessels under parietal pleura
17 Sympathetic trunk
18 Right superior intercostal vein

● The right vagus nerve passes obliquely downwards and backwards across the trachea which is covered by mediastinal pleura.
● The right phrenic nerve passes downwards under cover of the mediastinal pleura and overlying the superior vena cava, right atrium and pericardium, and inferior vena cava.
● The pleura on the right is in close contact with the trachea, but on the left the subclavian and common carotid arteries intervene.

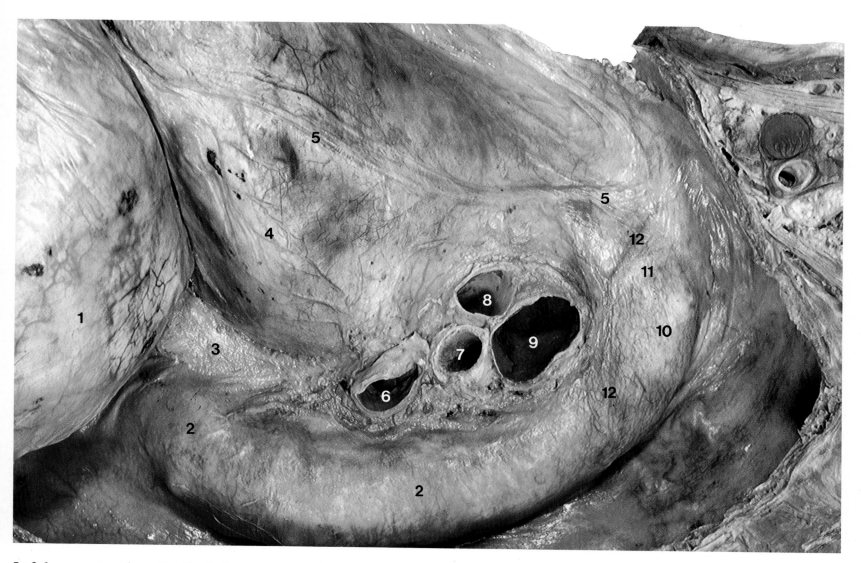

Left lung root and mediastinal pleura

1 Diaphragm
2 Thoracic aorta
3 Oesophagus
4 Mediastinal pleura and pericardium overlying left ventricle
5 Left phrenic nerve and pericardiacophrenic vessels
6 Left inferior pulmonary vein
7 Left principal bronchus
8 Left superior pulmonary vein
9 Left pulmonary artery
10 Arch of aorta
11 Left vagus nerve
12 Left superior intercostal vein

● The left vagus and phrenic nerves pass downwards over the arch of the aorta, the phrenic in front of the vagus.
● The left superior intercostal vein crosses the upper part of the aortic arch, and passes superficial to the vagus but deep to the phrenic nerve.
● In both lung roots the order of the main structures is: vein, artery, bronchus from before backwards, with the inferior pulmonary vein being the lowest structure (see page 184). Other structures in the lung roots are the bronchial vessels, lymph nodes and vessels and autonomic nerves.
● On the left side above the diaphragm, the oesophagus lies in a triangle bounded by the diaphragm, heart and aorta.

The medial surface of the upper part of the right lung.
Impressions of adjacent structures
1 Groove for first rib
2 Groove for subclavian vein
3 Groove for subclavian artery
4 Oesophageal and tracheal area
5 Groove for azygos vein
6 Groove for superior vena cava
7 Right pulmonary veins
8 Branches of right pulmonary artery
9 Branches of right principal bronchus

The medial surface of the upper part of the left lung.
Impressions of adjacent structures
1 Groove for aorta
2 Groove for left subclavian artery
3 Groove for left subclavian and brachiocephalic vein
4 Groove for first rib
5 Left pulmonary veins
6 Branches of left principal bronchus
7 Branches of left pulmonary artery

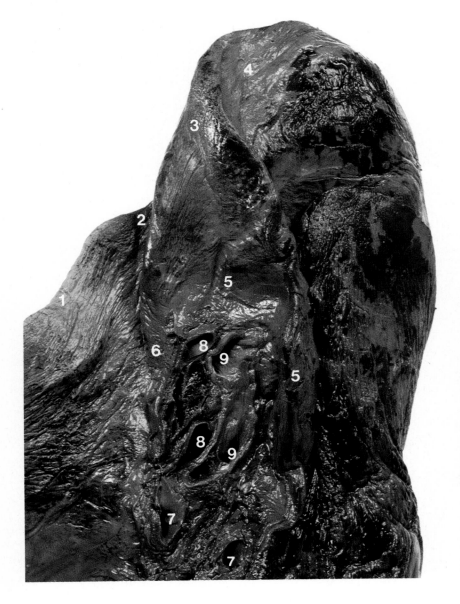

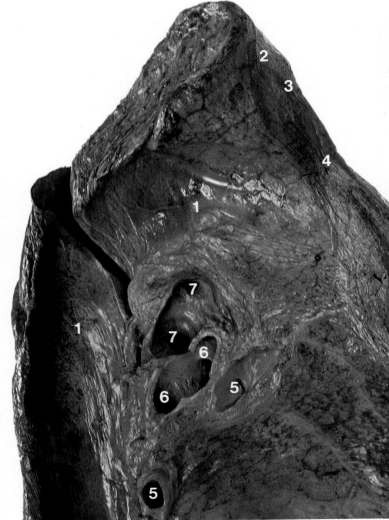

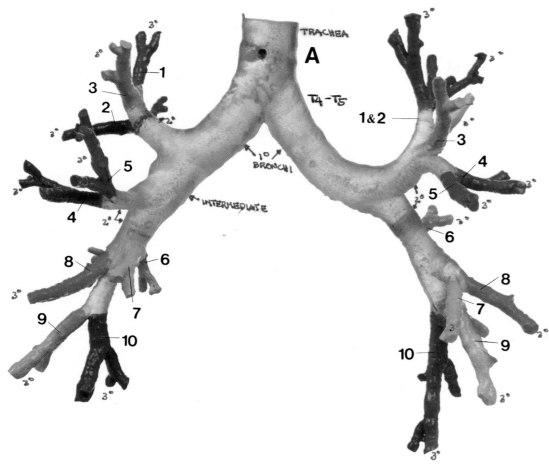

- The trachea divides into right and left principal bronchi. (T4–T5)
- The right principal bronchus is shorter, wider and more vertical than the left.
- The left principal bronchus is longer and narrower and lies more transversely than the right. Foreign bodies are therefore more likely to enter the right principal bronchus than the left.
- The right principal bronchus gives off a superior lobe bronchus and then enters the hilum of the right lung before dividing into middle and inferior lobe bronchi.
- The left principal bronchus enters the hilum of the lung before dividing into superior and inferior lobe bronchi.
- The branches of the lobar bronchi are called segmental bronchi and each supplies a segment of lung tissue – bronchopulmonary segment. The segmental bronchi and the bronchopulmonary segments have similar names, and the ten segments of each lung are officially numbered (as on pages 176–183) as well as being named. The bronchi here have been numbered to conform with those of the segments.
- The lobar bronchi of the left and right lungs are essentially similar except that (a) the apical and posterior bronchi of the superior lobe of the left lung arise from a common stem, thus called the apicoposterior bronchus and labelled here as 1 and 2; (b) there is no middle lobe in the left lung – the superior and inferior lingular bronchi of its superior lobe correspond to the lateral and medial bronchi of the middle lobe of the right lung, and so the corresponding segments bear similar numbers; and (c) the medial basal bronchus of the left lung usually arises in common with the anterior basal (but in the specimen illustrated it arises from the lateral basal bronchus).
- The apical (superior) bronchus of the inferior lobe (6) of both lungs is the first or highest bronchus to arise from the *posterior* surface of the bronchial tree. When lying on the back fluid may therefore be aspirated into this bronchus.

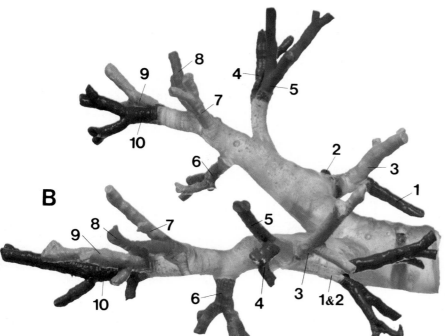

Right lung
Superior lobe
1 Apical
2 Posterior
3 Anterior

Middle lobe
4 Lateral
5 Medial

Inferior lobe
 6 Apical (superior)
 7 Medial basal
 8 Anterior basal
 9 Lateral basal
10 Posterior basal

Left lung
Superior lobe
1 & 2 Apicoposterior
3 Anterior
4 Superior lingular
5 Inferior lingular

Inferior lobe
 6 Apical (superior)
 7 Medial basal (cardiac)
 8 Anterior basal
 9 Lateral basal
10 Posterior basal

Cast of the lower trachea, principal bronchi and lobar bronchi, A from the front, B from the left as with the subject lying down (*a slightly anterior oblique view, with the right side higher than the left*)

Cast of the bronchial tree, from the front, with bronchopulmonary segments named and numbered

Right lung

Superior lobe
1 Apical
2 Posterior
3 Anterior

Middle lobe
4 Lateral
5 Medial

Inferior lobe
 6 Apical (superior)
 7 Medial basal
 8 Anterior basal
 9 Lateral basal
10 Posterior basal

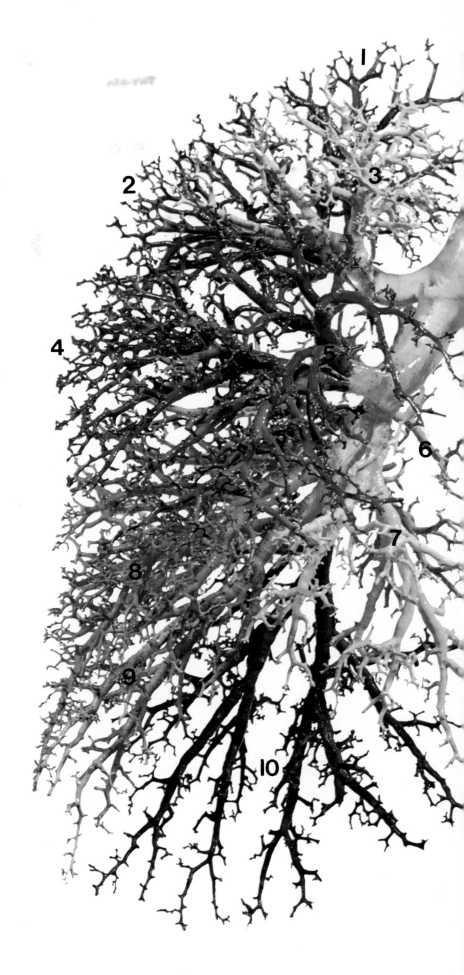

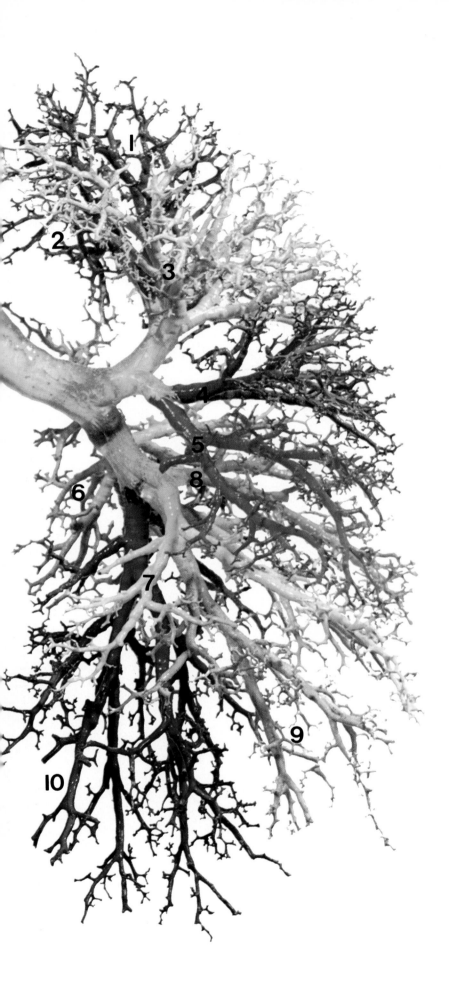

Left lung

Superior lobe
1 Apical
2 Posterior
3 Anterior
4 Superior lingular
5 Inferior lingular

Inferior lobe
 6 Apical (superior)
 7 Medial basal (cardiac)
 8 Anterior basal
 9 Lateral basal
10 Posterior basal

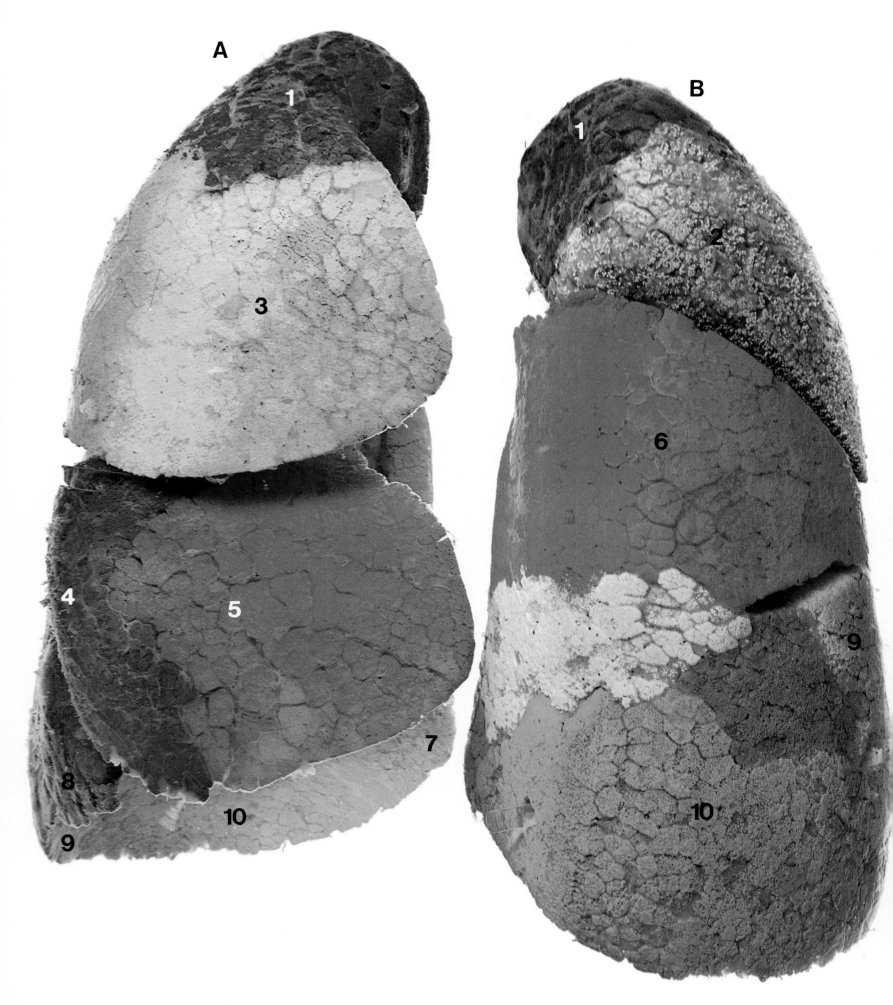

Bronchopulmonary segments of the right lung, A from the front, B from behind, C from the medial side

Superior lobe
1 Apical
2 Posterior
3 Anterior

Middle lobe
4 Lateral
5 Medial

Inferior lobe
 6 Apical (superior)
 7 Medial basal
 8 Anterior basal
 9 Lateral basal
10 Posterior basal

● A subapical (subsuperior) lobar bronchus and bronchopulmonary segment are present in over 50% of lungs; in this specimen this additional segment is shown in white.

● The posterior basal segment (10) is coloured with two different shades of green.

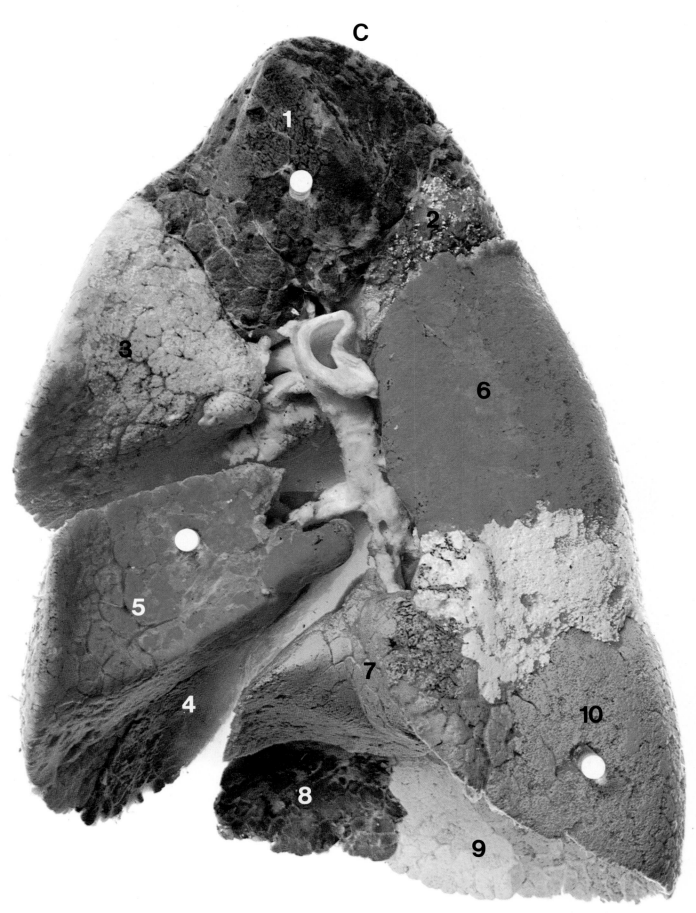

179

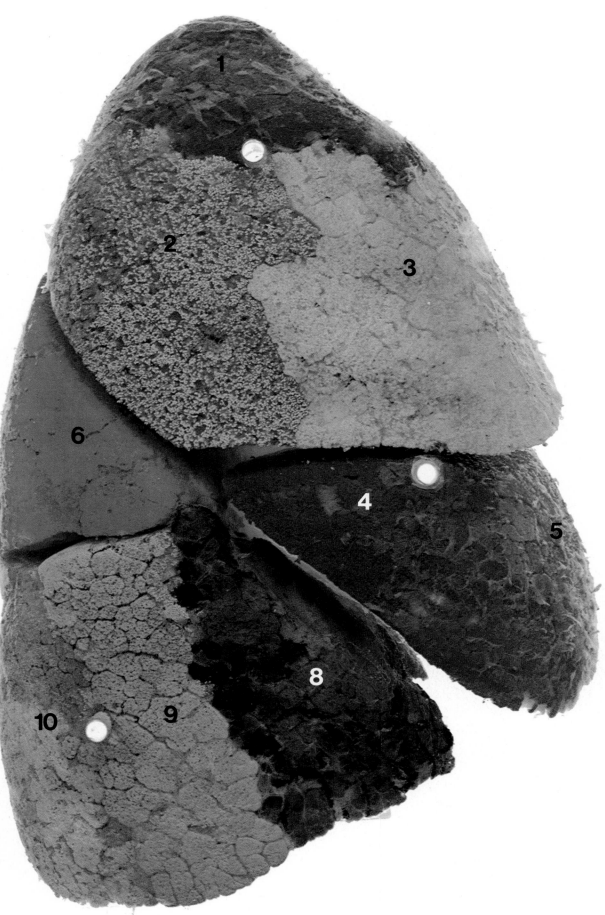

Bronchopulmonary segments of the right lung, costal surface

Superior lobe
1 Apical
2 Posterior
3 Anterior

Middle lobe
4 Lateral
5 Medial

Inferior lobe
6 Apical (superior)
7 Medial basal
8 Anterior basal
9 Lateral basal
10 Posterior basal

● The medial basal segment (7) is not seen in this view.
● The posterior basal segment (10) is coloured with two different shades of green.

Bronchopulmonary segments of the left lung, costal surface

Superior lobe
1 Apical
2 Posterior
3 Anterior
4 Superior lingular
5 Inferior lingular

Inferior lobe
 6 Apical (superior)
 7 Medial basal (cardiac)
 8 Anterior basal
 9 Lateral basal
10 Posterior basal

● The apical and posterior segments (1 & 2) are both coloured green, having been filled from the common apicoposterior bronchus (see page 175).

● The medial basal segment (7) is not seen in this view.

● See note on page 179 for the white segment.

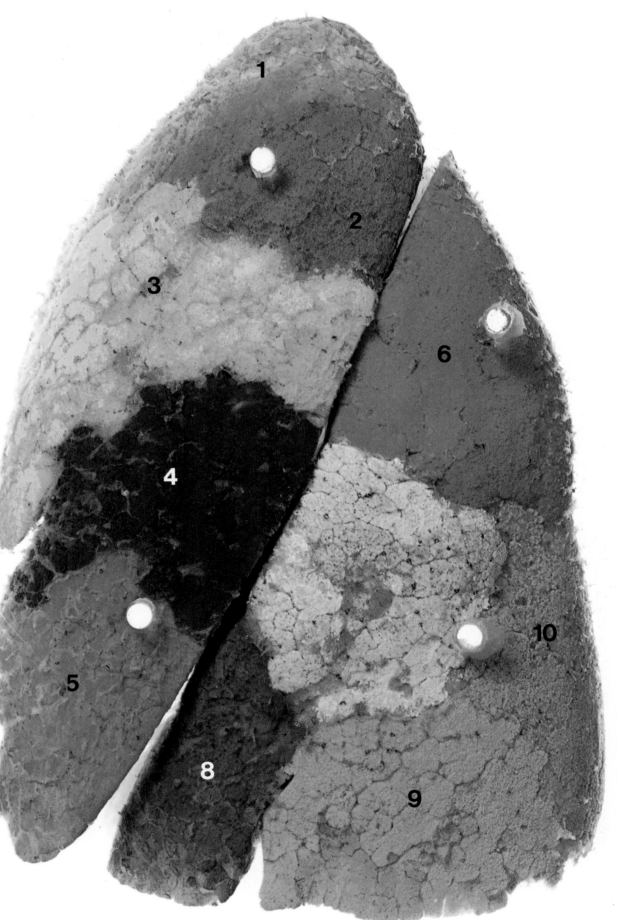

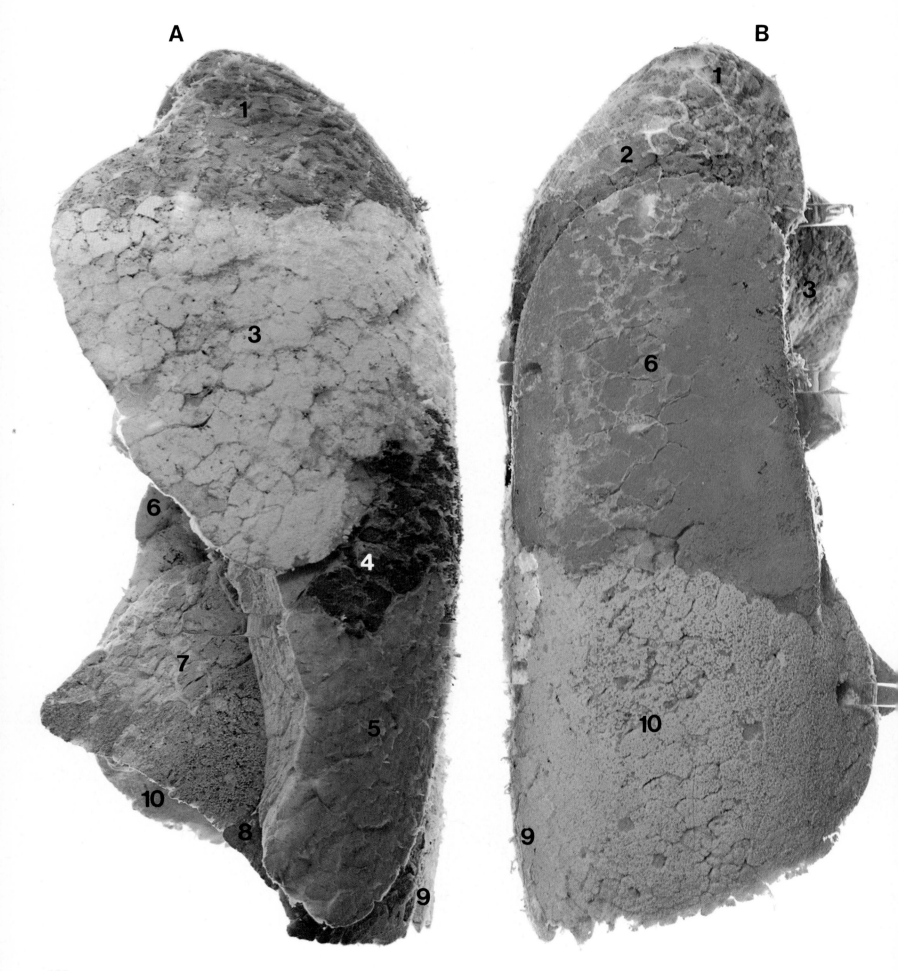

Bronchopulmonary segments of the left lung, A from the front, B from behind, C from the medial side

Superior lobe
1 Apical
2 Posterior
3 Anterior
4 Superior lingular
5 Inferior lingular

Inferior lobe
6 Apical (superior)
7 Medial basal (cardiac)
8 Anterior basal
9 Lateral basal
10 Posterior basal

● The apical and posterior segments (1 & 2) are both coloured green, having been filled from the common apicoposterior bronchus (see page 175).

● See note on page 179 for the white segment in B.

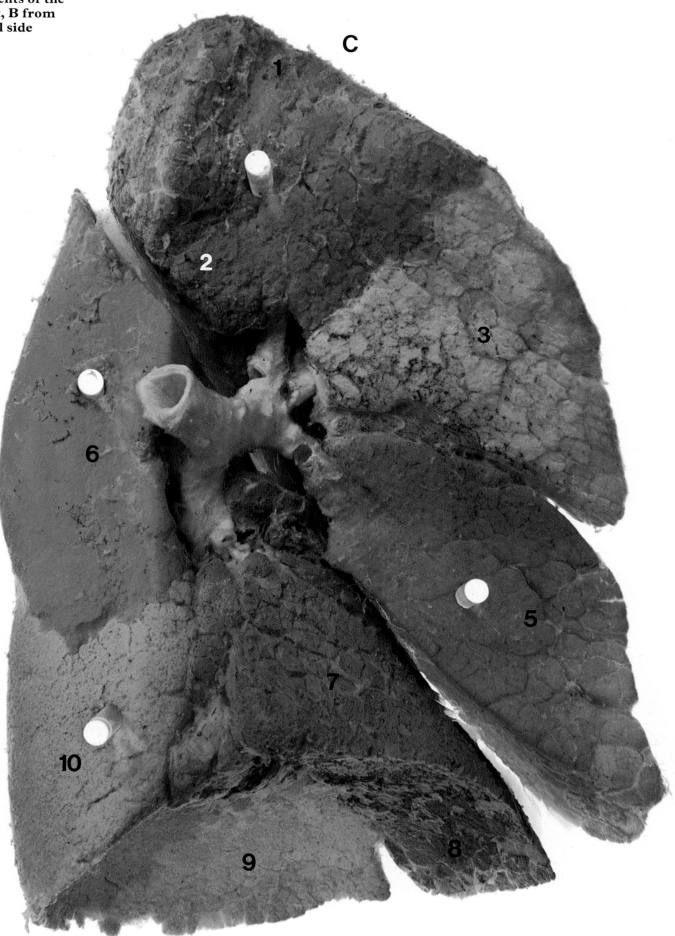

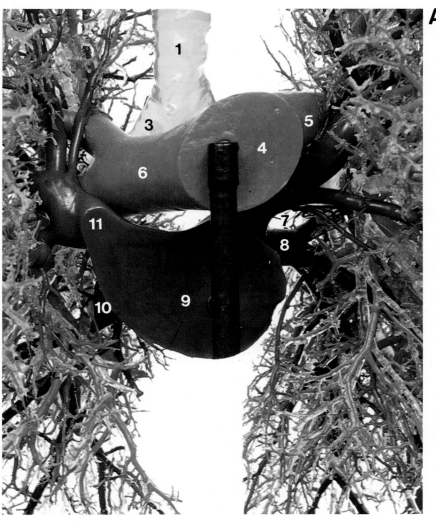

A

**Cast of the bronchi and pulmonary vessels, A
from the front, B from behind, C from the
right and behind**

1 Trachea
2 Left ⎫
3 Right ⎬ principal bronchus
4 Pulmonary trunk
5 Left ⎫
6 Right ⎬ pulmonary artery
7 Superior ⎫
8 Inferior ⎬ left pulmonary vein
9 Left atrium
10 Inferior ⎫
11 Superior ⎬ right pulmonary vein

● The order of the main structures entering the hilum of the
lung at the lung root is: vein, artery, bronchus from before
backwards, as in A (see pages 172 and 173).
● The lowest structure in the lung root is the inferior
pulmonary vein, as in B.
● The right pulmonary artery passes to the right immediately
below the bifurcation of the trachea, as in C.

B

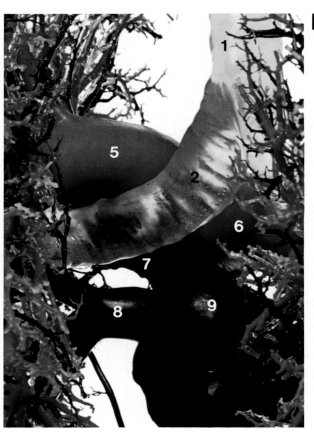

C

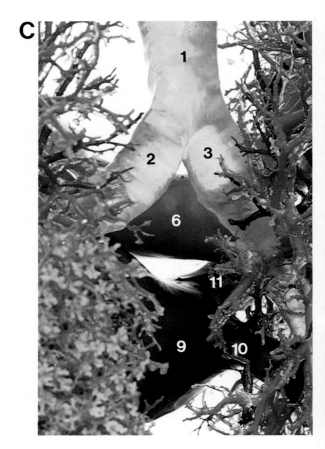

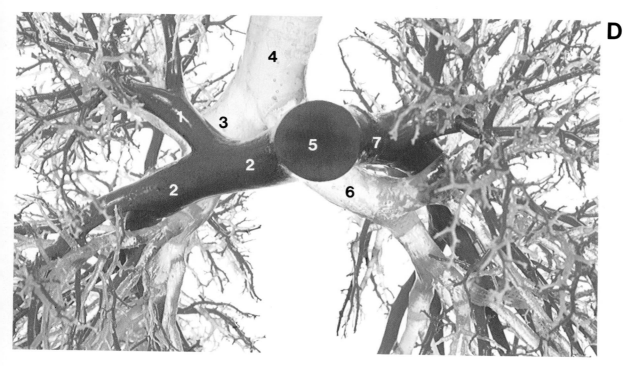

D Cast of the pulmonary arteries and bronchi, from the front

1 Branch of right pulmonary artery to
   superior lobe
2 Right pulmonary artery
3 Right principal bronchus
4 Trachea
5 Pulmonary trunk
6 Left principal bronchus
7 Left pulmonary artery

● The pulmonary trunk bifurcates in front of the left
principal bronchus.

● The left pulmonary artery hooks over the left
principal bronchus and descends behind the lobar
bronchi.

● The right pulmonary artery passes below the
bifurcation of the trachea and hooks over the right
principal bronchus but its branch to the superior lobe
remains in front of the superior lobe bronchus.

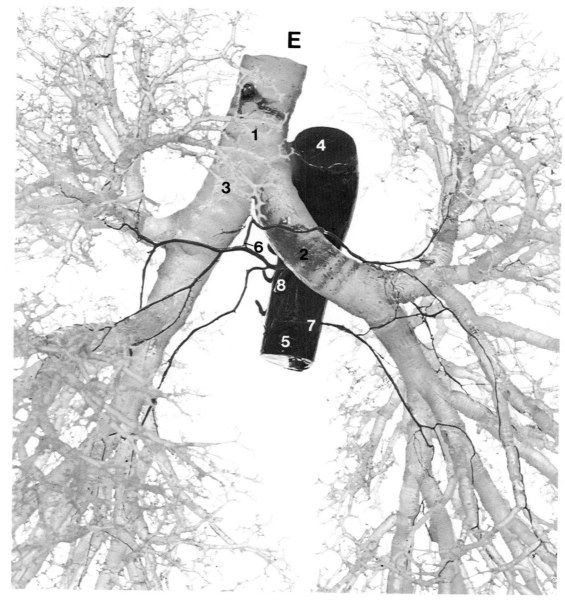

E Cast of the bronchi and bronchial arteries, from the front

1 Trachea
2 Left ⎫
3 Right ⎬ principal bronchus
4 Arch of aorta
5 Thoracic aorta
6 Origin of upper left bronchial artery
7 Origin of lower left bronchial artery
8 Origin of right bronchial artery

● There are usually two left bronchial arteries (from
the aorta) and one right artery (from the right third
posterior intercostal or upper left bronchial artery). This
specimen is unusual in that the upper left artery arises
from the right bronchial artery.

● The bronchial arteries normally lie behind the
bronchi, not in front as in this specimen.

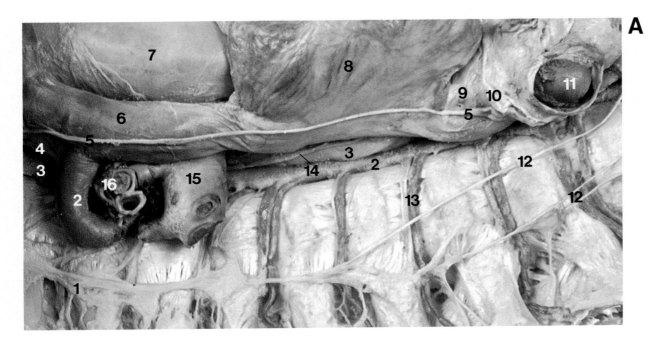

A

A The mediastinum from the right, with the pleura and diaphragm removed

1 Sympathetic trunk and ganglia
2 Azygos vein
3 Oesophagus
4 Trachea
5 Right phrenic nerve
6 Superior vena cava
7 Ascending aorta
8 Right atrium
9 Inferior vena cava
10 Cut edge of diaphragm
11 Right hepatic vein
12 Splanchnic nerves
13 Posterior intercostal vessels
14 Part of oesophageal plexus
15 Right pulmonary artery
16 Right principal bronchus

● For detail of the trachea above the azygos vein, see B.
● For a similar specimen before removal of the mediastinal pleura, see page 172.

B Superior vena cava and trachea, from the right

1 Oesophagus
2 Trachea
3 Right vagus nerve
4 Cardiac branches of vagus nerve
5 Superior vena cava
6 Right phrenic nerve
7 Arch of aorta
8 Second right costal cartilage
9 Right atrium
10 Branches of right pulmonary artery
11 Right bronchial artery
12 Superior lobe bronchus
13 Azygos vein

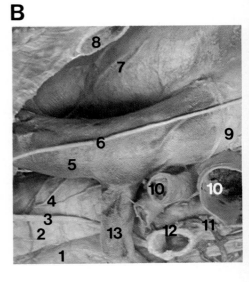

B

The arch of the aorta and associated structures, from the left

(The specimen has been removed from the thorax but the sternum has been retained)

1 Ascending aorta
2 Arch of aorta
3 Brachiocephalic trunk
4 Left common carotid artery
5 Left phrenic nerve
6 Left vagus nerve
7 Lower cervical cardiac branch of vagus nerve
8 Left subclavian artery
9 Cardiac branch of left superior cervical ganglion
10 Trachea
11 Upper cervical cardiac branch (double) of left vagus
12 Left recurrent laryngeal nerve
13 Oesophagus
14 Ligamentum arteriosum
15 Left pulmonary artery
16 Pulmonary trunk
17 Pulmonary vein
18 Branches of left principal bronchus
19 Descending (thoracic) aorta
20 Pericardium overlying left ventricle
21 Pericardium overlying right ventricle

● For a similar specimen before removal of the mediastinal pleura, see page 173.
● The sympathetic and vagal branches that cross the arch of the aorta between the phrenic nerve (in front) and the vagus form the superficial part of the cardiac plexus, situated to the right of the ligamentum arteriosum.
● The deep part of the cardiac plexus, situated in front of the bifurcation of the trachea, is formed by the cardiac branches from cervical sympathetic ganglia and from the vagus and recurrent laryngeal nerves.

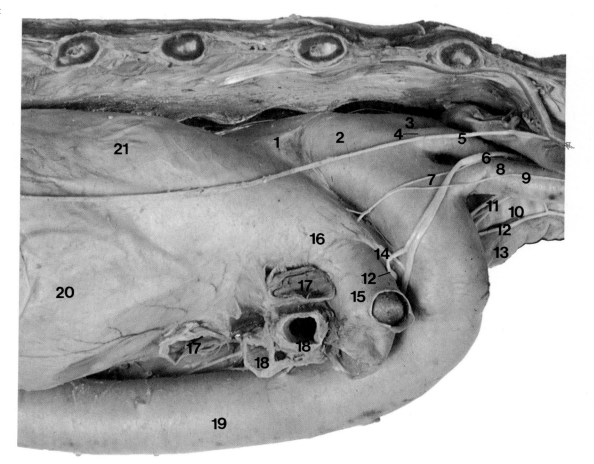

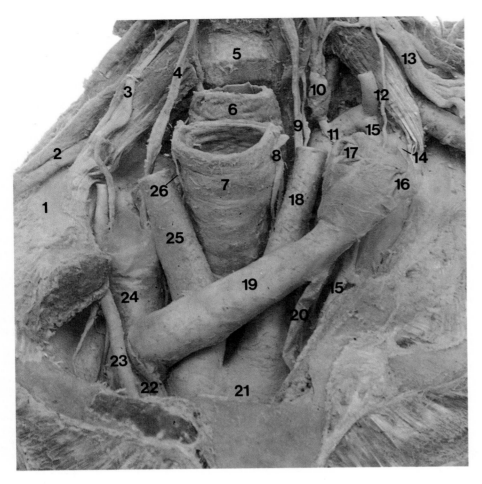

The thoracic inlet, after removal of the manubrium and first right costal cartilage

1 First rib
2 Lowest roots of brachial plexus
3 Right phrenic nerve and scalenus anterior
4 Right vagus nerve
5 Cervical vertebral column
6 Oesophagus
7 Trachea
8 Left recurrent laryngeal nerve
9 Left vagus nerve
10 Middle cervical sympathetic ganglion
11 Ansa subclavia and left subclavian artery
12 Left thyrocervical trunk, phrenic nerve and scalenus anterior
13 Upper trunk of brachial plexus (displaced downwards)
14 Apex of lung
15 Left internal thoracic artery
16 Left subclavian vein
17 Left internal jugular vein
18 Left common carotid artery
19 Left brachiocephalic vein
20 Left internal thoracic vein
21 Arch of aorta
22 Superior vena cava
23 Right internal thoracic artery
24 Right brachiocephalic vein
25 Brachiocephalic trunk
26 Right recurrent laryngeal nerve

Thoracic inlet, upper thorax and neck, from the front

(With the sternum, clavicles and costal cartilages and their attached muscles removed)

1 Subclavian artery
2 Scalenus anterior
3 Suprascapular artery
4 Superficial cervical artery
5 Phrenic nerve
6 Vagus nerve
7 Internal thoracic artery
8 Ansa subclavia
9 Apex of lung
10 Lateral lobe of thyroid gland
11 Superior thyroid artery
12 Common carotid artery
13 External carotid artery
14 Hyoid bone
15 Laryngeal prominence
16 Thyrohyoid
17 Cricothyroid
18 Arch of cricoid cartilage
19 Isthmus of thyroid gland
20 Trachea
21 Thyroidea ima artery
22 Recurrent laryngeal nerve
23 Brachiocephalic trunk
24 Left brachiocephalic vein
25 Right brachiocephalic vein
26 Superior vena cava
27 Internal thoracic vein
28 Fifth ⎤ cervical
29 Sixth ⎟ nerve
30 Seventh ⎟ ventral
31 Eighth ⎦ ramus
32 First rib
33 Cervicothoracic (stellate) ganglion
34 Upper trunk of brachial plexus
35 Suprascapular nerve

● Further details of the neck in this specimen have been given on page 39.

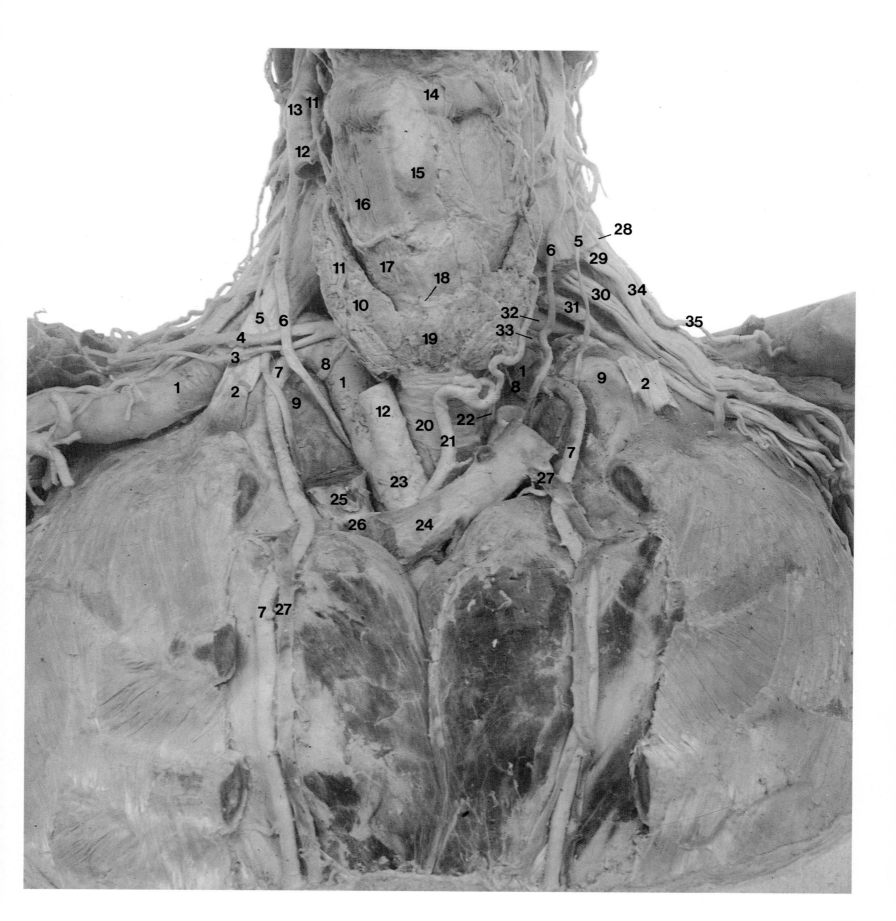

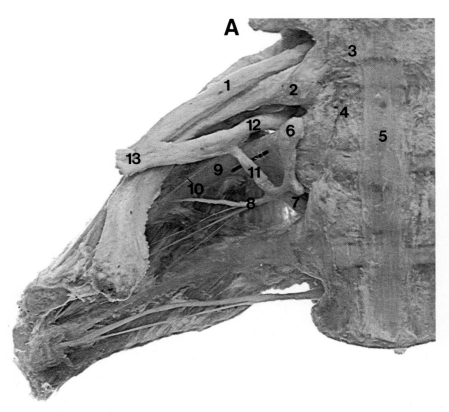

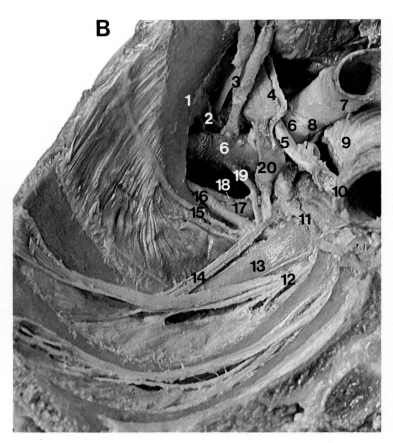

A Right first and second ribs. Nerve relations
1 Ventral ramus of eighth cervical nerve
2 Head of first rib
3 Seventh cervical vertebra
4 First thoracic vertebra
5 Anterior longitudinal ligament
6 Sympathetic trunk and ganglion
7 Ventral ramus of second thoracic nerve
8 Second intercostal nerve
9 Second rib
10 First intercostal nerve
11 Communication with first thoracic nerve
12 Ventral ramus of first thoracic nerve
13 Lower trunk of brachial plexus

● In this specimen the second thoracic nerve makes a large contribution (in front of the red marker) to the brachial plexus.

B Relations of the right cervical pleura, from below
1 First rib
2 Subclavian vein
3 Internal thoracic vessels
4 Brachiocephalic vein
5 Vagus nerve
6 Subclavian artery
7 Brachiocephalic trunk
8 Recurrent laryngeal nerve
9 Trachea
10 Right principal bronchus
11 Sympathetic trunk
12 Second intercostal nerve
13 Second rib
14 Superior intercostal vein
15 First intercostal nerve
16 Ventral ramus of first thoracic nerve
17 Neck of first rib
18 Ventral ramus of eighth cervical nerve
19 Superior intercostal artery
20 Vertebral vein

● The neck of the first rib is in contact with (in order from medial to lateral): the sympathetic trunk, the supreme intercostal vein (not seen in this specimen), the superior intercostal artery and the contribution of the first thoracic nerve to the brachial plexus.

C The thoracic duct, from the right after removal of thoracic and abdominal viscera and most of the diaphragm and pleura
1 Sympathetic trunk underlying pleura
2 Azygos vein
3 Thoracic duct
4 Thoracic aorta
5 Right crus of diaphragm
6 Coeliac trunk
7 Superior mesenteric artery
8 Right renal artery
9 Abdominal aorta
10 Cisterna chyli
11 Greater splanchnic nerve
12 Medial arcuate ligament
13 Psoas major
14 Diaphragm
15 First lumbar artery and first lumbar vertebra
16 Twelfth thoracic vertebra and subcostal artery

C

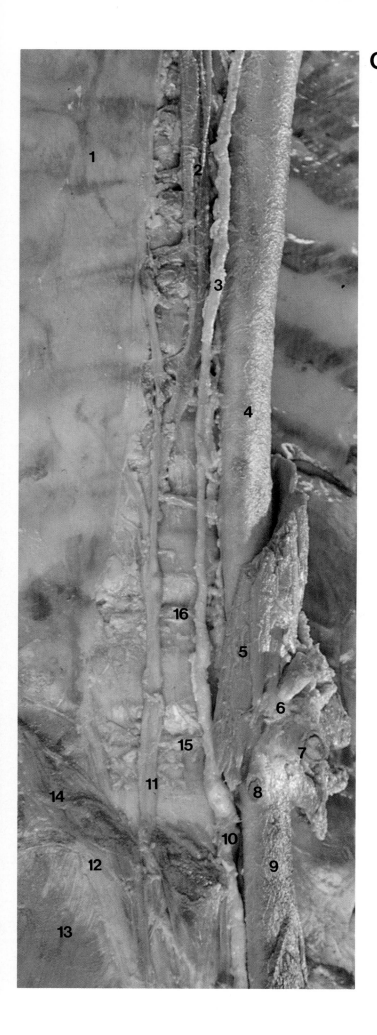

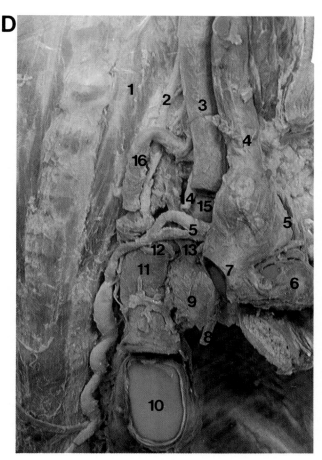

D Termination of the thoracic duct. Deep dissection of the thoracic inlet on the left, from the front

1 Longus colli
2 Sympathetic trunk
3 Common carotid artery
4 Internal jugular vein
5 Thoracic duct
6 Subclavian vein
7 Brachiocephalic vein
8 Phrenic nerve
9 Pleura
10 Arch of aorta
11 Subclavian artery
12 Ansa subclavia
13 Internal thoracic artery
14 Vagus nerve
15 Origin of vertebral artery
16 Inferior thyroid artery

● From the cisterna chyli, situated under cover of the left margin of the right crus of the diaphragm at the level of the first and second lumbar vertebrae, the thoracic duct passes upwards (through the aortic opening in the diaphragm) on the right side of the front of the thoracic vertebral column, crossing to the left at the level of the fifth thoracic vertebra and ending by opening into the left side of the union of the left internal jugular and subclavian veins after passing between the common carotid artery (in front) and the vertebral artery (behind).

The diaphragm, from above, removed from the body with the adjacent part of the trunk

1 Costodiaphragmatic recess
2 Central tendon
3 Vertebral column
4 Position of right phrenic nerve
5 Foramen for inferior vena cava
6 Thoracic aorta passing into aortic opening
7 Oesophageal opening
8 Cut edge of fibrous pericardium
9 Position of left phrenic nerve
10 Costomediastinal recess

● In this specimen the aorta is unusually large and the three principal openings in the diaphragm appear to be at approximately the same level, but in most subjects the aortic opening is in the midline at the level of the twelfth thoracic vertebra, the oesophageal opening to the left of the midline at the level of the tenth thoracic vertebra, and the foramen for the vena cava in the central tendon to the right of the midline at the level of the disc between the eighth and ninth thoracic vertebrae.

● The central tendon of the diaphragm has the shape of a trefoil leaf and has no bony attachment.

● The right phrenic nerve passes through the vena caval foramen of the central tendon, with a few filaments piercing the tendon immediately to the right of the foramen.

● The left phrenic nerve pierces the muscular part of the diaphragm in front of the central tendon just lateral to the overlying pericardium.

● The phrenic nerves are *the only motor* nerves to the diaphragm; the supply from the lower intercostal nerves is purely afferent.

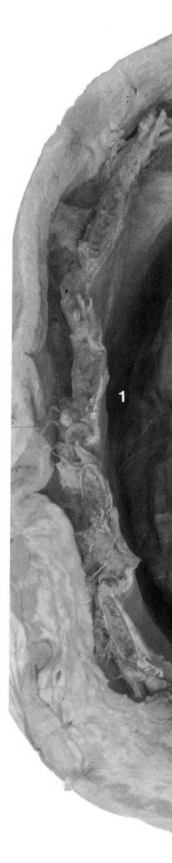

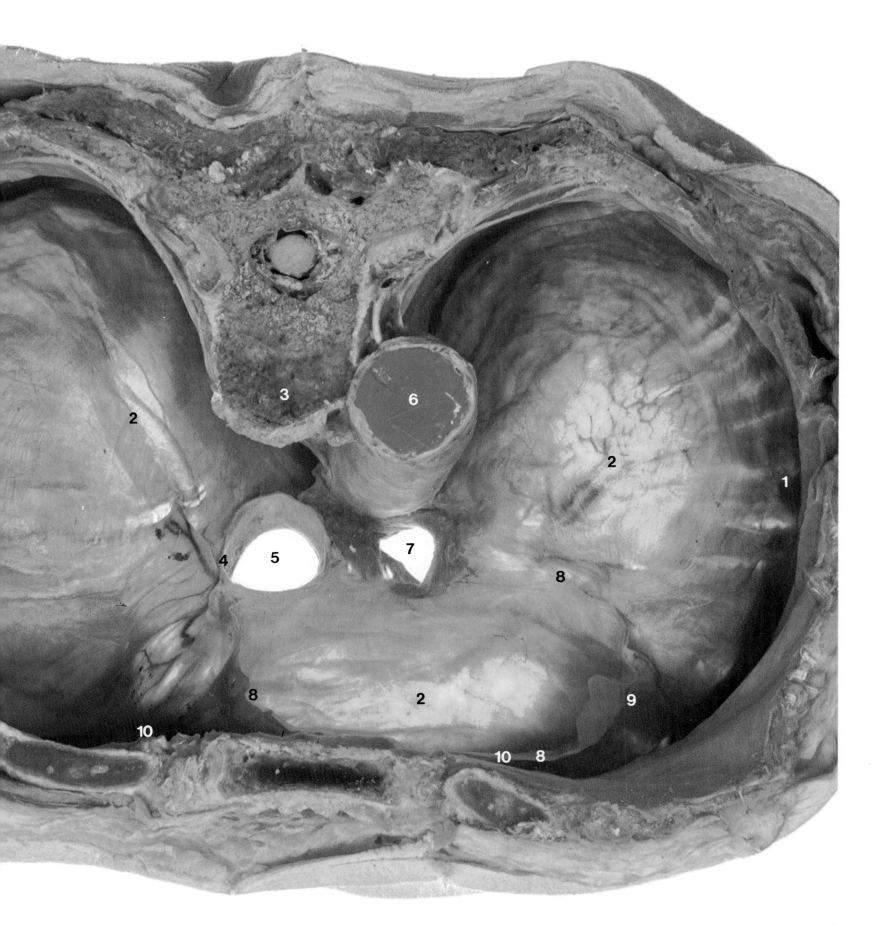

The oesophagus and thoracic aorta, from behind

1 Left subclavian artery
2 Upper cervical cardiac branches of left vagus nerve
3 Left phrenic nerve
4 Left common carotid artery
5 Left recurrent laryngeal nerve
6 Oesophagus
7 Right subclavian artery and ansa subclavia
8 Right recurrent laryngeal nerve
9 Right brachiocephalic vein
10 Superior vena cava
11 Right phrenic nerve
12 Right internal thoracic vessels
13 Azygos vein
14 Third right posterior intercostal artery
15 Right bronchial artery
16 Right vagus nerve
17 Right principal bronchus
18 Right inferior pulmonary vein
19 Oesophageal plexus (right and left vagus nerves)
20 Right atrium
21 Inferior vena cava
22 Thoracic aorta and origins of left posterior intercostal arteries
23 Left inferior pulmonary vein
24 Left principal bronchus
25 Left superior pulmonary vein
26 Left pulmonary artery
27 Arch of aorta

● After forming the oesophageal plexus, the vagi become reconstituted as the anterior and posterior vagal trunks which enter the abdomen with the oesophagus on its anterior and posterior surfaces respectively (page 240). The anterior vagal trunk consists mainly of fibres from the left vagus nerve, the posterior trunk being formed mainly by the right vagus, but there is some mixture of fibres in each trunk.

Intercostal spaces with vessels and nerves, on the right adjacent to the vertebral column, from the front with the pleura removed

1 Subcostal muscle
2 Eighth rib
3 Eighth posterior intercostal vein
4 Eighth posterior intercostal artery
5 Eighth intercostal nerve
6 Sympathetic trunk and ganglia
7 Body of ninth thoracic vertebra
8 Greater splanchnic nerve

● The expected order of structures beneath a rib is: vein, artery, nerve from above downwards.

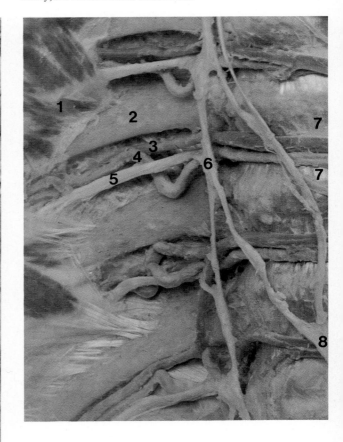

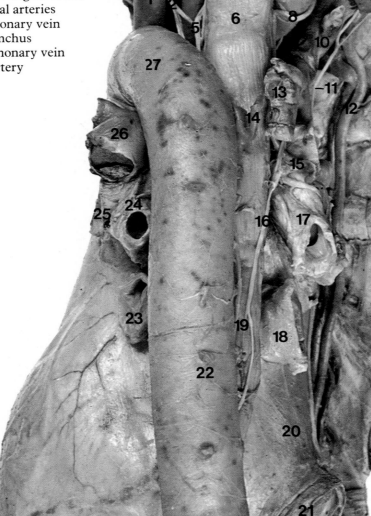

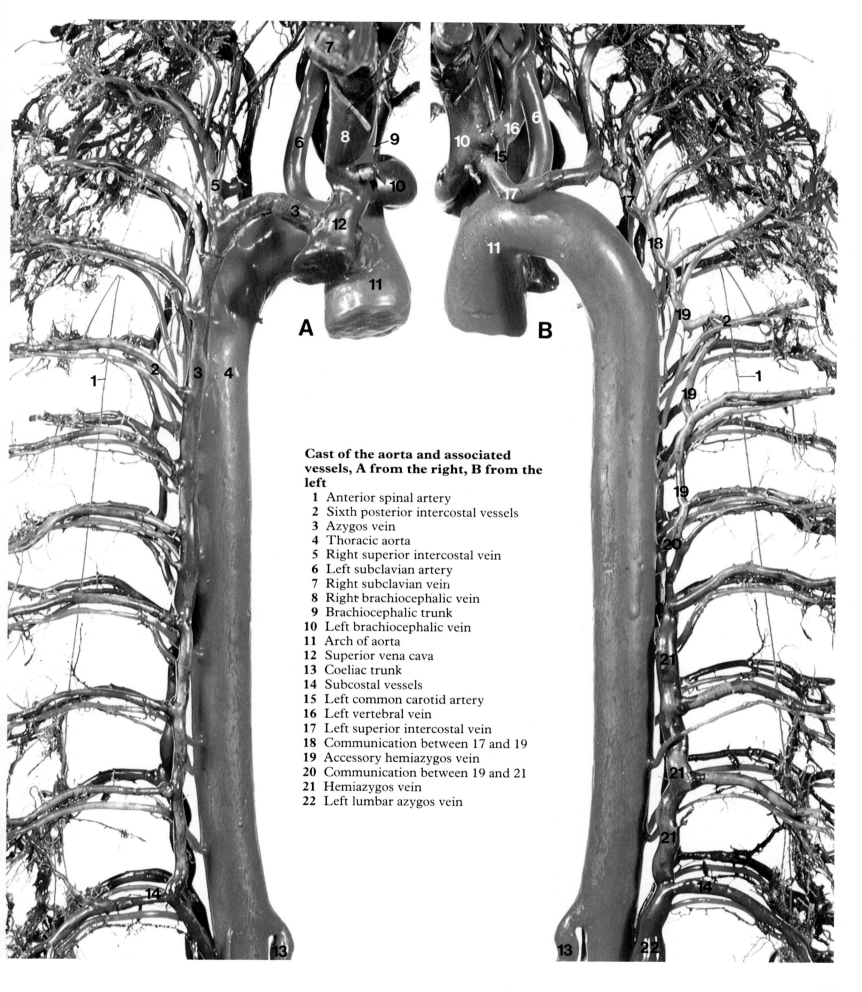

Cast of the aorta and associated vessels, A from the right, B from the left

1 Anterior spinal artery
2 Sixth posterior intercostal vessels
3 Azygos vein
4 Thoracic aorta
5 Right superior intercostal vein
6 Left subclavian artery
7 Right subclavian vein
8 Right brachiocephalic vein
9 Brachiocephalic trunk
10 Left brachiocephalic vein
11 Arch of aorta
12 Superior vena cava
13 Coeliac trunk
14 Subcostal vessels
15 Left common carotid artery
16 Left vertebral vein
17 Left superior intercostal vein
18 Communication between 17 and 19
19 Accessory hemiazygos vein
20 Communication between 19 and 21
21 Hemiazygos vein
22 Left lumbar azygos vein

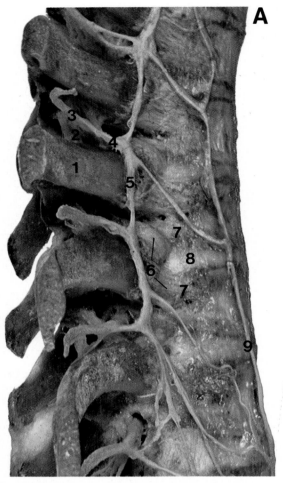

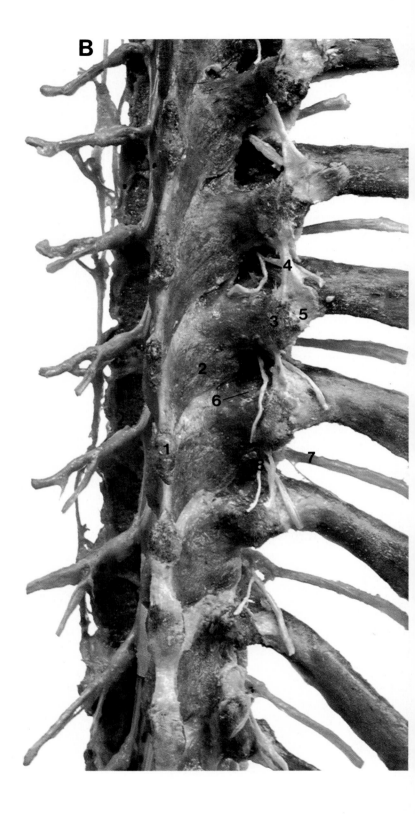

A Right costovertebral joints, from the right
1 Neck of rib
2 Superior costotransverse ligament
3 Ventral ramus of spinal nerve
4 Rami communicantes
5 Sympathetic trunk
6 Radiate ligament of joint of head of rib
7 Vertebral body
8 Intervertebral disc
9 Greater splanchnic nerve

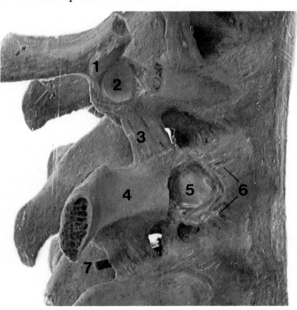

C Disarticulated right costovertebral joints, from the right
1 Articular facet of tubercle of rib
2 Articular facet of transverse process
3 Superior costotransverse ligament
4 Neck of rib
5 Cavity of joint of head of rib
6 Radiate ligament
7 Marker between anterior and posterior parts of superior costotransverse ligament

B Right costotransverse ligaments and the rami of spinal nerves, from behind

1 Spinous process
2 Lamina
3 Transverse process
4 Superior ⎱ costotransverse
5 Lateral ⎰ ligament
6 Costotransverse ligament
7 Ventral ⎱ ramus of
8 Dorsal ⎰ spinal nerve

● The dorsal rami of spinal nerves pass backwards *medial* to the superior costotransverse ligaments, dividing into medial and lateral branches.

● The ventral rami of spinal nerves pass laterally *in front of* the superior costotransverse ligaments.

● There are two types of costovertebral joint – the joints of the heads of the ribs with the facets on the vertebral bodies, and the costotransverse joints between the articular facets on the tubercles of the ribs and the facets on the transverse processes.

● There are three kinds of costotransverse ligament: *the* costotransverse ligament between the back of the neck of a rib and the front of the corresponding transverse process; the *lateral* costotransverse ligament, between the tip of a transverse process and the non-articular part of the tubercle of the corresponding rib; and the *superior* costotransverse ligament, having anterior and posterior layers and passing from the (upper) crest of the neck of a rib to the transverse process of the vertebra above.

D Radiograph of the heart, from the front

1 Anterior end of second rib
2 Arch of aorta (aortic knuckle)
3 Left pulmonary artery
4 Auricle of left atrium
5 Hilar shadows
6 Left ventricle
7 Dome of diaphragm
8 Right atrium
9 Superior vena cava
10 Pleural line (see note below)

● The shadow of the right border of the heart extends from the third to the sixth costal cartilage, forming a curved line (slightly convex laterally) just beyond the right border of the sternum.

● The shadow of the left border of the heart extends from the second costal cartilage at the lateral border of the sternum to the fifth intercostal space about 8.5 cm from the midline.

● The hilar shadows (and markings in the lung fields) are due mainly to the arteries and veins.

● The linear shadow occasionally seen in the upper part of the right lung field is due to a pleural fold (containing the azygos vein) that becomes invaginated into the upper lobe. The lung tissue medial to the fold is known as the azygos lobe.

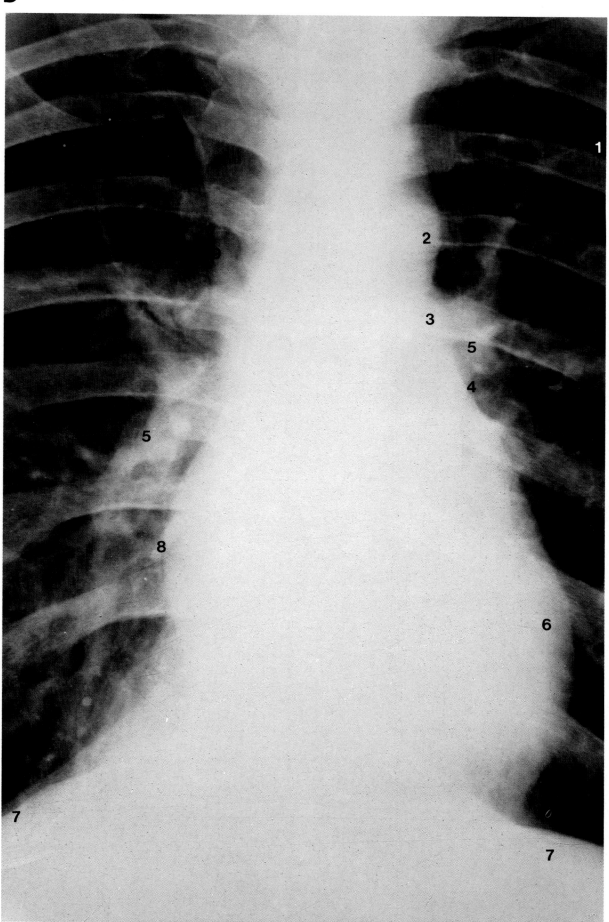

D

Bronchogram of the right lung after injection of contrast medium into the trachea
1 Superior vena cava
2 Principal bronchus

3 Superior ⎫
4 Middle ⎬ lobe bronchus
5 Inferior ⎭
6 Right border of heart
7 Dome of diaphragm

● Compare with the cast of the bronchial tree on pages 176 and 177.

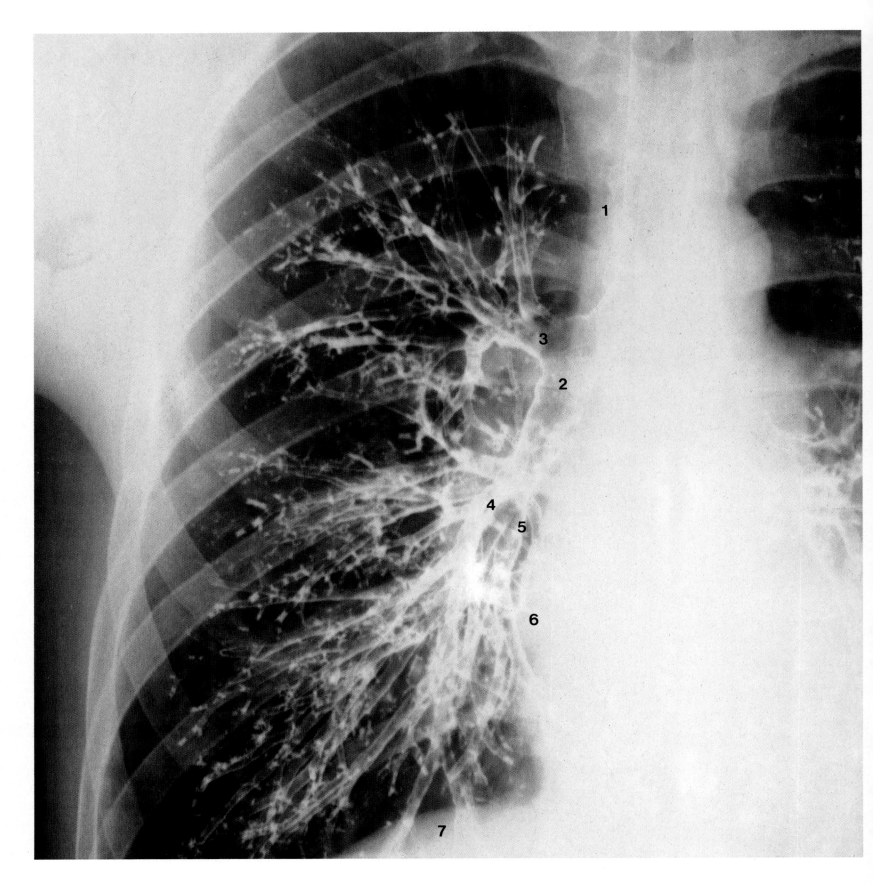

Bronchogram of the left lung

1 Arch of aorta
2 Left pulmonary artery
3 Principal bronchus
4 Left border of heart
5 Dome of diaphragm

● On the left side the shadow of the heart obscures bronchial detail.

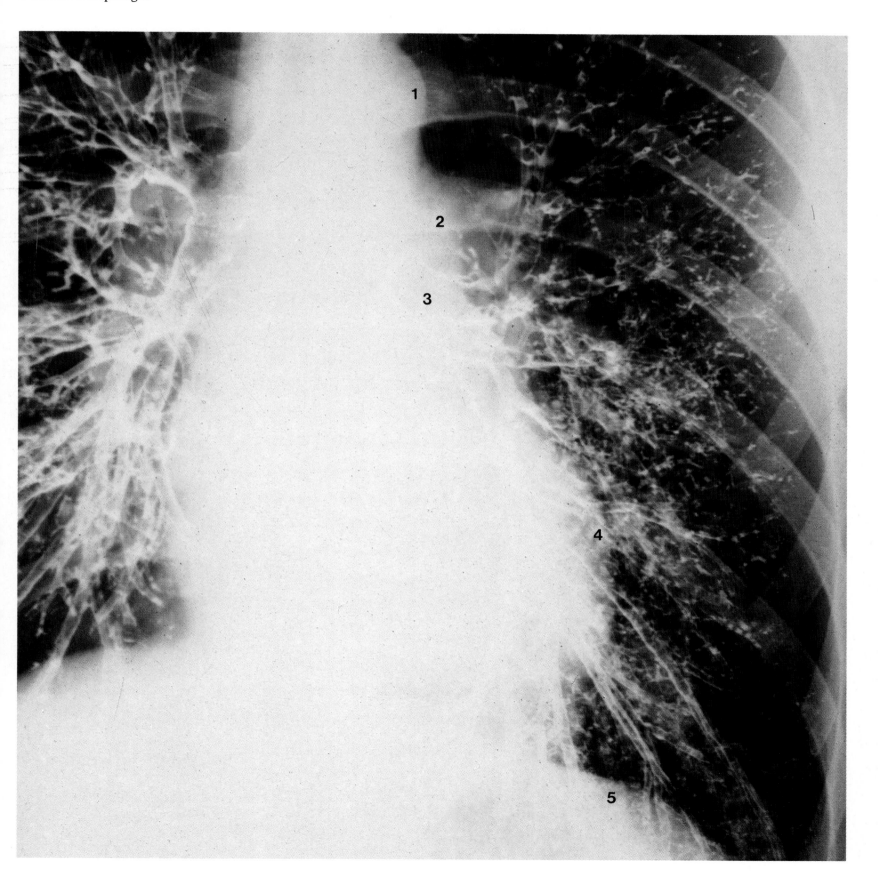

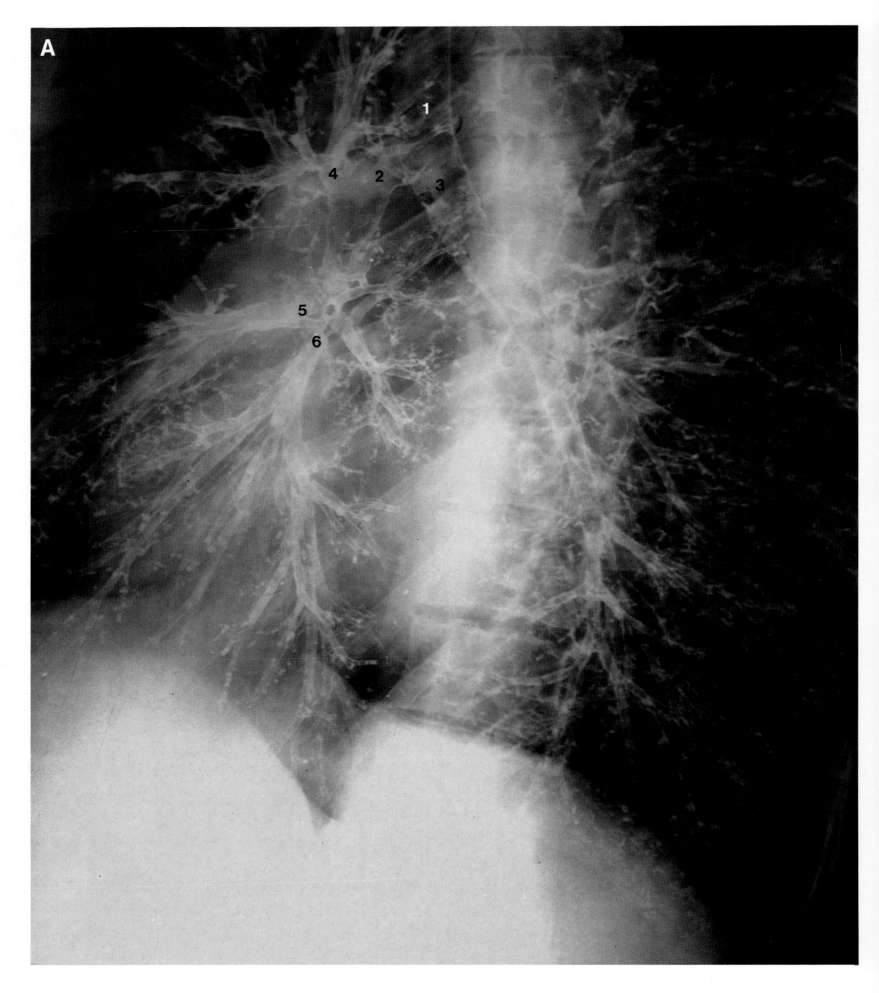

A Bronchogram of the right lung, oblique view

1 Trachea
2 Right ⎫
3 Left ⎬ principal bronchus
4 Superior ⎫
5 Middle ⎬ lobe bronchus
6 Inferior ⎭ of right lung

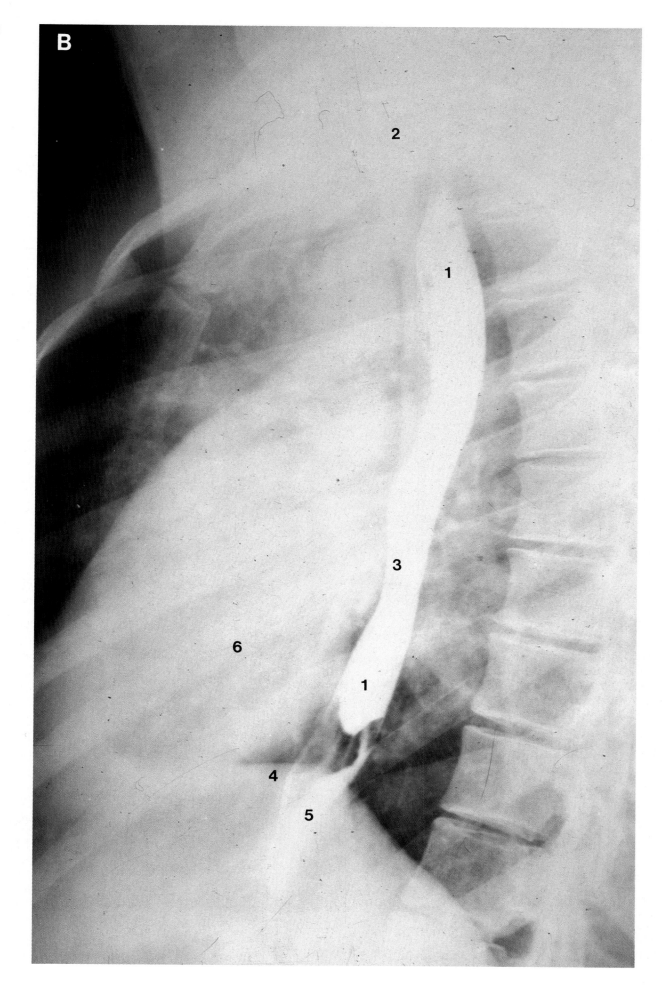

B Radiograph of the oesophagus, after swallowing barium paste (oblique view)

1 Oesophagus
2 Level of arch of aorta
3 Shallow indentation by left atrium
4 Dome of diaphragm
5 Level of cardio-oesophageal junction
6 Heart shadow

201

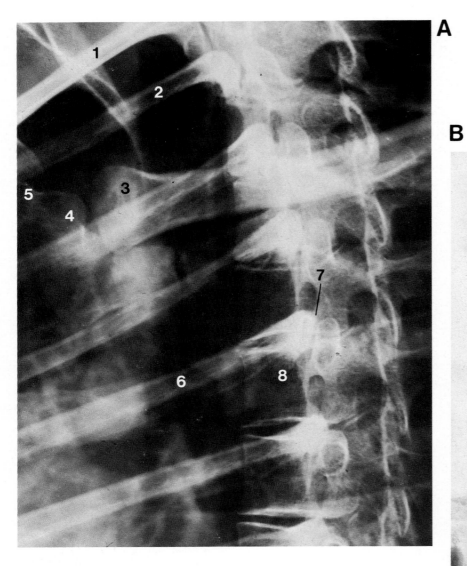

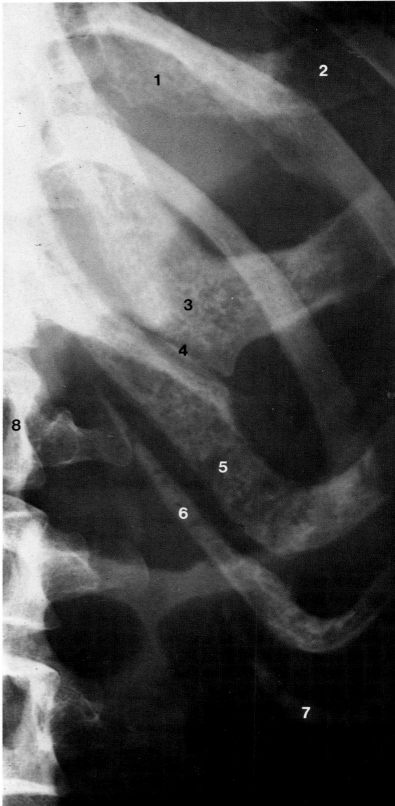

A Radiograph of upper thoracic vertebrae and ribs, from the left and behind

1 Left first rib
2 Left second rib
3 Sternal end of right clavicle
4 Manubrium
5 Sternal end of left clavicle
6 Left fifth rib
7 Costotransverse joint
8 Fifth thoracic vertebra

B Radiograph of left costal margin

1 Sixth costal cartilage
2 Anterior end of sixth rib
3 Seventh costal cartilage
4 Interchondral joint
5 Eighth ⎫
6 Ninth ⎬ costal cartilage
7 Tenth ⎭
8 First lumbar vertebra

Abdomen and Pelvis

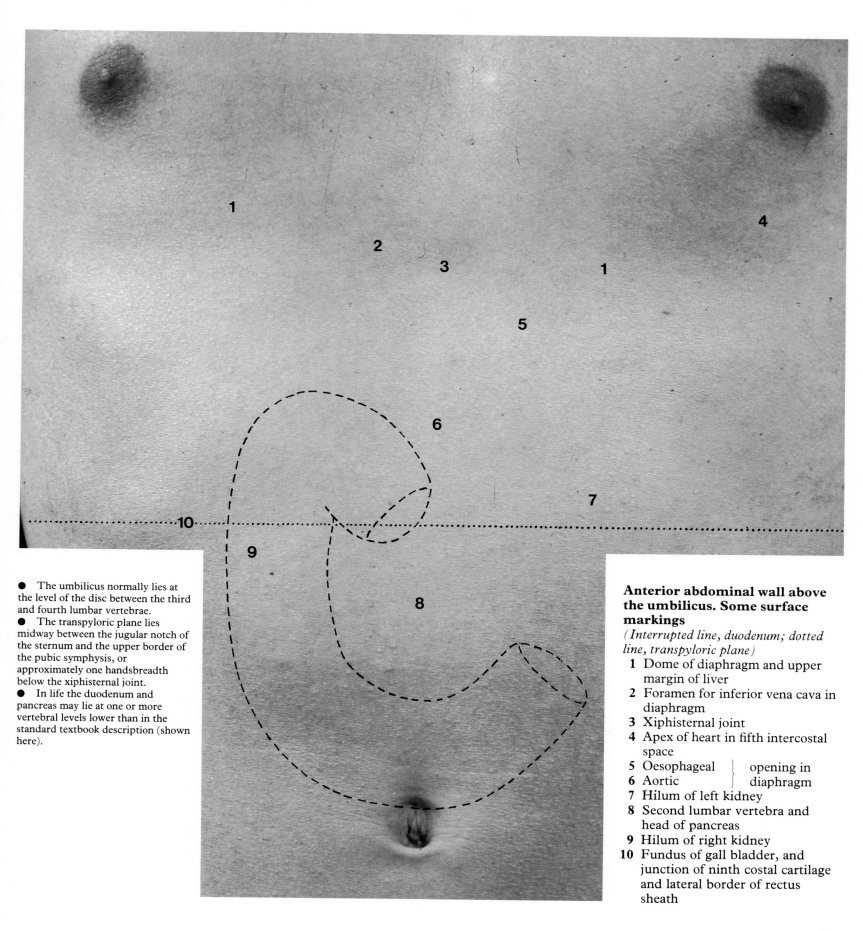

● The umbilicus normally lies at the level of the disc between the third and fourth lumbar vertebrae.

● The transpyloric plane lies midway between the jugular notch of the sternum and the upper border of the pubic symphysis, or approximately one handsbreadth below the xiphisternal joint.

● In life the duodenum and pancreas may lie at one or more vertebral levels lower than in the standard textbook description (shown here).

Anterior abdominal wall above the umbilicus. Some surface markings
(Interrupted line, duodenum; dotted line, transpyloric plane)

1 Dome of diaphragm and upper margin of liver
2 Foramen for inferior vena cava in diaphragm
3 Xiphisternal joint
4 Apex of heart in fifth intercostal space
5 Oesophageal ⎫ opening in
6 Aortic ⎭ diaphragm
7 Hilum of left kidney
8 Second lumbar vertebra and head of pancreas
9 Hilum of right kidney
10 Fundus of gall bladder, and junction of ninth costal cartilage and lateral border of rectus sheath

Anterior abdominal wall above the umbilicus. Muscles and rectus sheath

1 External oblique
2 Anterior wall of rectus sheath
3 Rectus abdominis
4 Tendinous intersections of rectus muscle
5 Linea alba
6 Xiphoid process
7 Seventh ⎤
8 Eighth ⎬ costal cartilage
9 Ninth ⎦
10 Superior epigastric artery
11 Branches of eighth intercostal nerve
12 Transversus abdominis
13 Posterior wall of rectus sheath

14 Internal oblique
15 Internal oblique aponeurosis
16 Branches of ninth intercostal nerve
17 Branches of tenth intercostal nerve
18 Umbilicus
19 Branch of tenth intercostal nerve
20 Lateral cutaneous branch of eleventh intercostal nerve

● The rectus sheath is formed by the internal oblique aponeurosis which splits at the lateral border of the rectus muscle into two layers, one passing behind the rectus to blend with the aponeurosis of the transverse muscle, the other passing in front of the rectus to blend with the external oblique aponeurosis. These reunite at the medial border of the rectus to form the midline linea alba. (For a note on the sheath below the umbilicus see page 211.)

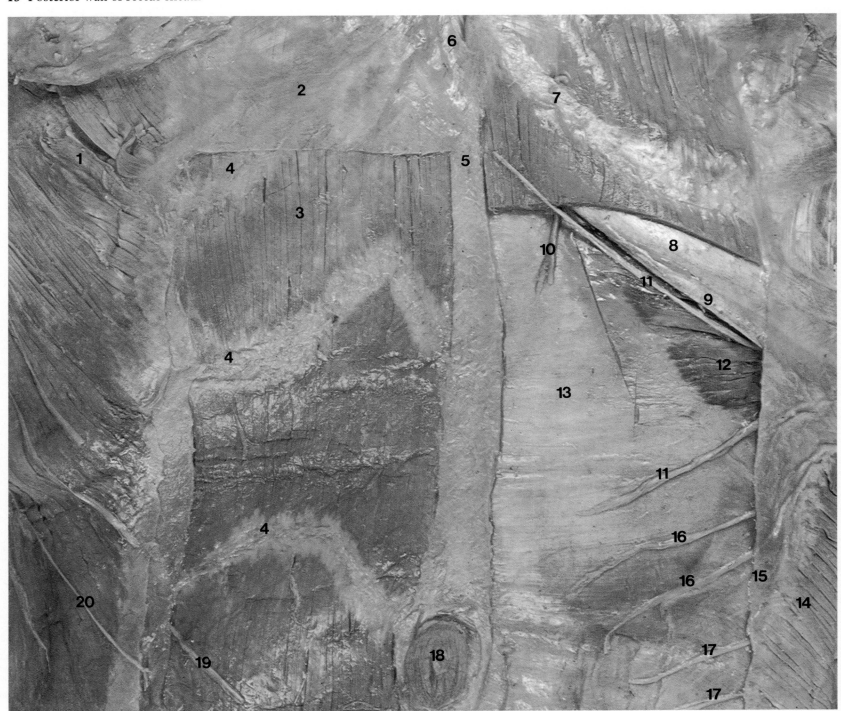

**Anterior abdominal wall. Upper part of the
right external and internal oblique muscles**
1 Serratus anterior digitation
2 External oblique
3 External oblique aponeurosis
4 Internal oblique aponeurosis
5 Rectus abdominis and tendinous intersection
6 Internal oblique
7 Tenth rib

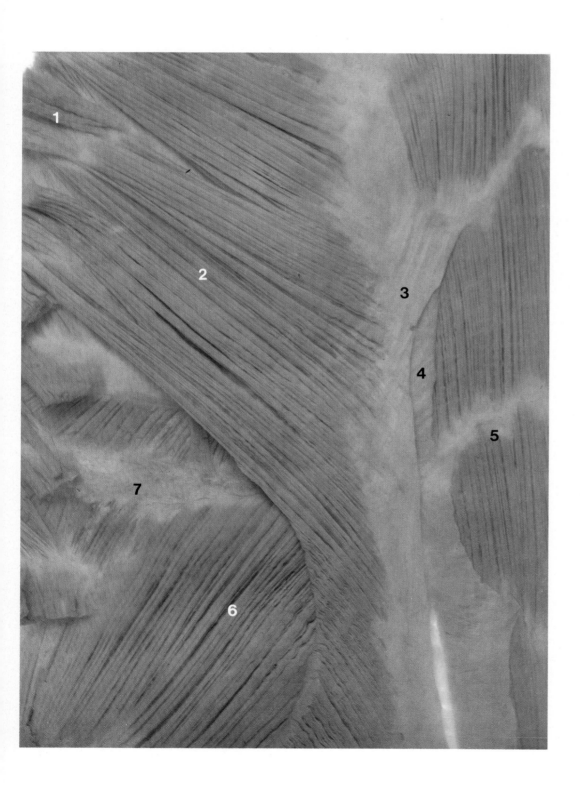

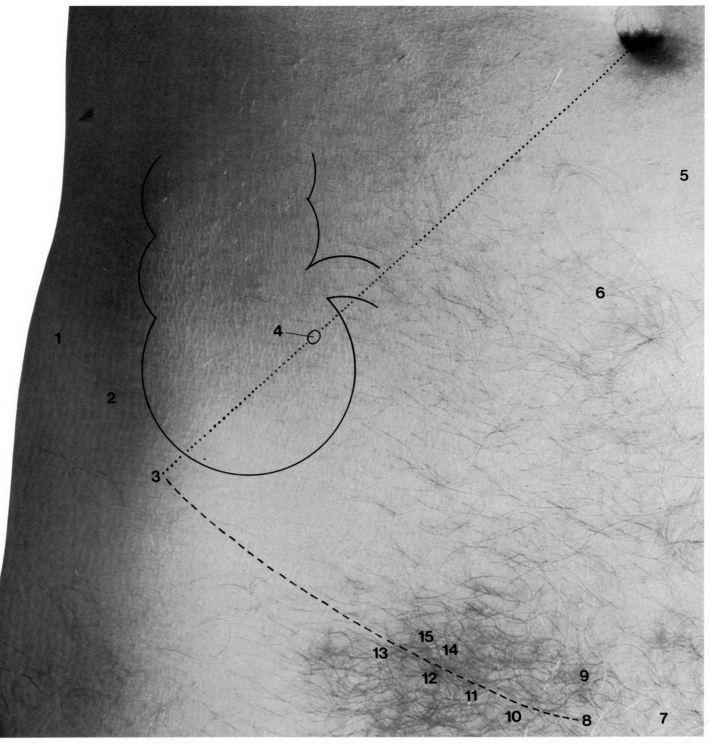

Right lower quadrant of the anterior abdominal wall and the inguinal region. Some surface markings
(Caecum, lower ascending colon and terminal ileum, continuous line; inguinal ligament, interrupted line; the dotted line joins the anterior superior iliac spine and the umbilicus)

1 Tubercle of iliac crest
2 Iliac crest
3 Anterior superior iliac spine
4 McBurney's point (see note below)
5 Bifurcation of aorta (fourth lumbar vertebra)
6 Lower end of inferior vena cava (fifth lumbar vertebra)

7 Pubic symphysis
8 Pubic tubercle
9 Superficial inguinal ring
10 Femoral canal
11 Femoral vein
12 Femoral artery
13 Femoral nerve
14 Inferior epigastric vessels
15 Deep inguinal ring

● McBurney's point indicates the opening of the appendix into the caecum, and lies at the junction of the lateral and middle thirds of a line drawn from the anterior superior iliac spine to the umbilicus.
● The superficial inguinal ring (at the medial end of the inguinal canal) lies 1 cm above the pubic tubercle.
● The deep inguinal ring (at the lateral end of the inguinal canal) lies 1 cm above the midpoint of the inguinal ligament.
● The femoral artery (whose pulsation should normally be palpable) enters the thigh midway between the pubic symphysis and the anterior superior iliac spine.

Anterior abdominal wall below the umbilicus, and superficial inguinal region, in the female

1 External oblique
2 External oblique aponeurosis
3 Internal oblique aponeurosis
4 Rectus abdominis
5 Transversalis fascia
6 Branch of tenth intercostal nerve
7 Posterior wall of rectus sheath
8 Arcuate line
9 Peritoneum
10 Medial umbilical ligament (fragmented into strands)
11 Inferior epigastric vessels (cut)
12 Internal oblique
13 Iliohypogastric nerve
14 Inguinal ligament
15 Sartorius
16 Cutaneous branches of femoral nerve
17 Superficial inguinal lymph nodes
18 Superficial epigastric vein
19 Ilio-inguinal nerve
20 Anterior wall of rectus sheath
21 Pubic symphysis
22 Round ligament of uterus
23 Superficial external pudendal vessels
24 Great saphenous vein
25 Femoral vein
26 Femoral artery
27 Femoral nerve
28 Superficial circumflex iliac vessels

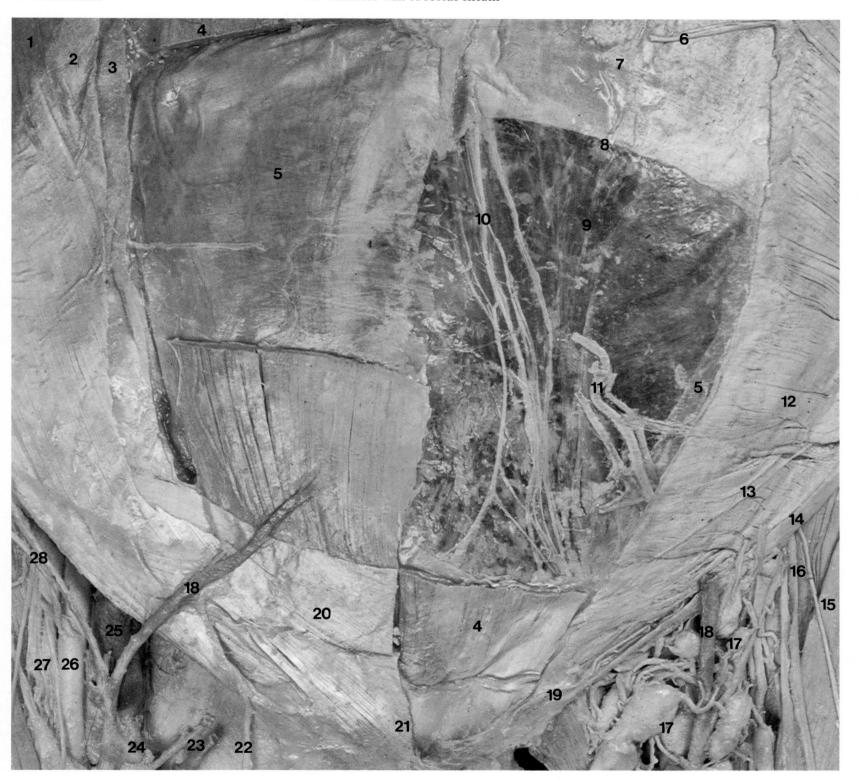

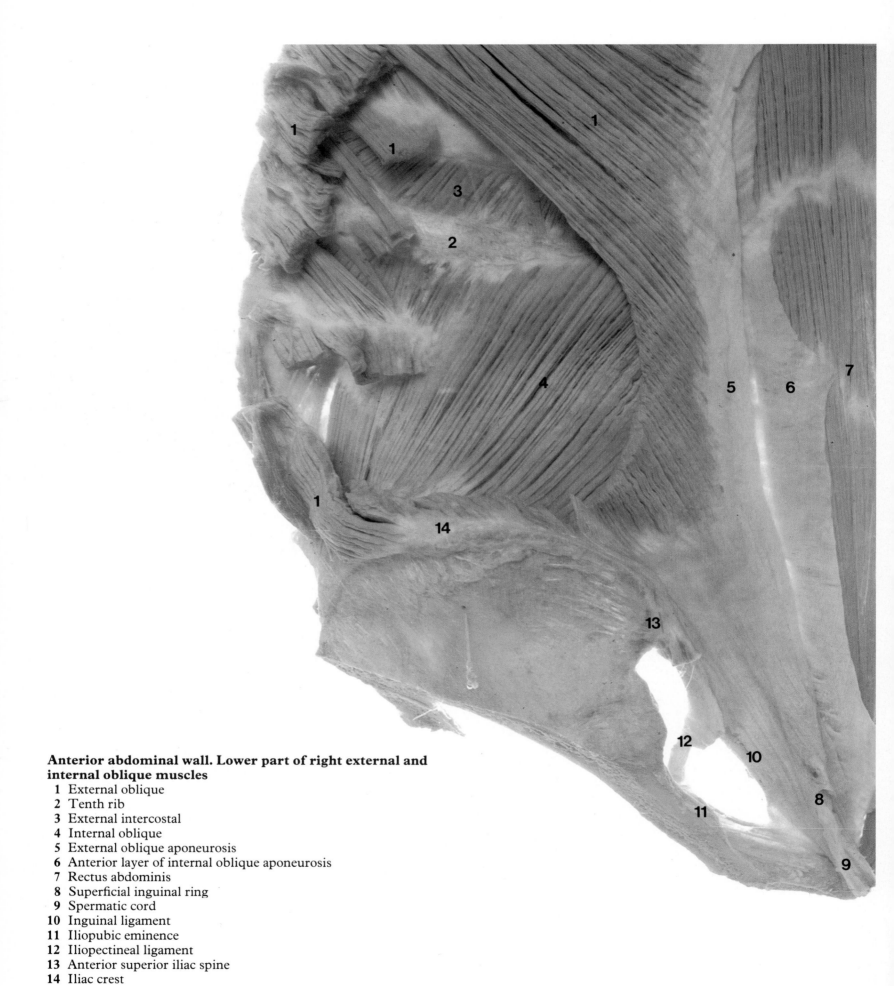

Anterior abdominal wall. Lower part of right external and internal oblique muscles

1 External oblique
2 Tenth rib
3 External intercostal
4 Internal oblique
5 External oblique aponeurosis
6 Anterior layer of internal oblique aponeurosis
7 Rectus abdominis
8 Superficial inguinal ring
9 Spermatic cord
10 Inguinal ligament
11 Iliopubic eminence
12 Iliopectineal ligament
13 Anterior superior iliac spine
14 Iliac crest

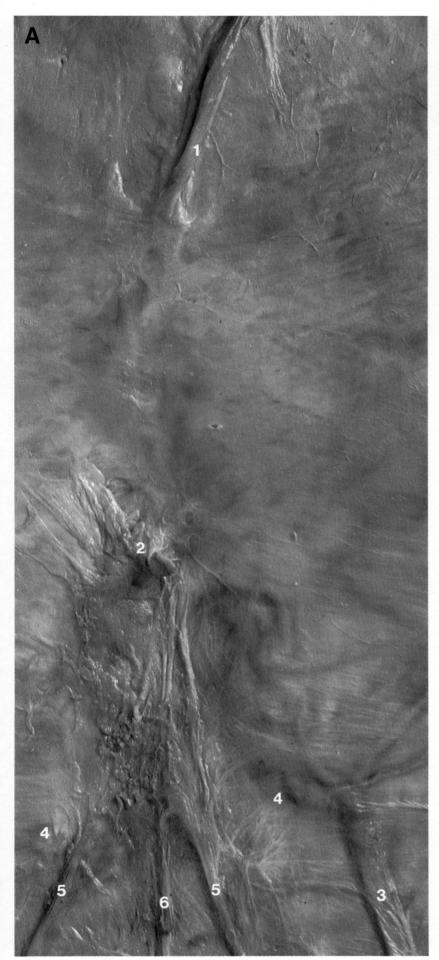

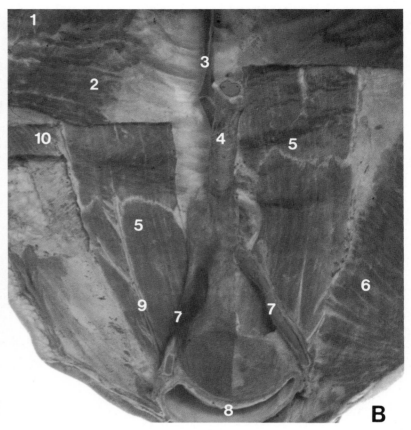

B Anterior abdominal wall, from behind, in a full-term fetus. Umbilical vessels

(With peritoneum and parts of muscles and rectus sheaths removed)

1 Diaphragm
2 Transversus abdominis
3 Falciform ligament
4 Left umbilical vein
5 Rectus abdominis
6 Internal oblique
7 Umbilical artery
8 Urinary bladder
9 Inferior epigastric vessels
10 External oblique

A Anterior abdominal wall, from behind. Umbilical folds

1 Falciform ligament
2 Umbilicus and remains of vitello-intestinal duct
3 Lateral umbilical fold
4 Arcuate line
5 Medial umbilical fold
6 Median umbilical fold

● The falciform ligament contains the ligamentum teres (the obliterated left umbilical vein).
● The median umbilical fold contains the median umbilical ligament (the remains of the urachus).
● The medial umbilical fold contains the medial umbilical ligament (the obliterated umbilical artery).
● The lateral umbilical fold, which does not reach the umbilicus, contains the inferior epigastric vessels before they enter the rectus sheath.
● In this specimen the ligamentum teres has not raised a falciform fold until some distance from the umbilicus.

Anterior abdominal wall. Upper part of the right transversus abdominis from behind

1 Rectus abdominis
2 Transversus abdominis
3 Diaphragm
4 Tenth rib
5 Transversus abdominis aponeurosis
6 Lateral border of rectus sheath

● The uppermost fibres of the transversus muscle interdigitate at their origin with fibres of the diaphragm, and then pass behind the upper part of the rectus muscle before becoming aponeurotic.

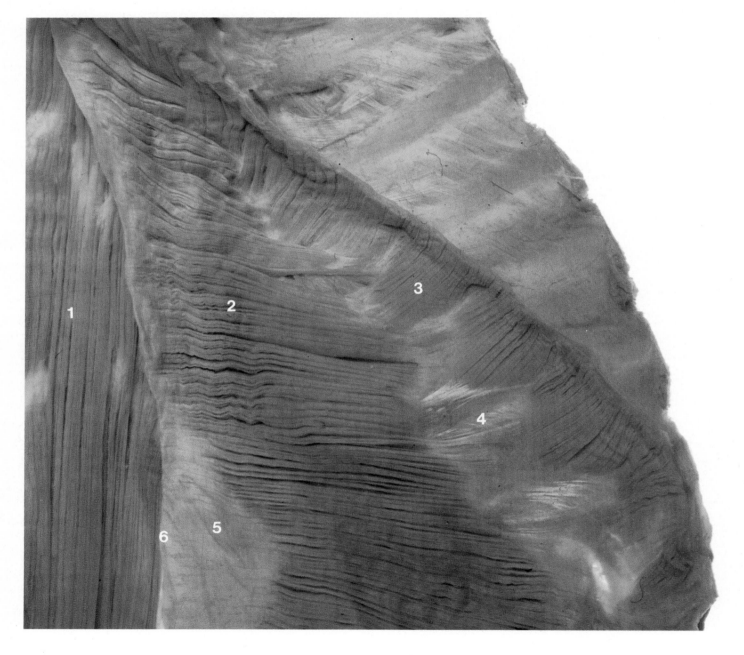

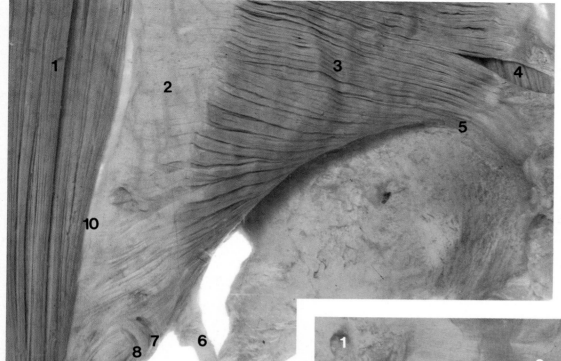

A Anterior abdominal wall. Lower part of the right transversus abdominis, from behind

**A Anterior abdominal wall. Lower part
of the right transversus abdominis,
from behind**

1 Rectus abdominis
2 Transversus abdominis aponeurosis
3 Transversus abdominis
4 Internal oblique (seen through incision in
   transversus abdominis)
5 Iliac crest
6 Iliopectineal ligament
7 Inguinal ligament
8 Position of deep inguinal ring
9 Spermatic cord
10 Lateral border of rectus sheath

● In contrast to the upper part, the lower part of the
transversus muscle becomes aponeurotic some distance
before reaching the rectus sheath.

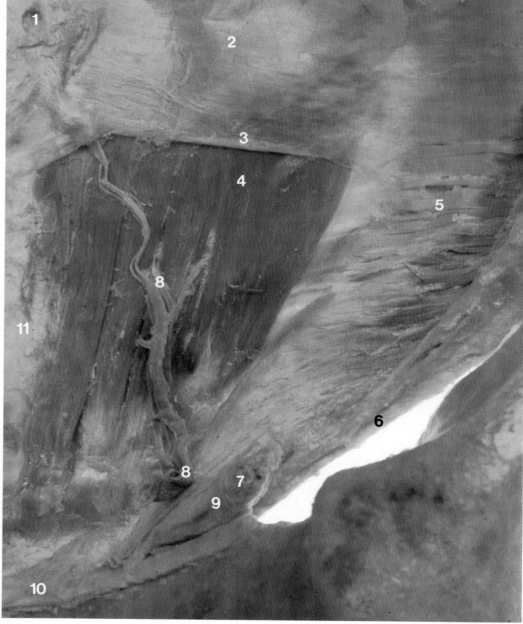

**B Anterior abdominal wall. Lower right
quadrant, from behind**

*(The transversalis fascia and peritoneum have
been removed)*

1 Umbilicus
2 Posterior wall of rectus sheath
3 Arcuate line
4 Rectus abdominis
5 Transversus abdominis
6 Inguinal ligament
7 Spermatic cord
8 Inferior epigastric vessels
9 Position of deep inguinal ring
10 Pubic crest
11 Linea alba

● A short distance below the level of the umbilicus the
posterior wall of the rectus sheath comes to an abrupt end at
the arcuate line. Below this level the aponeuroses of the
external and internal oblique and transversus muscles all lie
in front of the rectus muscle. The inferior epigastric vessels
enter the sheath by passing under the arcuate line.

A Upper abdominal viscera in situ

(After removal of the anterior abdominal wall, part of the diaphragm and lower thoracic wall)

1 Lower lobe of right lung
2 Pericardial fat
3 Diaphragm
4 Falciform ligament
5 Right lobe of liver
6 Left lobe of liver
7 Stomach

8 Lower lobe of left lung
9 Greater omentum
10 Superior (first) part of duodenum
11 Gall bladder
12 Transverse colon

● In this obese subject there is a large amount of pericardial and peritoneal fat.

B Greater omentum

1 Right lobe of liver
2 Falciform ligament
3 Left lobe of liver
4 Stomach
5 Greater omentum
6 Small intestine
7 Caecum
8 Ascending colon
9 Right colic flexure
10 Transverse colon
11 Fundus of gall bladder
12 Superior (first) part of duodenum

● The greater omentum hangs down from the greater curvature of the stomach, covering most of the small and large intestine.

A

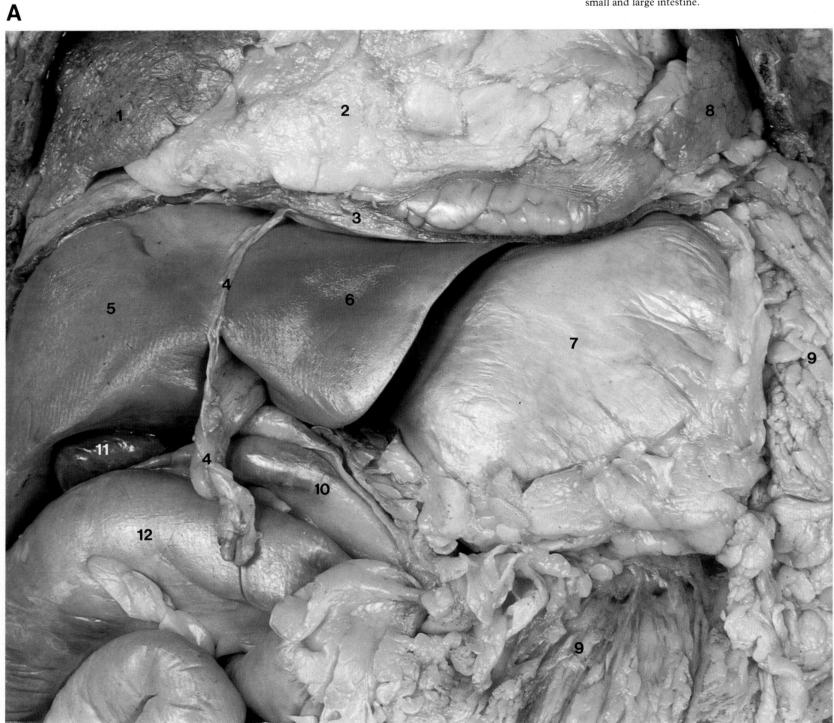

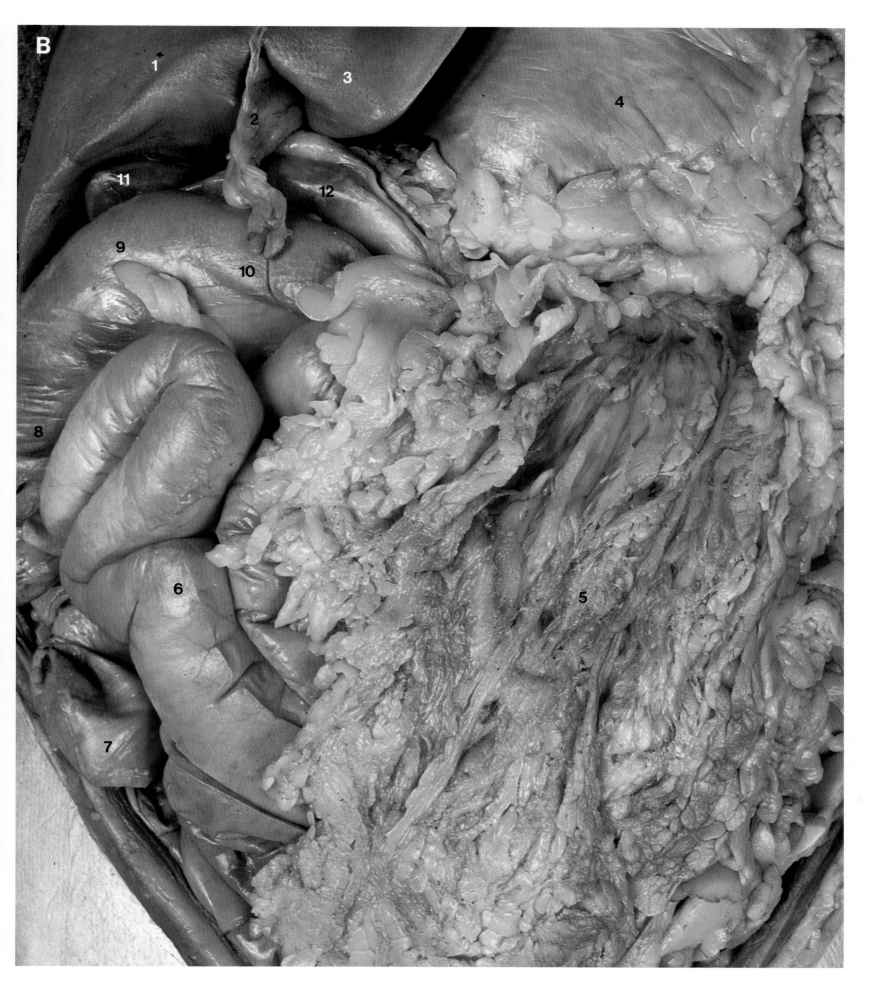

Upper abdominal viscera, with greater omentum lifted upwards

1 Right lobe of liver
2 Falciform ligament
3 Left lobe of liver
4 Posterior surface of greater omentum
5 Transverse colon
6 Appendices epiploicae
7 Small intestine
8 Superior (first) part of duodenum

● For further details of the peritoneum and greater omentum in a less obese subject, see pages 216–218.

● The appendices epiploicae are fat-filled appendages of peritoneum on the various parts of the colon (ascending, transverse, descending and sigmoid). They are not present on the small intestine or the rectum, and may be rudimentary on the caecum and appendix. In abdominal operations they are one feature that helps to distinguish colon from other parts of the intestine.

● In strict anatomical nomenclature the term 'small intestine' includes the duodenum, jejunum and ileum, but clinically it is frequently used to mean jejunum and ileum, with the duodenum being referred to by its own name.

● The parts of the duodenum are properly called superior, descending, horizontal and ascending, but are more commonly known as the first, second, third and fourth parts respectively.

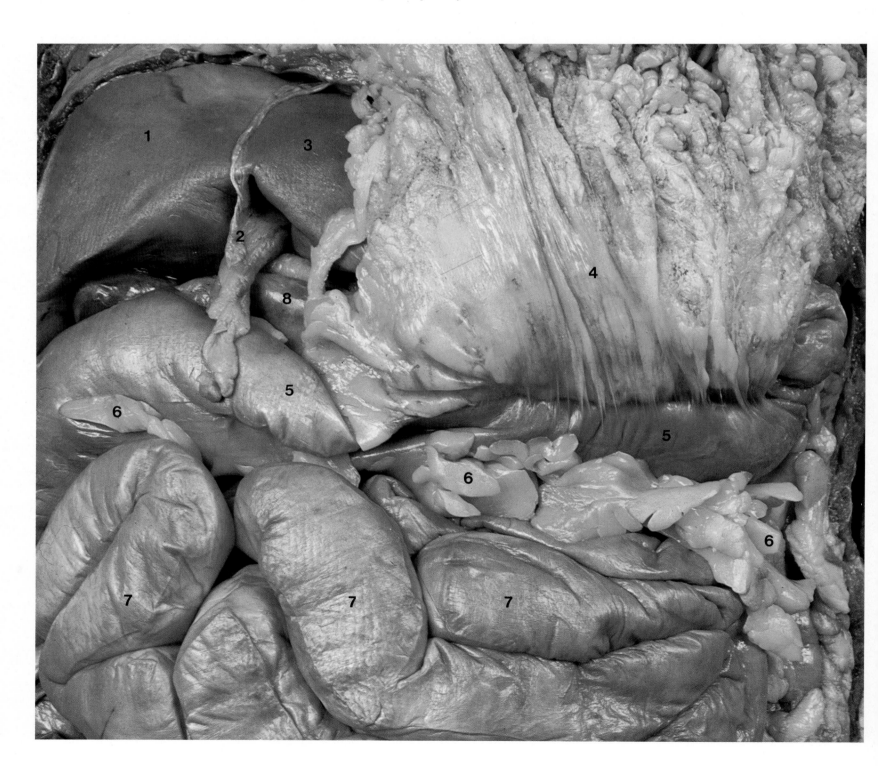

Lesser omentum and epiploic foramen, A from the front, B from the right

1 Falciform ligament
2 Left lobe of liver
3 Diaphragm
4 Pericardium
5 Lesser curvature of stomach
6 Lesser omentum
7 Right free margin of lesser omentum
8 Superior (first) part of duodenum
9 Gall bladder
10 Quadrate lobe of liver
11 Epiploic foramen
12 Descending (second) part of duodenum
13 Upper pole of right kidney
14 Inferior vena cava
15 Right lobe of liver

● The epiploic foramen (of Winslow) is bounded behind by the inferior vena cava, in front by the right free margin of the lesser omentum (which contains posteriorly the portal vein with in front of it the bile duct to the right and the hepatic artery to the left), below by the first part of the duodenum (which passes *backwards* as well as to the right), and above by the caudate process of the liver (overlapped in B by a bulbous upper end of the gall bladder). See also page 219.

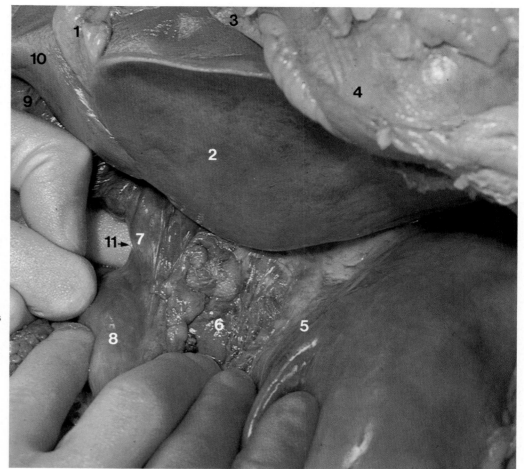

A

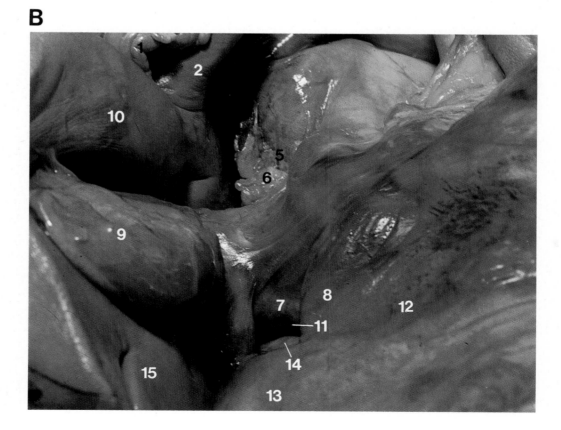

B

A Upper abdominal viscera in situ
1 Gall bladder
2 Left lobe of liver
3 Lesser omentum overlying pancreas
4 Body ⎫
5 Lesser curvature ⎪
6 Greater curvature ⎬ of stomach
7 Pyloric part ⎭

8 Greater omentum overlying transverse mesocolon and transverse colon
9 Descending colon
10 Small intestine and mesentery
11 Ascending colon
12 Transverse colon
13 Descending (second) part of duodenum

● In this specimen there is less adipose tissue than in that on page 213, and the stomach is more contracted, lying at a lower level and enabling part of the body of the pancreas to be seen through the lesser omentum.
● The transverse colon is often more tortuous, and may lie at a lower level, than its name would suggest.
● The pyloric *part* of the stomach consists of the pyloric *antrum* and pyloric *canal*.

A

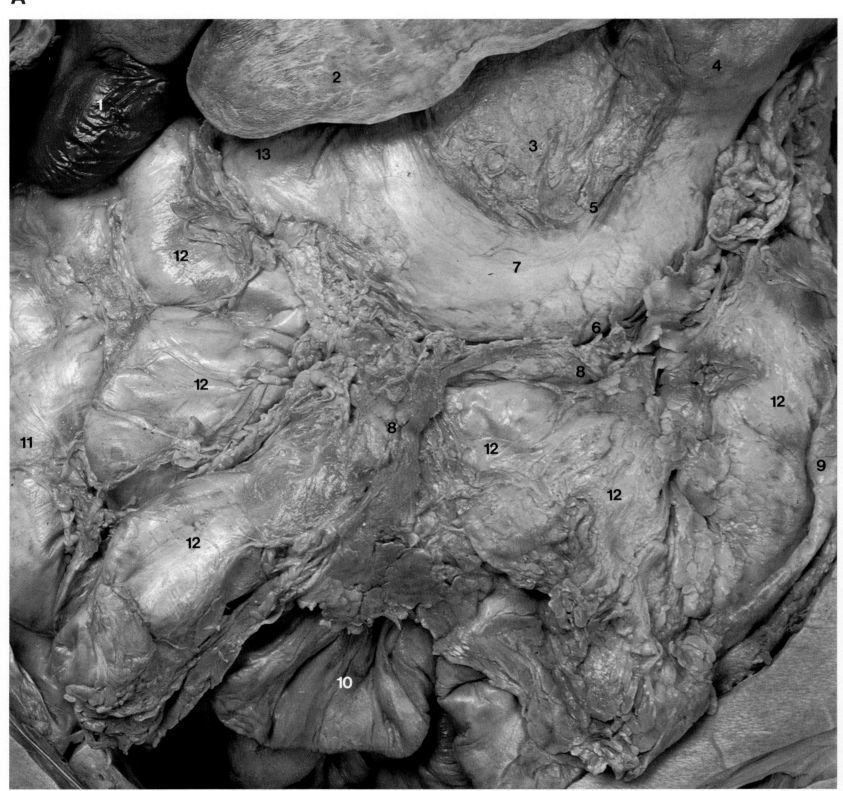

B Upper abdominal viscera, from the left and below

(The greater omentum, transverse colon and mesocolon and stomach have been lifted upwards)

1 Greater omentum
2 Transverse colon
3 Transverse mesocolon
4 Greater ⎫
5 Lesser ⎬ curvature of stomach
6 Lower border of pancreas
7 Jejunum
8 Duodenojejunal flexure
9 Ascending ⎫
10 Horizontal ⎬ part of duodenum
11 Mesentery

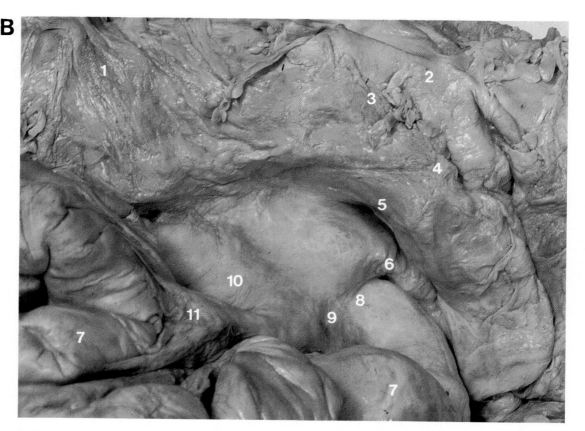

C Lesser sac and transverse mesocolon

(The greater omentum has been separated from the transverse colon and mesocolon, and lifted up with the stomach, so opening up the cavity known as the lesser sac)

1 Greater omentum
2 Greater ⎫
3 Lesser ⎬ curvature of stomach
4 Lesser omentum
5 Peritoneum of lesser sac overlying pancreas
6 Transverse mesocolon
7 Transverse colon
8 Mesentery
9 Coils of jejunum and ileum

● The greater omentum hanging down from the greater curvature of the stomach overlies the transverse mesocolon and transverse colon and fuses with them (as in A), so that when the greater omentum is lifted up the transverse colon is lifted also (as in B). When the greater omentum is dissected off the transverse colon and mesocolon and lifted up (as in C), the transverse colon is left behind, suspended from the lower border of the pancreas by its mesocolon.

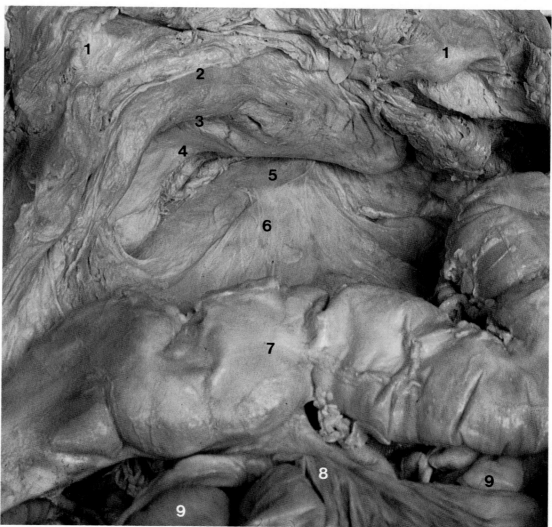

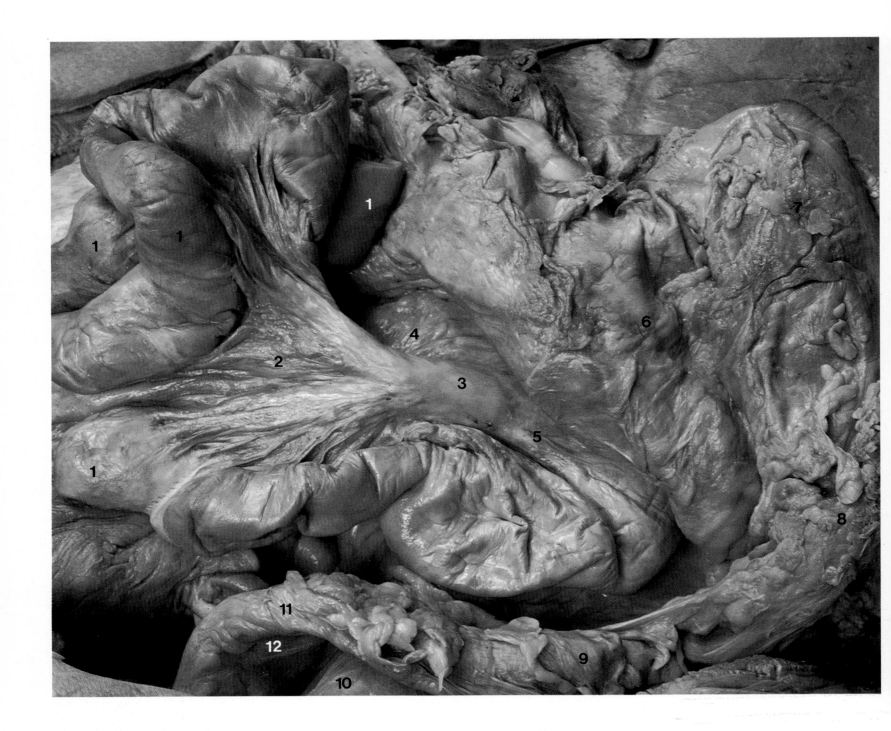

Mesentery and sigmoid colon, from the left
(The stomach and transverse colon have been lifted upwards)

1　Coils of jejunum and ileum
2　Mesentery
3　Root of mesentery
4　Horizontal (third) part of duodenum
5　Duodenojejunal flexure
6　Greater curvature of stomach
7　Transverse colon
8　Left colic flexure
9　Descending colon
10　Peritoneum overlying external iliac vessels
11　Sigmoid colon
12　Sigmoid mesocolon

● The root of the mesentery begins at the duodenojejunal flexure and passes downwards and to the right, crossing the horizontal part of the duodenum; the superior mesenteric vessels enter the mesentery at this point (see page 221).
● The sigmoid colon, like the transverse colon, has its own mesentery, the sigmoid mesocolon.

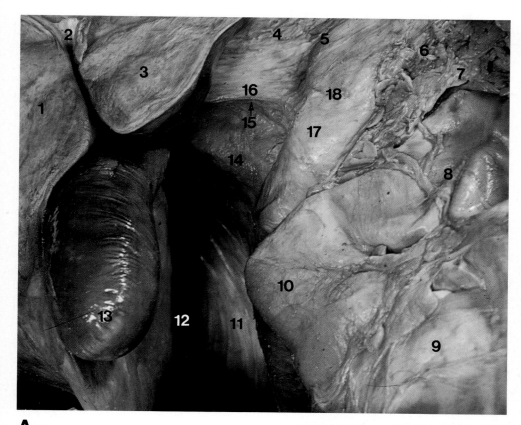

A The hepatorenal pouch of peritoneum, from the right and below

(The liver has been displaced upwards and to the right to open up the space between the liver and right kidney)

1 Right lobe of liver
2 Falciform ligament
3 Left lobe of liver
4 Lesser omentum overlying pancreas
5 Lesser } curvature ot stomach
6 Greater }
7 Greater omentum
8 Transverse colon
9 Ascending colon
10 Right colic flexure
11 Upper pole of right kidney
12 Hepatorenal (Morison's) pouch
13 Gall bladder
14 Inferior vena cava
15 Epiploic foramen
16 Right free margin of lesser omentum
17 Superior part of duodenum
18 Gastroduodenal junction

● The upper boundary of the hepatorenal pouch is the inferior layer of the coronary ligament, where the peritoneum is reflected from the lower margin of the bare area of the liver to the upper pole of the right kidney (see page 227).

B Duodenojejunal flexure, from the left

(With the mesentery and intestine lifted to the right)

1 Jejunum
2 Mesentery
3 Root of mesentery
4 Duodenojejunal flexure
5 Transverse colon
6 Ascending part of duodenum
7 Inferior duodenal recess
8 Peritoneum and retroperitoneal fat of posterior abdominal wall
9 Appendices epiploicae of descending colon
10 Horizontal part of duodenum

● The number and size of peritoneal recesses related to the duodenum are variable. This specimen shows one of the commonest, a small inferior recess.

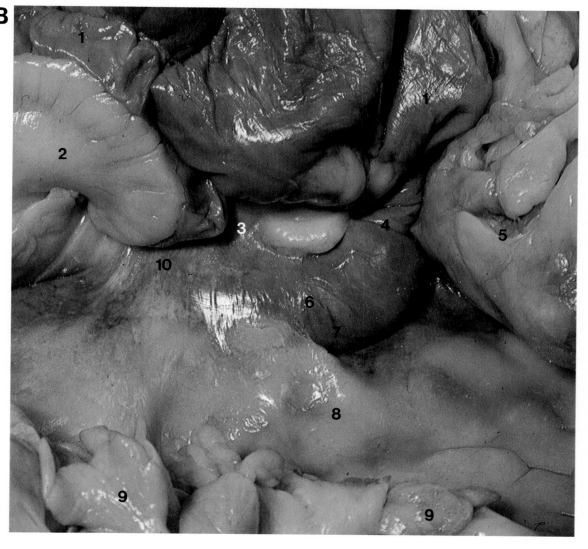

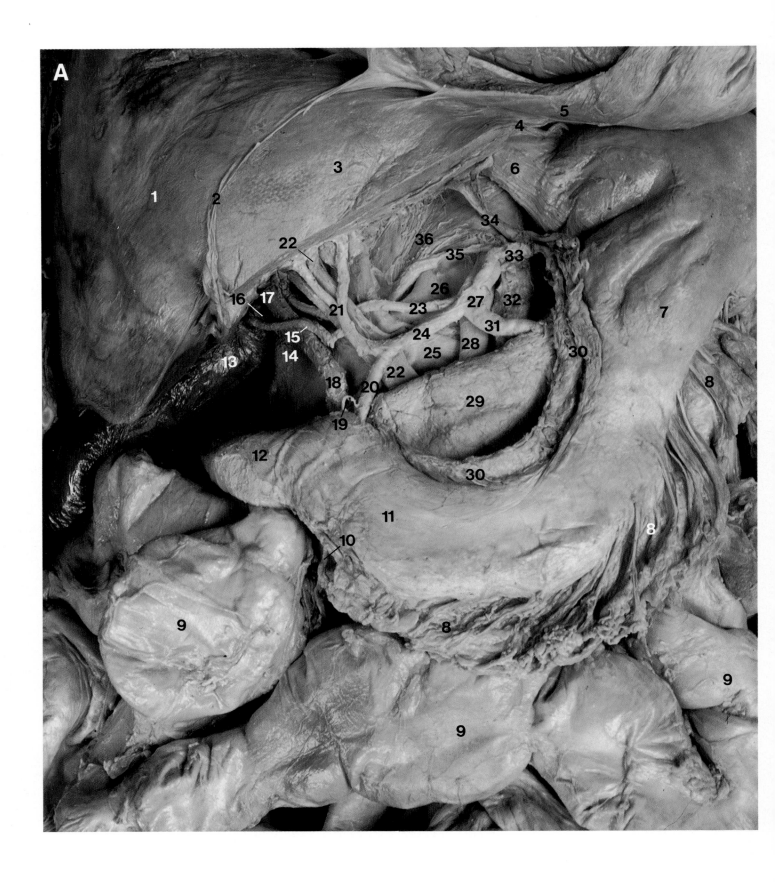

A Coeliac trunk and its branches

(Most of the left lobe of the liver, lesser omentum and greater omentum have been removed)

1 Right lobe of liver
2 Falciform ligament
3 Left lobe of liver
4 Left triangular ligament
5 Diaphragm
6 Abdominal part of oesophagus
7 Body of stomach
8 Branches of left and right gastro-epiploic arteries in greater omentum
9 Transverse colon
10 Right gastro-epiploic artery
11 Pyloric part of stomach
12 Superior (first) part of duodenum
13 Gall bladder
14 Inferior vena cava
15 Cystic artery
16 Cystic duct
17 Common hepatic duct
18 Bile duct
19 Right gastric artery
20 Gastroduodenal artery
21 Hepatic artery and right and left branches
22 Portal vein
23 Accessory hepatic artery
24 Common hepatic artery
25 Left renal vein
26 Abdominal aorta
27 Coeliac trunk
28 Superior mesenteric artery
29 Body of pancreas
30 Lesser omentum containing right and left gastric arteries
31 Splenic artery
32 Left crus of diaphragm
33 Left gastric artery
34 Oesophageal branch of left gastric artery
35 Median arcuate ligament
36 Right crus of diaphragm

● The portal vein, hepatic artery and bile duct are contained within the right free margin of the lesser omentum, the duct being the structure farthest to the right.

● The cystic artery is normally derived from the right branch of the hepatic artery and passes behind the common hepatic and cystic ducts. Here it comes from the hepatic artery itself and passes in front of the bile duct.

● If an accessory hepatic artery is present (as in this specimen) it passes *behind* the portal vein, not in front like the normal artery.

● It is normal for the right gastric artery to be much smaller than the left.

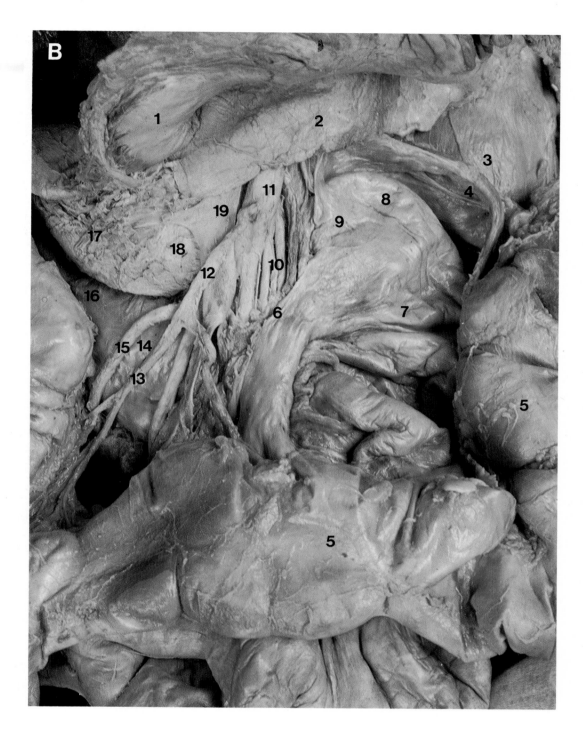

B Superior mesenteric vessels

(The stomach has been lifted upwards but the transverse colon is in its normal position although its mesocolon has been removed)

1 Posterior surface of pyloric part of stomach
2 Body of pancreas
3 Lower pole of left kidney
4 Branches of left colic vessels
5 Transverse colon
6 Cut edge of peritoneum at root of mesentery
7 Jejunum
8 Duodenojejunal flexure
9 Ascending (fourth) part of duodenum
10 Jejunal and ileal arteries
11 Superior mesenteric artery
12 Middle colic artery
13 Right colic artery
14 Horizontal (third) part of duodenum
15 Ileocolic artery
16 Descending (second) part of duodenum
17 Head of pancreas
18 Uncinate process of head of pancreas
19 Superior mesenteric vein

● The right colic artery is normally a branch of the superior mesenteric artery but often (as here) arises from its middle colic branch.

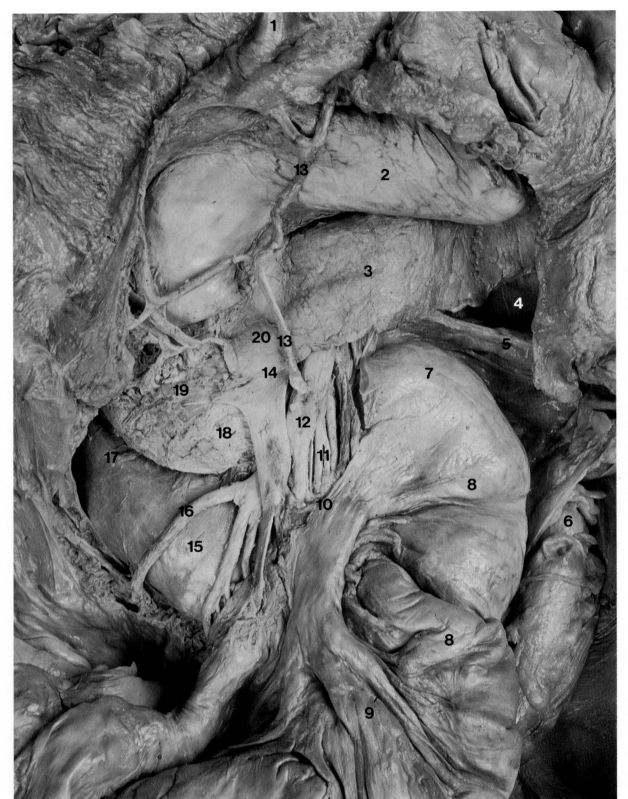

Superior mesenteric vessels

(The stomach and transverse colon have been lifted upwards, and most of the peritoneum removed)

1 Transverse colon
2 Posterior surface of body of stomach
3 Body of pancreas
4 Left kidney
5 Left colic vessels
6 Descending colon
7 Duodenojejunal flexure
8 Jejunum
9 Mesentery
10 Cut edge of peritoneum at root of mesentery
11 Jejunal and ileal arteries
12 Superior mesenteric artery
13 Middle colic artery
14 Superior mesenteric vein
15 Horizontal (third) part of duodenum
16 Ileocolic artery
17 Descending (second) part of duodenum
18 Uncinate process of head of pancreas
19 Head ⎱ of pancreas
20 Neck ⎰

● In its normal position the middle colic artery passes downwards from its superior mesenteric origin to the transverse colon, but obviously when the transverse colon is lifted upwards the vessel appears to be passing upwards also (textbook drawings often illustrate it in this position).

Inferior mesenteric vein and associated structures on the posterior abdominal wall, from the left

(Most of the peritoneum has been removed, the duodenum reflected to the right, and the lower border of the pancreas, transverse colon and stomach reflected upwards)

 1 Mesentery
 2 Horizontal (third)
 3 Ascending (fourth) } part of duodenum
 4 Duodenojejunal flexure
 5 Inferior mesenteric artery
 6 Abdominal aorta
 7 Suspensory muscle of duodenum (muscle of Treitz)
 8 Superior mesenteric artery
 9 Superior mesenteric vein
10 Splenic vein
11 Body of pancreas
12 Middle colic artery
13 Posterior surface of pyloric part of stomach

14 Left renal vein
.15 Transverse colon
16 Splenic artery
17 Left renal artery
18 Lower pole of left kidney
19 Branches of left colic vessels
20 Descending colon
21 Pelvis of kidney
22 Testicular artery
23 Testicular vein
24 Inferior mesenteric vein
25 Psoas major
26 Genitofemoral nerve
27 Ureter
28 Left colic artery
29 Cut edge of peritoneum

● In this specimen (as in that on page 241) the testicular artery arises from the renal artery and not from the aorta.

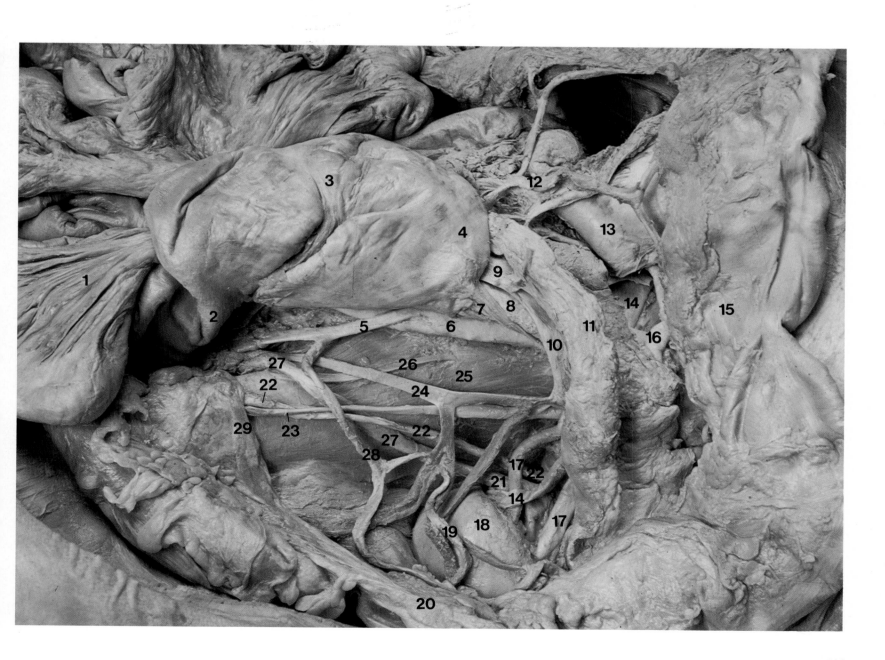

A Stomach and its arteries, from the front

1 Cardio-oesophageal junction
2 Fundus
3 Greater curvature
4 Body
5 Left gastro-epiploic artery
6 Right gastro-epiploic artery
7 Pyloric antrum
8 Pyloric canal
9 Gastroduodenal junction
10 Right gastric artery
11 Lesser curvature
12 Left gastric artery

● In this museum specimen the left and right gastro-epiploic arteries anastomose along the greater curvature, as in the standard textbook description, but often a direct anastomotic connexion is not obvious.

● The left and right gastric arteries normally anastomose along the lesser curvature.

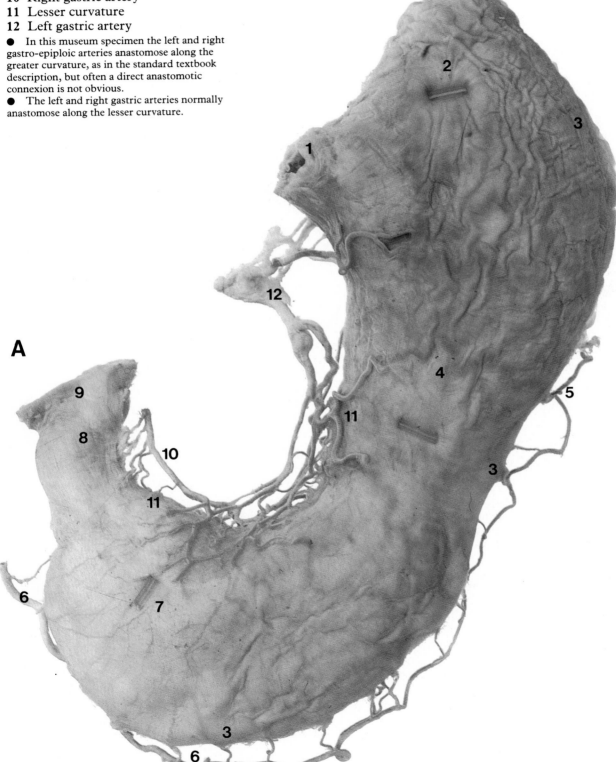

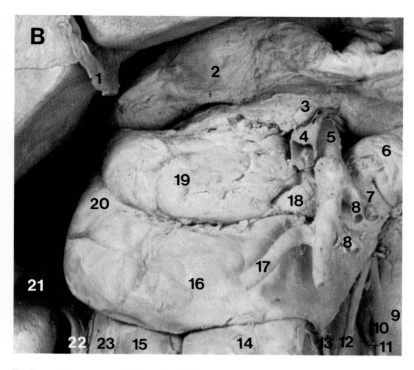

B Duodenum and head of the pancreas
(*With the peritoneum removed and the pyloric part of the stomach lifted upwards*)

1 Falciform ligament
2 Pyloric part of stomach
3 Neck of pancreas
4 Superior mesenteric vein
5 Superior mesenteric artery
6 Duodenojejunal flexure
7 Ascending (fourth) part of duodenum
8 Jejunal and ileal arteries
9 Lower pole of left kidney
10 Left testicular (ovarian) vein
11 Left ureter
12 Inferior mesenteric vein
13 Left testicular (ovarian) artery

14 Abdominal aorta
15 Inferior vena cava
16 Horizontal (third) part of duodenum
17 Middle colic artery
18 Uncinate process of head of pancreas
19 Head of pancreas
20 Descending (second) part of duodenum
21 Hilum of right kidney
22 Right ureter
23 Right testicular (ovarian) vein

● The head of the pancreas lies within the C-shaped curve of the duodenum, often referred to clinically and radiogically as the 'duodenal loop'.

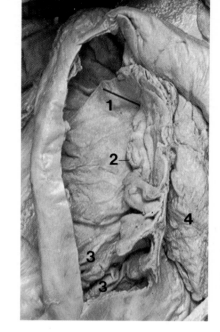

C Duodenal papillae
(*The anterior wall of the descending part of the duodenum has been removed*)

1 Bristle in minor duodenal papilla
2 Major duodenal papilla
3 Circular folds of mucous membrane
4 Head of pancreas

● The hepatopancreatic ampulla, formed by the union of the bile and pancreatic ducts, opens on the summit of the major papilla. The smooth muscle that surrounds the ampulla and the ends of the two ducts constitutes the ampullary sphincter (of Oddi).

● The accessory pancreatic duct opens on the summit of the minor papilla.

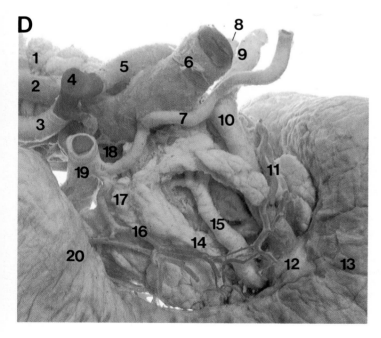

D Duodenum and head of pancreas, from behind

1 Body of pancreas
2 Splenic vein
3 Splenic artery
4 Coeliac trunk
5 Common hepatic artery
6 Portal vein
7 Accessory hepatic artery
8 Common hepatic duct
9 Cystic duct
10 Bile duct
11 Posterior branch of superior pancreaticoduodenal artery
12 Bile and pancreatic ducts entering duodenal wall

13 Descending (second) part of duodenum
14 Head of pancreas
15 Pancreatic duct
16 Posterior branch of inferior pancreaticoduodenal artery
17 Uncinate process of head
18 Superior mesenteric vein
19 Superior mesenteric artery
20 Ascending (fourth) part of duodenum

The liver, from above (with part of the diaphragm attached)
1 Right triangular ligament
2 Diaphragm overlying bare area
3 Superior layer of coronary ligament
4 Inferior vena cava
5 Fibrous pericardium
6 Diaphragm overlying left triangular ligament
7 Superior ⎱ surface of left lobe
8 Anterior ⎰
9 Falciform ligament
10 Anterior ⎱ surface of right lobe
11 Superior ⎰
12 Right surface

● The main surfaces of the liver are named as diaphragmatic and visceral; the diaphragmatic surface has superior, right, anterior and posterior parts (surfaces) and the bare area.
● The caudate and quadrate lobes are classified *anatomically* as part of the right lobe, but *functionally* they belong to the left lobe, since they receive blood from the left branches of the hepatic artery and portal vein, and drain bile to the left hepatic duct.
● The caudate *process* joins the caudate lobe to the right lobe. It is the caudate process (not the caudate lobe) that forms the upper boundary of the epiploic foramen.

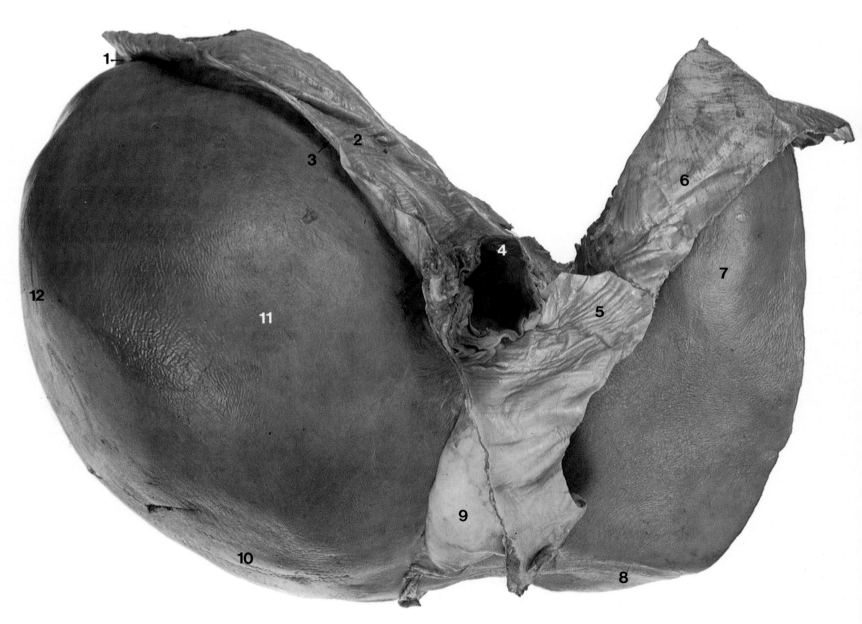

The liver, from above and behind (with part of the diaphragm attached)
1 Left triangular ligament
2 Diaphragm
3 Left lobe
4 Gastric impression
5 Oesophageal groove
6 Lesser omentum in fissure for ligamentum venosum
7 Inferior vena cava
8 Caudate lobe
9 Diaphragm on part of bare area
10 Bare area
11 Inferior layer of coronary ligament
12 Right triangular ligament
13 Renal impression
14 Right lobe
15 Colic impression
16 Duodenal impression
17 Suprarenal impression
18 Caudate process
19 Right free margin of lesser omentum in porta hepatis
20 Portal vein
21 Hepatic artery
22 Bile duct
23 Gall bladder
24 Quadrate lobe
25 Ligamentum teres and falciform ligament in fissure for ligamentum teres
26 Omental tuberosity

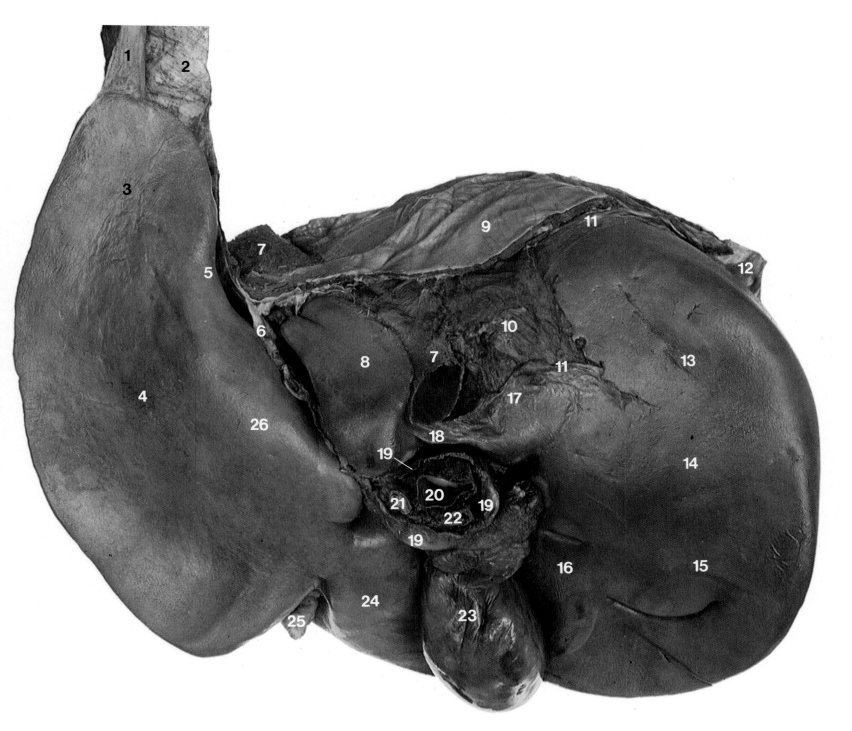

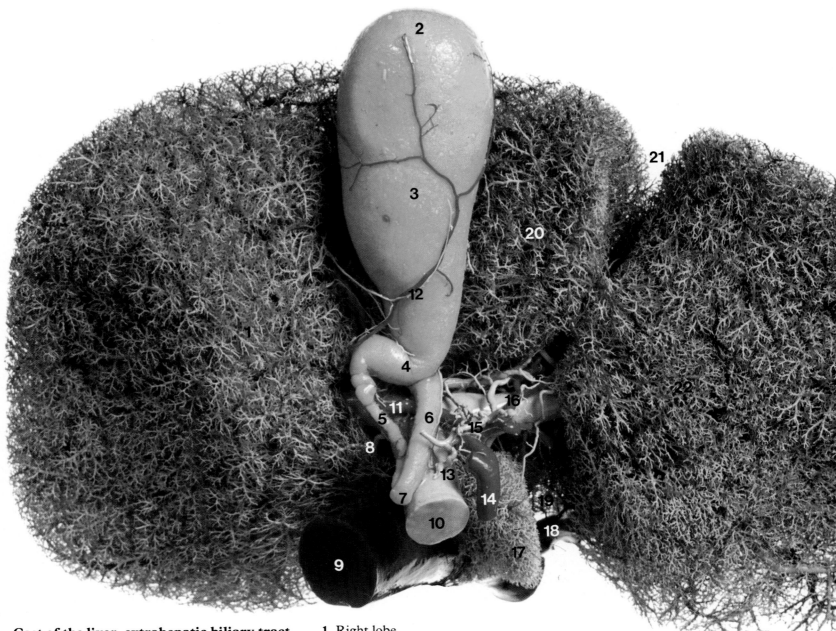

Cast of the liver, extrahepatic biliary tract and associated vessels, from behind
(Yellow, gall bladder and biliary tract; red, hepatic artery and branches; light blue, portal vein and tributaries; dark blue, inferior vena cava, hepatic veins and tributaries)

1 Right lobe
2 Fundus ⎫
3 Body ⎬ of gall bladder
4 Neck ⎭
5 Cystic duct
6 Common hepatic duct
7 Bile duct
8 Caudate process
9 Inferior vena cava
10 Portal vein
11 Right branch of hepatic artery and portal vein
12 Cystic artery and veins
13 Right gastric vein
14 Hepatic artery
15 Left gastric vein
16 Left branch of hepatic artery and portal vein and left hepatic duct
17 Caudate lobe
18 Left hepatic vein
19 Fissure for ligamentum venosum
20 Quadrate lobe
21 Fissure for ligamentum teres
22 Left lobe

Cast of the duodenum, biliary tract and associated vessels, from the front

(Yellow, biliary tract, pancreatic duct and urinary tract; red, arteries; blue, portal venous system)

1 Right branch of portal vein and hepatic artery and right hepatic duct
2 Gall bladder
3 Bile duct
4 Hepatic artery
5 Portal vein
6 Left branch of portal vein and hepatic artery and left hepatic duct
7 Left gastric artery
8 Left gastric vein
9 Splenic artery
10 Splenic vein
11 Short gastric vessels
12 Left gastro-epiploic vessels
13 Vessels of left kidney
14 Pancreatic duct
15 Duodenojejunal flexure
16 Superior mesenteric artery
17 Superior mesenteric vein
18 Horizontal (third) part of duodenum
19 Right gastro-epiploic vessels
20 Pyloric canal
21 Pylorus
22 Superior (first) part of duodenum
23 Right gastric vessels
24 Branches of superior and inferior pancreaticoduodenal vessels
25 Descending (second) part of duodenum
26 Vessels of right kidney

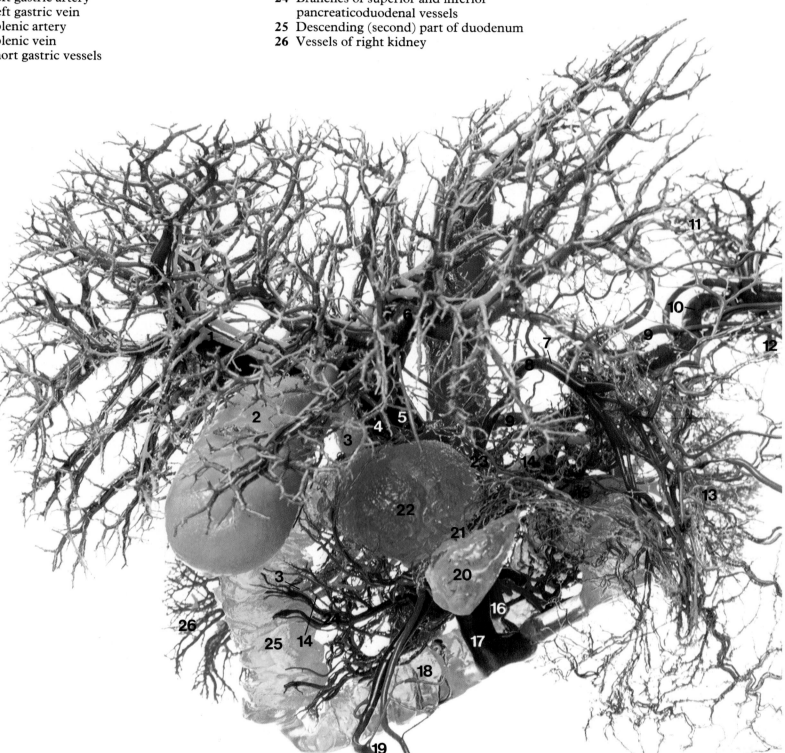

229

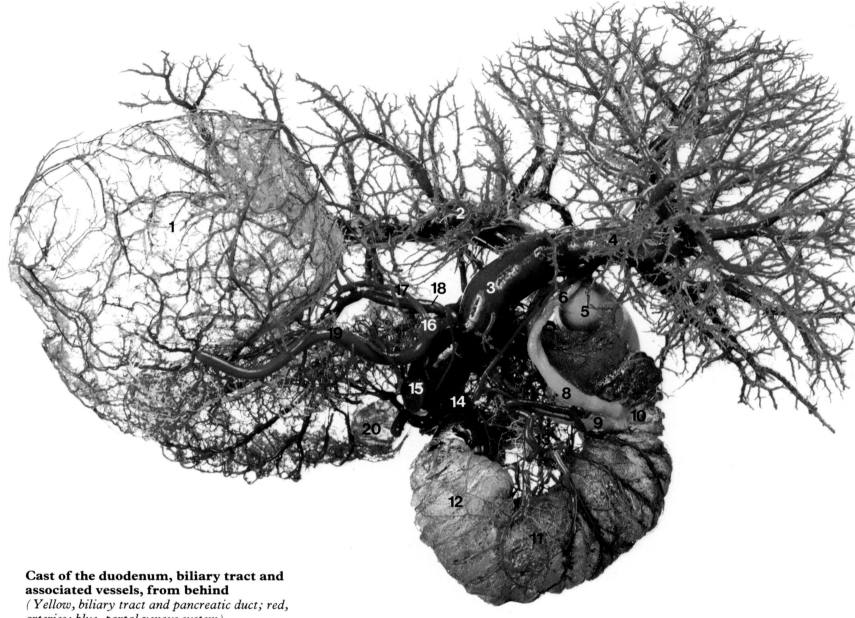

Cast of the duodenum, biliary tract and associated vessels, from behind
(Yellow, biliary tract and pancreatic duct; red, arteries; blue, portal venous system)

1 Stomach outlined by its vessels
2 Left branch of portal vein and hepatic artery and left hepatic duct
3 Portal vein
4 Right branch of portal vein and hepatic artery and right hepatic duct
5 Gall bladder
6 Cystic duct
7 Common hepatic duct
8 Bile duct
9 Pancreatic duct
10 Descending (second) ⎫
11 Horizontal (third) ⎬ part of duodenum
12 Ascending (fourth) ⎭
13 Branches of pancreaticoduodenal vessels
14 Superior mesenteric vein
15 Splenic vein
16 Coeliac trunk
17 Left gastric artery
18 Left gastric vein
19 Splenic artery
20 Pyloric canal

Cast of the liver and associated structures, from above and behind. Hepatic segments (indicated by interrupted lines)

(Green, biliary tract; yellow, pancreatic ducts; red, arteries; blue, portal venous system)

1 Left lateral ⎤
2 Left medial ⎥
3 Right anterior ⎥ segments
4 Right posterior ⎦
5 Gall bladder
6 Descending (second) part of duodenum
7 Accessory pancreatic duct
8 Bile duct
9 Pancreatic duct

10 Inferior pancreaticoduodenal vessels
11 Superior mesenteric vein
12 Superior mesenteric artery
13 Portal vein
14 Left gastric vein
15 Common hepatic artery
16 Gastroduodenal artery
17 Coeliac trunk
18 Left gastric artery
19 Accessory hepatic artery
20 Splenic artery
21 Splenic vein

● The left lateral segment corresponds to the left lobe, and the left medial segment to the caudate and quadrate lobes.

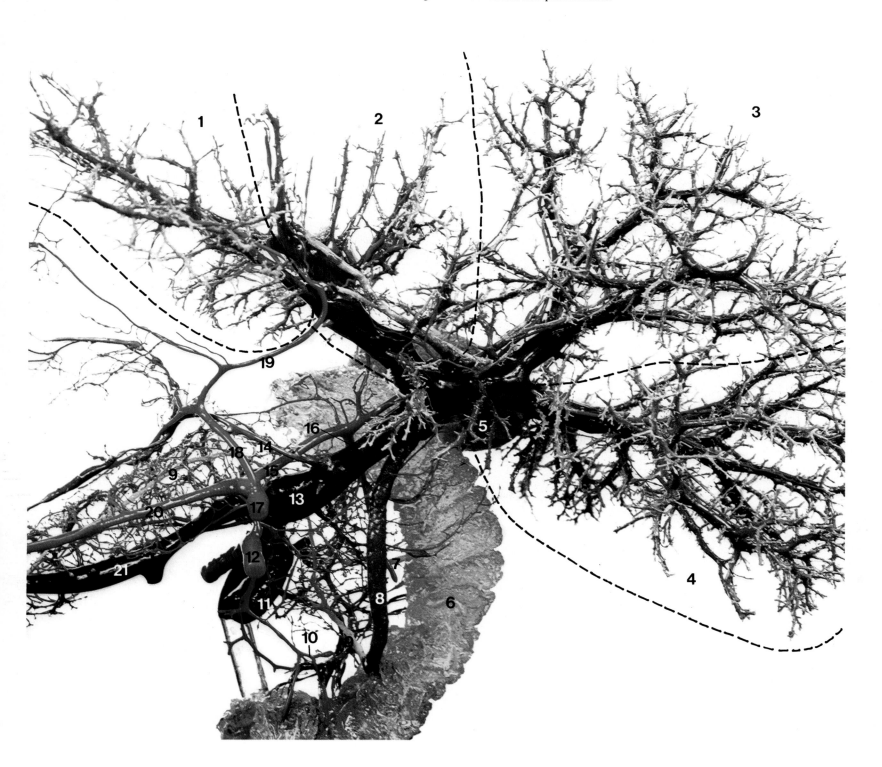

231

Cast of the portal vein and tributaries, from behind

(Yellow, biliary tract and pancreatic ducts; red, arteries; blue, portal venous system)

 1 Pancreatic duct
 2 Splenic vein
 3 Splenic artery
 4 Coeliac trunk
 5 Left gastric artery and vein
 6 Left ⎤ branch of
 7 Right ⎦ hepatic artery
 8 Portal vein
 9 Left ⎤
10 Right ⎦ branch of portal vein
11 Bile duct
12 Pancreaticoduodenal vessels
13 Pancreatic ducts in head of pancreas
14 Branches of middle colic vessels
15 Right colic vessels
16 Ileocolic vessels
17 Inferior mesenteric artery
18 Sigmoid vessels
19 Inferior mesenteric vein
20 Left colic vessels
21 Superior mesenteric artery
22 Superior mesenteric vein

● The inferior mesenteric vein normally drains into the splenic vein behind the body of the pancreas, but it may join the splenic vein nearer the union with the superior mesenteric vein or (as in this specimen) enter the superior mesenteric vein itself.

● The colic arteries anastomose with one another near the colonic wall forming what is often called the marginal artery (as at the arrows).

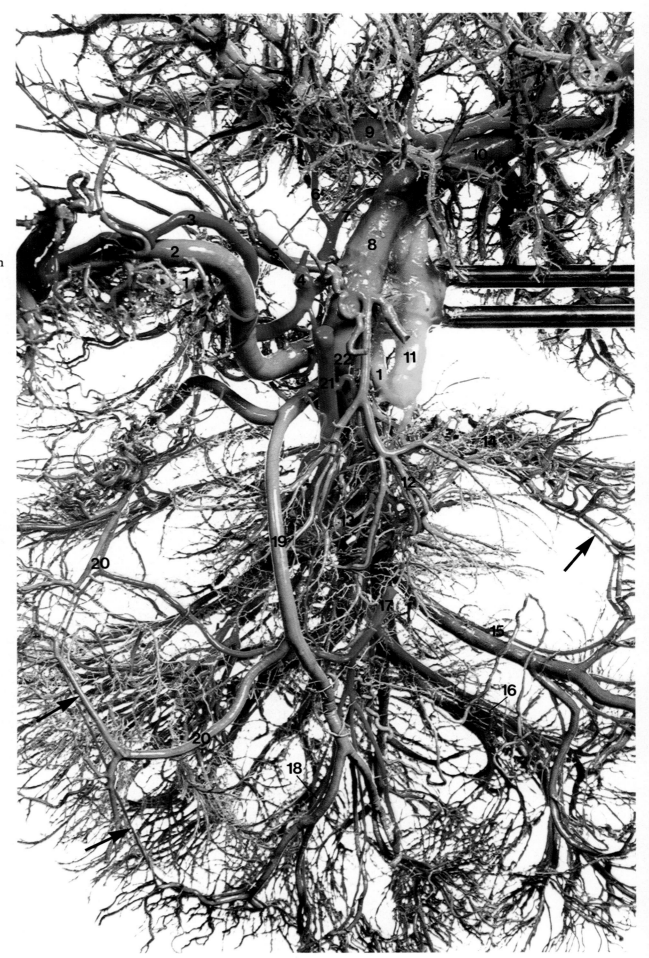

232

The spleen in situ
(The stomach has been pulled towards the right and part of the diaphragm detached and lifted upwards)

1 Diaphragm
2 Stomach
3 Gastrosplenic ligament
4 Gastric impression
5 Superior border
6 Notch
7 Diaphragmatic surface
8 Inferior border
9 Left colic flexure
10 Costodiaphragmatic recess
11 Thoracic wall

● The spleen lies in the long axis of the tenth rib.
● The gastrosplenic ligament contains the short gastric and left gastro-epiploic branches of the splenic vessels.
● The lienorenal ligament contains the tail of the pancreas and the splenic vessels.

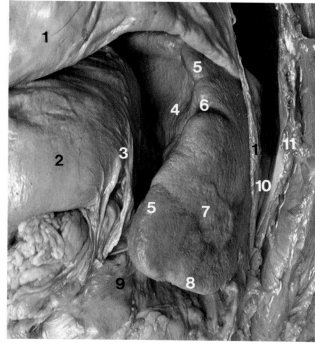

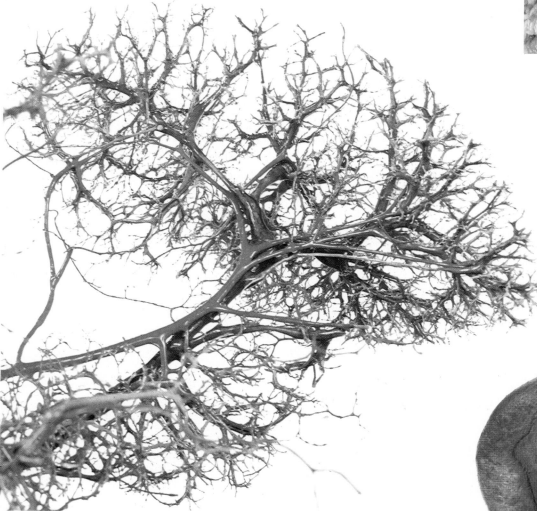

Cast of the splenic vessels, from above and in front. Many pancreatic vessels are also displayed. The pancreatic duct is in yellow

The spleen, visceral surface
1 Superior border
2 Gastric impression
3 Gastrosplenic ligament
4 Notch
5 Colic impression
6 Tail of pancreas and splenic vessels in lienorenal ligament
7 Renal impression
8 Inferior border

233

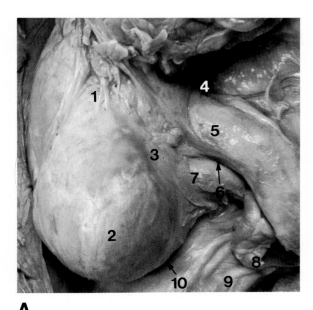

A The appendix in situ

1 Ascending colon
2 Caecum
3 Anterior taenia coli
4 Superior ileocaecal recess
5 Terminal ileum
6 Inferior ileocaecal recess
7 Base ⎱ of appendix
8 Tip ⎰
9 Peritoneum overlying external iliac vessels
10 Retrocaecal recess

● The position of the *base* of the appendix (properly called the vermiform appendix) is constant, opening just below and behind the ileocaecal valve, but the *tip* may lie in a variety of positions – over the pelvic brim, behind the caecum or ascending colon, below the caecum, or behind the terminal part of the ileum.

● The three taeniae coli of the ascending colon and caecum converge on the base of the appendix, and serve as useful guides to the base.

B Interior of the caecum
(After opening the anterior wall)

1 Ascending colon
2 Lips of ileocaecal valve
3 Opening of appendix

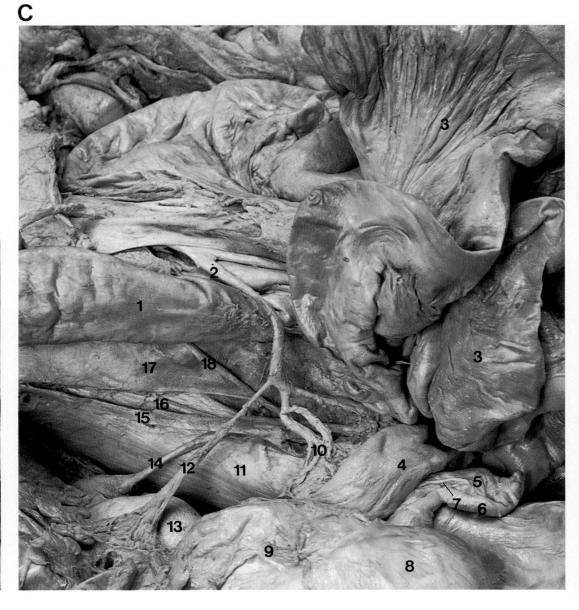

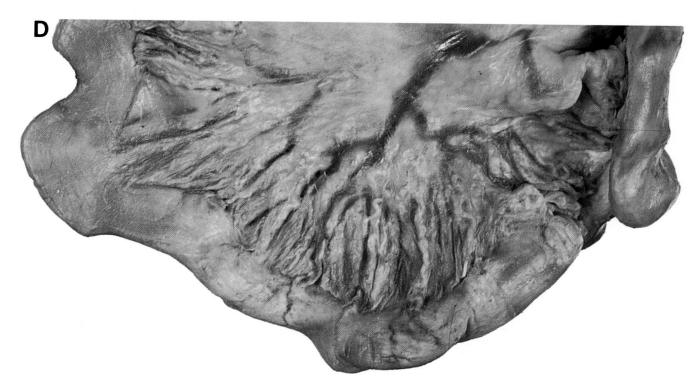

D Part of the mesentery and jejunum

● The vessels are largely obscured by fat in the mesentery

C Ileocolic artery and appendix, from the right

(The peritoneum on the posterior abdominal wall has been removed and the descending part of the duodenum reflected medially)

1 Descending (second) part of the duodenum
2 Ileocolic artery
3 Mesentery and coils of jejunum and ileum
4 Terminal part of ileum
5 Mesoappendix
6 Appendix
7 Appendicular artery in mesoappendix
8 Caecum
9 Ascending colon
10 Ileal and caecal vessels
11 Psoas major
12 Right colic artery
13 Lower pole of kidney
14 Ureter
15 Testicular vein
16 Genitofemoral nerve
17 Inferior vena cava
18 Testicular artery

E Part of the sigmoid colon and mesocolon

● In all parts of the colon (and in the caecum) the outer longitudinal muscle layer is largely collected into three bands, the taeniae coli, one of which is clearly seen here. The taeniae probably give rise to the sacculated appearance of the colon (well illustrated in the radiograph on page 260).

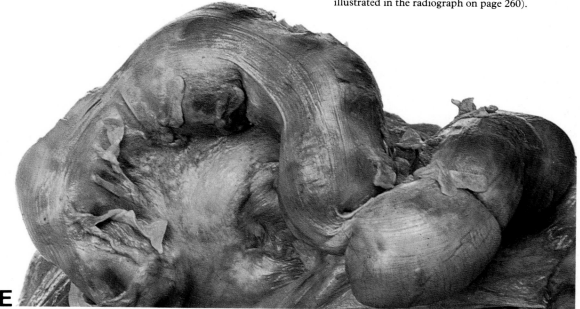

Kidneys and suprarenal glands, in position on the posterior abdominal wall

1 Kidney
2 Suprarenal gland
3 Renal vein
4 Renal artery
5 Inferior vena cava
6 Inferior phrenic artery
7 Crus of diaphragm
8 Left gastric artery
9 Oesophagus
10 Coeliac trunk and coeliac plexus
11 Common hepatic artery
12 Splenic artery
13 Superior mesenteric artery
14 Sympathetic trunk
15 Testicular artery
16 Testicular vein
17 Ureter
18 Subcostal nerve
19 Iliohypogastric nerve
20 Ilio-inguinal nerve
21 Quadratus lumborum
22 Psoas major
23 Inferior mesenteric artery
24 Abdominal aorta and aortic plexus

● In this specimen the testicular arteries arise from the renal arteries instead of the normal origin from the front of the aorta below the origin of the renal arteries.

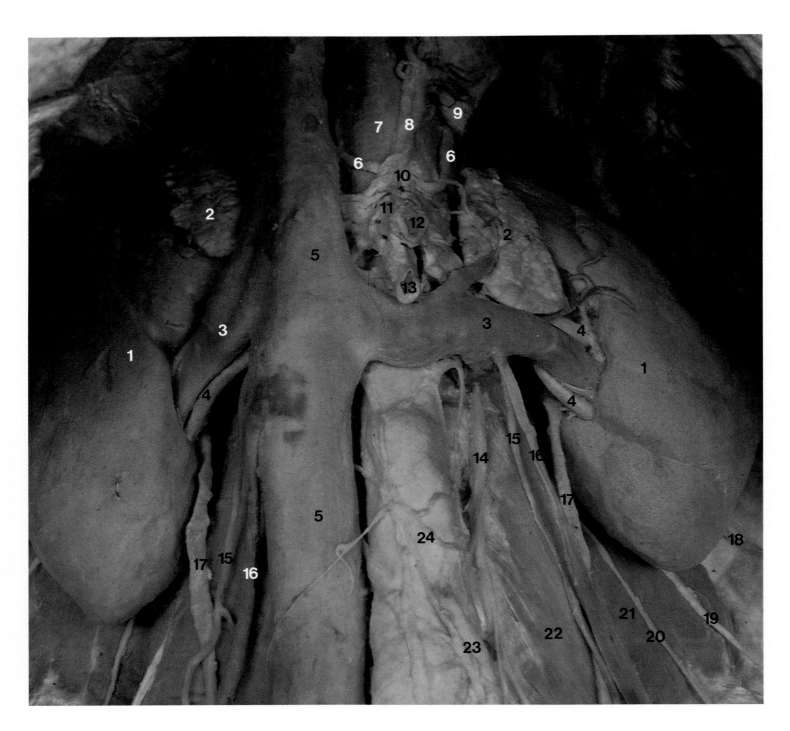

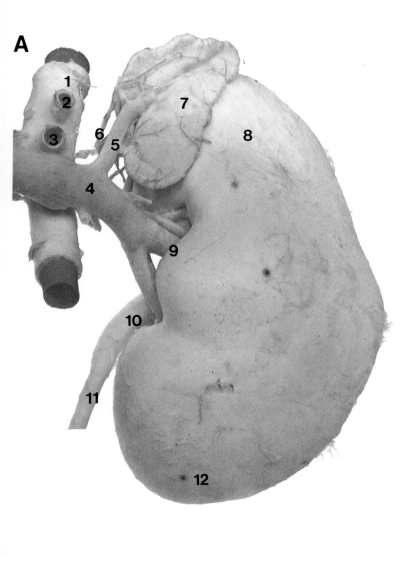

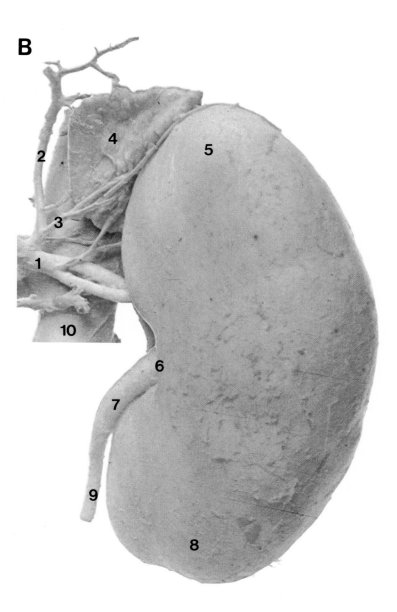

A **Left kidney and suprarenal gland with related vessels, from the front**
1 Abdominal aorta
2 Coeliac trunk
3 Superior mesenteric artery
4 Left renal vein overlying renal artery
5 Left suprarenal vein
6 Suprarenal arteries
7 Suprarenal gland
8 Upper pole of kidney
9 Hilum of kidney
10 Pelvis of kidney
11 Ureter
12 Lower pole of kidney

B **Right kidney and suprarenal gland with related vessels, from behind**
1 Right renal artery
2 Right inferior phrenic artery
3 Suprarenal arteries
4 Suprarenal gland
5 Upper pole of kidney
6 Hilum of kidney
7 Pelvis of kidney
8 Lower pole of kidney
9 Ureter
10 Inferior vena cava

● In the hilum of each kidney the order of structures is: vein, artery, pelvis from before backwards. (Compare with vein, artery, bronchus in the hilum of the lung).

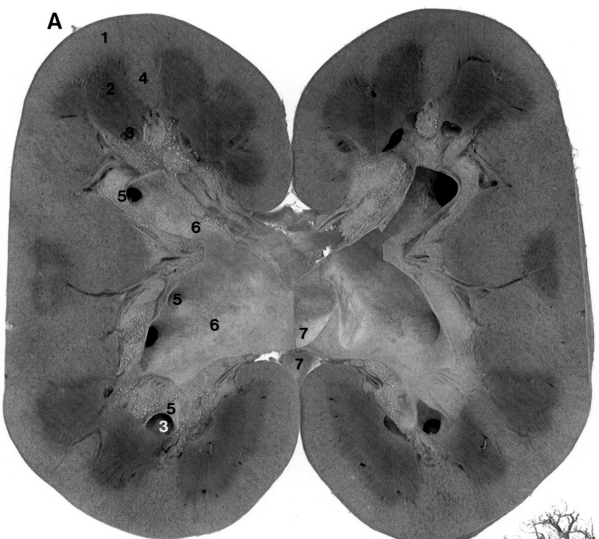

A (label in image)

A The kidney in longitudinal section

1 Cortex
2 Medullary pyramid
3 Papilla
4 Renal column
5 Minor calyx
6 Major calyx
7 Pelvis of kidney

● The renal medulla is composed of the medullary pyramids, whose apices form the renal papillae which project into the minor calyces. The renal columns are the parts of the cortex that intervene between the pyramids. (The granular appearance in part of this preserved specimen is a fixation artefact).

C Cast of the aorta and renal arteries, from the front, with double ureters on the right

1 Early branching of right renal artery
2 Coeliac trunk
3 Superior mesenteric artery
4 Accessory left renal artery
5 Left renal artery

● Accessory renal arteries represent segmental vessels that arise directly from the aorta. In this specimen, the left accessory vessel supplies the superior and anterior superior segments, leaving the 'normal' vessel to supply the posterior, anterior inferior and inferior segments.

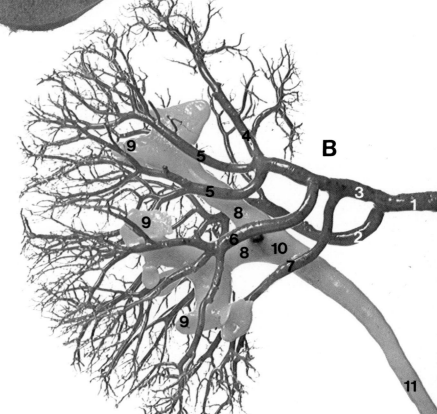

B (label in image)

B Cast of the right renal artery, calyces, pelvis and ureter, from the front

1 Renal artery
2 Posterior division (forming posterior segment artery)
3 Anterior division
4 Superior segment artery
5 Anterior superior segment artery (double)
6 Anterior inferior segment artery
7 Inferior segment artery
8 Major calyx
9 Minor calyx
10 Pelvis of kidney
11 Ureter

● The kidney has five arterial segments, named posterior, superior, anterior superior, anterior inferior and inferior. Typically the renal artery divides into anterior and posterior divisions; the posterior supplies the posterior segment and the anterior supplies the remainder. However, the pattern of branching displays many variations.

● This specimen shows a fairly typical pattern, although the superior segment obtains a small additional branch from the posterior division, and the anterior superior segment receives two major branches.

● The pelvis of the kidney is the funnel-shaped upward continuation of the ureter, and it divides into two (or three) major calyces, each of which receives minor calyces (which range from seven to thirteen in number).

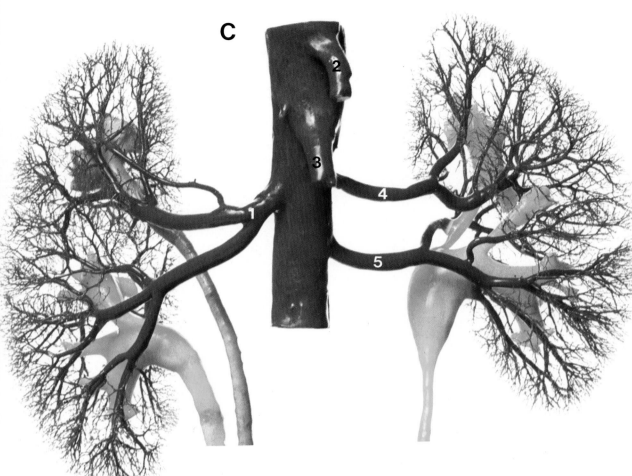

C

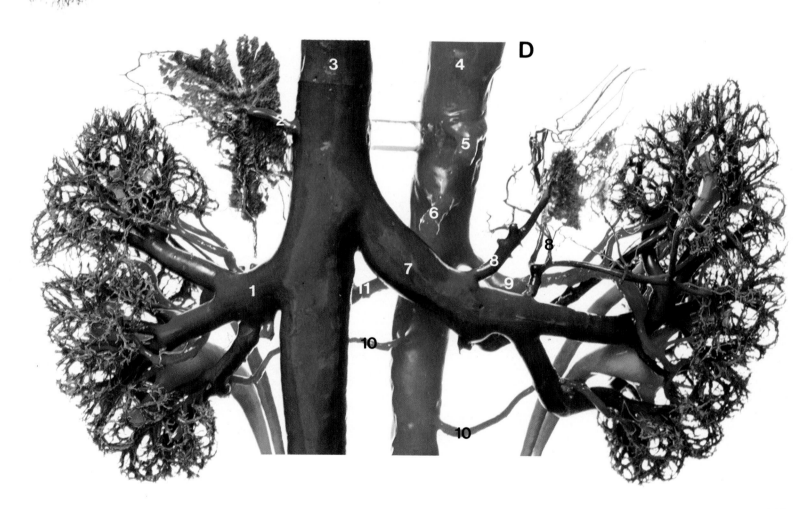

D

D Cast of the aorta, inferior vena cava, renal and supra-renal vessels, from the front, with kidneys with double ureters and accessory arteries

 1 Right renal vein
 2 Right suprarenal vein
 3 Inferior vena cava
 4 Aorta
 5 Coeliac trunk
 6 Superior mesenteric artery
 7 Left renal vein
 8 Left suprarenal veins
 9 Left renal artery
10 Accessory renal arteries
11 Right renal artery

● The left suprarenal vein is double in this specimen. Although the suprarenal glands receive numerous arterial vessels (from the aorta, inferior phrenic and renal arteries), there is normally only one vein from each gland – on the left it drains into the left renal vein, on the right directly into the inferior vena cava.

● The left renal vein crosses the aorta *below* the origin of the superior mesenteric artery. (The splenic vein crosses the aorta *above* the origin of that artery and below the coeliac trunk).

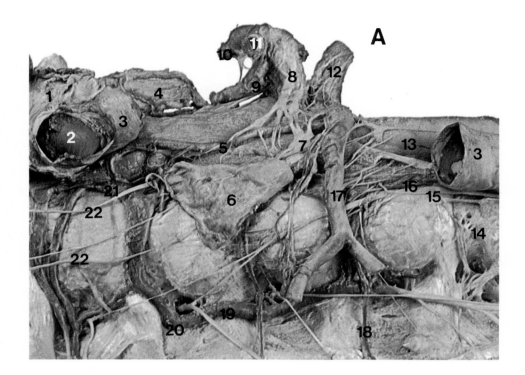

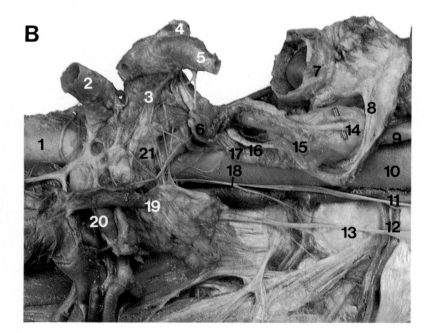

● The two coeliac ganglia lie one on each side of the origin of the coeliac trunk, and form part of the coeliac plexus whose branches pass down in front of the aorta and along all its major branches.

● The anterior and posterior vagal trunks are sometimes known as the gastric nerves, since they provide secretory and motor fibres to the stomach. In the operation of vagotomy, they are cut to diminish gastric secretion and motility.

C Posterior abdominal wall. Crura of the diaphragm after removal of viscera and vessels

1 Right crus
2 Oesophageal opening
3 Left crus
4 Median arcuate ligament
5 Coeliac trunk
6 Aorta
7 Sympathetic trunk
8 Psoas major
9 Medial arcuate ligament
10 Diaphragm
11 Lateral arcuate ligament
12 Quadratus lumborum
13 Subcostal nerve
14 Lumbar part of thoracolumbar fascia
15 Third lumbar artery
16 Second lumbar intervertebral disc
17 Second lumbar vertebra
18 Second lumbar artery
19 First lumbar artery
20 Abnormal communication between crura (superficial to marker)
21 Subcostal artery

● The right crus of the diaphragm has a more extensive origin (from the upper three lumbar vertebrae) than the left (from the upper two) because of the greater bulk of the liver on the right; the crura help to pull the liver downwards when the diaphragm contracts.

● Fibres of the *right* crus form the *right and left* boundaries of the oesophageal opening.

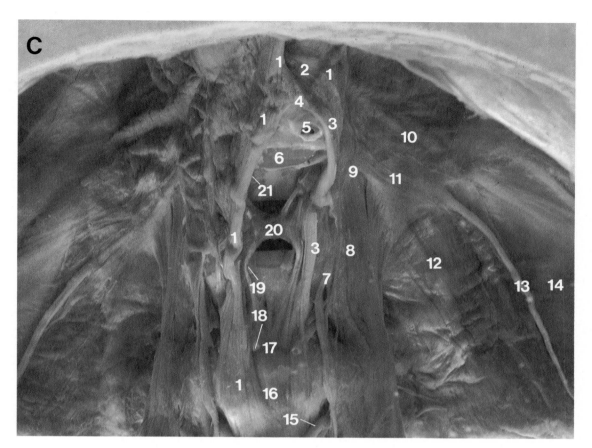

D Posterior abdominal wall. Left side, with the lower part of the kidney, vessels and nerves

1 Suprarenal vein
2 Suprarenal gland
3 Renal vein
4 Renal artery
5 Ureter
6 Lower pole of kidney
7 Ilio-inguinal nerve
8 Quadratus lumborum
9 Iliohypogastric nerve
10 Lumbar part of thoracolumbar fascia
11 Subcostal nerve
12 Transversus abdominis
13 Iliac crest
14 Fourth lumbar artery
15 Testicular vein
16 Testicular artery
17 Psoas major
18 Genitofemoral nerve
19 Inferior mesenteric artery
20 Aorta and aortic plexus
21 Sympathetic trunk and ganglion

● In this specimen the testicular artery arises from the renal artery and not from the aorta which is its normal origin.

● For the lower part of this specimen see the next page.

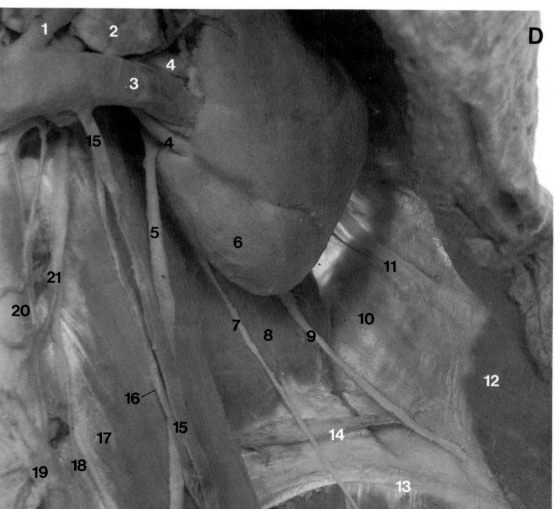

**A Posterior abdominal wall and pelvis.
Vessels and nerves**
1 Psoas major
2 Testicular vessels
3 Ureter
4 Genitofemoral nerve
5 Inferior vena cava
6 Aorta and aortic plexus
7 Inferior mesenteric artery and plexus
8 Sympathetic trunk and ganglia
9 Femoral ⎱ branch of genito-
10 Genital ⎰ femoral nerve
11 Quadratus lumborum
12 Fourth lumbar artery
13 Ilio-inguinal nerve
14 Iliohypogastric nerve
15 Lumbar part of thoracolumbar fascia
16 Iliolumbar ligament
17 Iliacus and branches from femoral nerve
and iliolumbar artery
18 Lateral cutaneous nerve of thigh arising
from femoral nerve
19 Deep circumflex iliac artery
20 Femoral nerve
21 External iliac artery
22 External iliac vein
23 Inguinal ligament

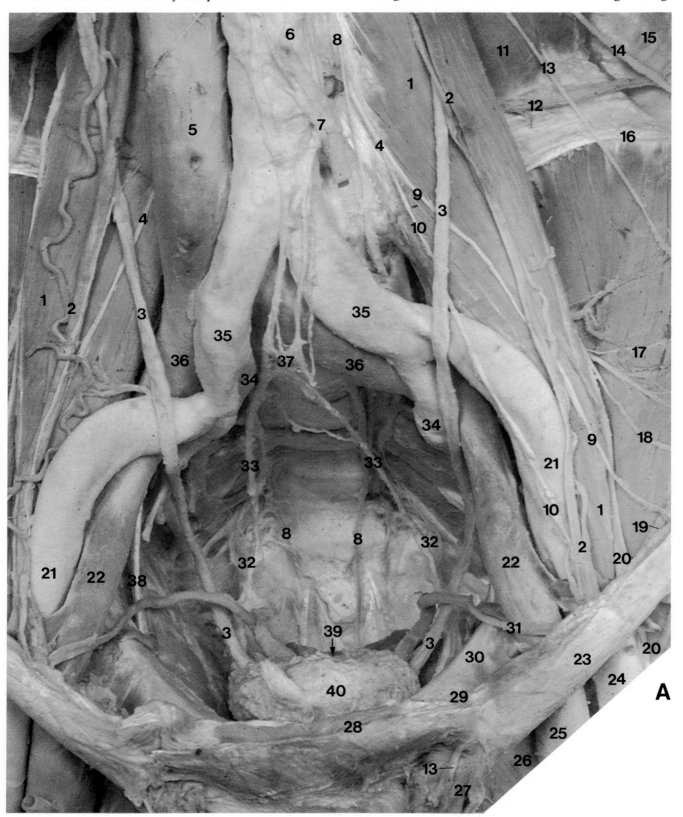

24 Femoral artery
25 Femoral vein
26 Position of femoral canal
27 Spermatic cord
28 Rectus abdominis
29 Lacunar ligament
30 Pectineal ligament
31 Ductus deferens
32 Inferior hypogastric (pelvic) plexus and pelvic splanchnic nerves
33 Hypogastric nerve
34 Internal iliac artery
35 Common iliac artery
36 Common iliac vein
37 Superior hypogastric plexus
38 Obturator nerve and vessels
39 Rectum (cut edge)
40 Bladder

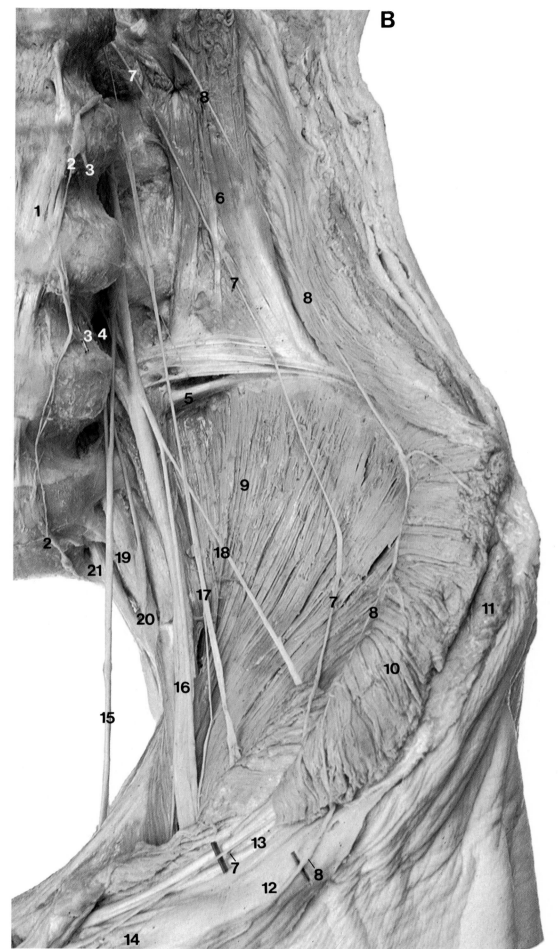

B Left lumbar plexus, from the front, after removal of psoas major

(The lowest parts of the internal oblique muscle and external oblique aponeurosis have been turned downwards)

  1 Third lumbar vertebra and anterior longitudinal ligament
  2 Sympathetic trunk and ganglia
  3 Rami communicantes
  4 Ventral ramus of fourth lumbar nerve
  5 Iliolumbar ligament
  6 Quadratus lumborum
  7 Ilio-inguinal nerve
  8 Iliohypogastric nerve
  9 Iliacus
 10 Internal oblique
 11 External oblique
 12 External oblique aponeurosis
 13 Upper surface of inguinal ligament
 14 Superficial inguinal ring
 15 Obturator nerve
 16 Femoral nerve
 17 Genitofemoral nerve
 18 Lateral cutaneous nerve of thigh
 19 Ventral ramus of fifth lumbar nerve
 20 Lumbosacral trunk
 21 Ventral ramus of first sacral nerve

● The lumbar plexus is embedded *within* the psoas major muscle. The ascending lumbar and lumbar veins lie *behind* the psoas muscle, in front of the vertebral transverse processes.

243

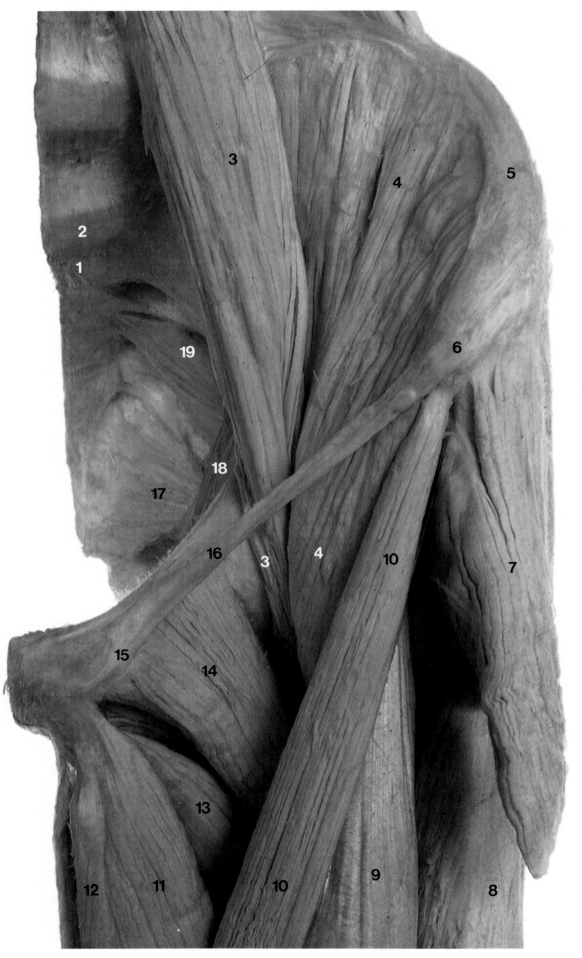

Muscles of the left half of the pelvis and upper thigh, from the front
1 Promontory of sacrum
2 Fifth lumbar intervertebral disc
3 Psoas major
4 Iliacus
5 Iliac crest
6 Anterior superior iliac spine
7 Tensor fasciae latae
8 Vastus lateralis
9 Rectus femoris
10 Sartorius
11 Adductor longus
12 Gracilis
13 Adductor brevis
14 Pectineus
15 Pubic tubercle
16 Inguinal ligament
17 Coccygeus
18 Obturator internus
19 Piriformis

Muscles of the left half of the pelvis, from the right

1 Coccyx
2 Coccygeus
3 Piriformis
4 Sacral canal
5 Promontory of sacrum
6 Psoas major
7 Iliacus
8 Anterior superior iliac spine
9 Inguinal ligament
10 Lacunar ligament
11 Pubic symphysis
12 Adductor longus
13 Gracilis
14 Adductor magnus
15 Gluteus maximus
16 Sacrotuberous ligament
17 Obturator internus
18 Levator ani (cut edge)

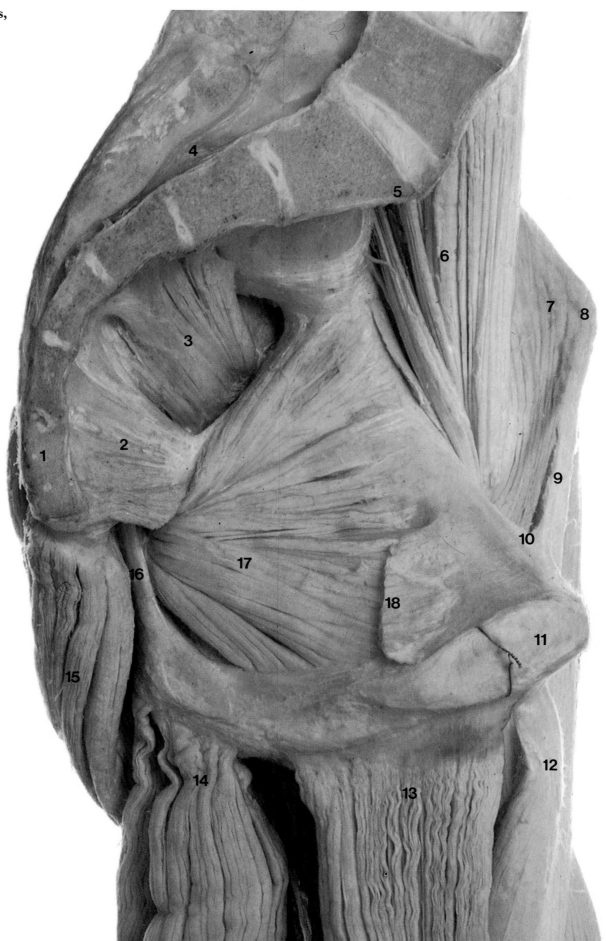

A Right inguinal region, in the male. Superficial dissection

1 External oblique aponeurosis
2 Inguinal ligament
3 Fascia lata
4 Upper margin of saphenous opening
5 Cribriform fascia
6 Great saphenous vein and tributaries
7 Upper margin of superficial inguinal ring
8 Spermatic cord
9 Ilio-inguinal nerve

● The spermatic cord consists of the ductus deferens, the obliterated remains of the processus vaginalis of peritoneum, three arteries (testicular, cremasteric and deferential), the pampiniform plexus of veins, the genital branch of the genitofemoral nerve, sympathetic nerve fibres (accompanying the arteries) from the testicular and pelvic plexuses, and lymph vessels from the testis.

● The *coverings* of the cord consist of the internal spermatic fascia (derived from the transversalis fascia at the deep inguinal ring), the cremasteric fascia (from the transversus and internal oblique muscles), and the external spermatic fascia (from the external oblique aponeurosis at the superficial inguinal ring).

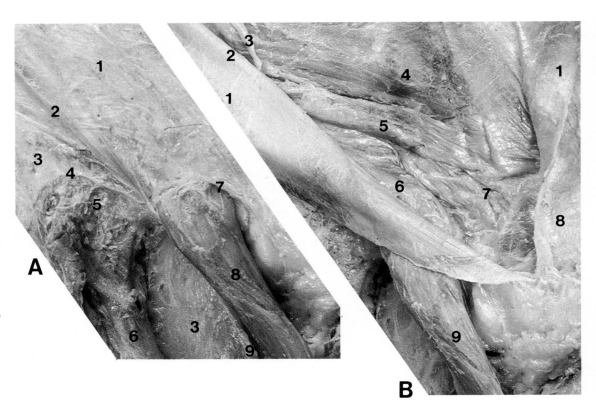

A

B

B Right inguinal canal, in the male

(The external oblique aponeurosis has been incised and reflected)

1 External oblique aponeurosis
2 Inguinal ligament
3 Ilio-inguinal nerve
4 Internal oblique
5 Lowest fibres of internal oblique
6 Spermatic cord covered by internal spermatic and cremasteric fasciae
7 Conjoint tendon
8 Rectus sheath
9 Spermatic cord in its three coverings

● The lowest fibres of the internal oblique muscle (together with those of the transversus abdominis) constitute the roof of the inguinal canal and arch over the spermatic cord to form the conjoint tendon.

● In the male the inguinal canal contains the spermatic cord and the ilio-inguinal nerve.

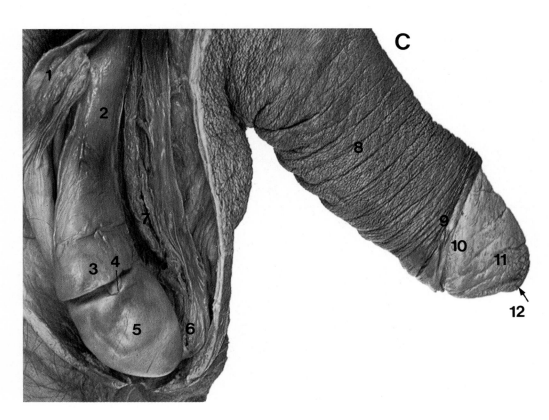

C

C Right testis and epididymis, and the penis

(The scrotum and the tunica vaginalis have been opened and the testis rotated – see note below)

1 Tunica vaginalis
2 Spermatic cord
3 Head of epididymis
4 Appendix of testis
5 Testis
6 Tail of epididymis
7 Ductus deferens
8 Body of penis
9 Foreskin (retracted)
10 Corona of glans
11 Glans penis
12 External urethral orifice

● In its normal position the epididymis adheres to the posterolateral aspect of the testis; in this illustration the testis has been rotated to show that the ductus deferens is the upward continuation of the tail of the epididymis.

D Right inguinal canal in the female

(The external oblique aponeurosis has been reflected downwards)

1 External oblique aponeurosis
2 Ilio-inguinal nerve
3 Internal oblique
4 Upper surface of inguinal ligament
5 Round ligament of uterus in inguinal canal
6 Posterior surface of superficial inguinal ring

● In the female the inguinal canal contains the round ligament of the uterus and the ilio-inguinal nerve.

● The processus vaginalis is normally obliterated, but if it remains patent within the female inguinal canal it is sometimes known as the canal of Nuck.

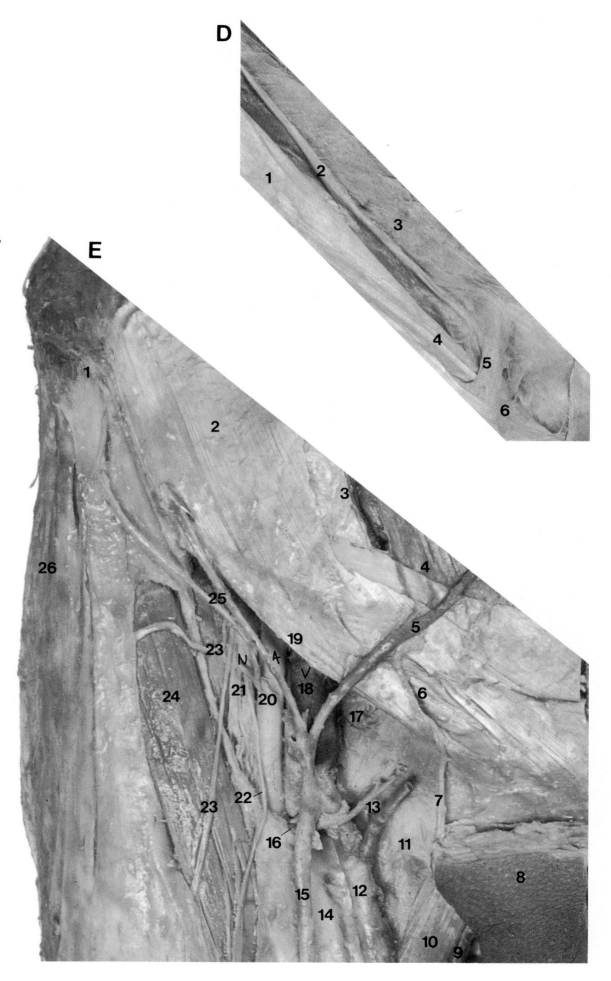

E Right inguinal region in the female. Superficial dissection

1 Anterior superior iliac spine
2 External oblique aponeurosis
3 Cut edge of rectus sheath
4 Rectus abdominis
5 Superficial epigastric vein
6 Superficial inguinal ring
7 Round ligament of uterus
8 Mons pubis
9 Gracilis
10 Adductor longus
11 Pectineus
12 Great saphenous vein
13 Superficial external pudendal vessels
14 Fascia lata
15 Accessory saphenous vein
16 Lower edge of saphenous opening
17 Position of femoral canal
18 Femoral vein
19 Inguinal ligament
20 Femoral artery
21 Femoral nerve
22 Medial   ⎫ cutaneous nerve
23 Intermediate ⎭ of thigh
24 Sartorius
25 Superficial circumflex iliac vessels
26 Fascia lata overlying tensor fasciae latae

● Part of the fascia lata over sartorius and over the upper part of the femoral nerve and vessels has been removed, including the fascia bordering the upper part of the saphenous opening, through which the great saphenous vein and other smaller vessels pass. Anteriorly the upper part of the fascia lata is attached to the inguinal ligament and superior ramus of the pubis.

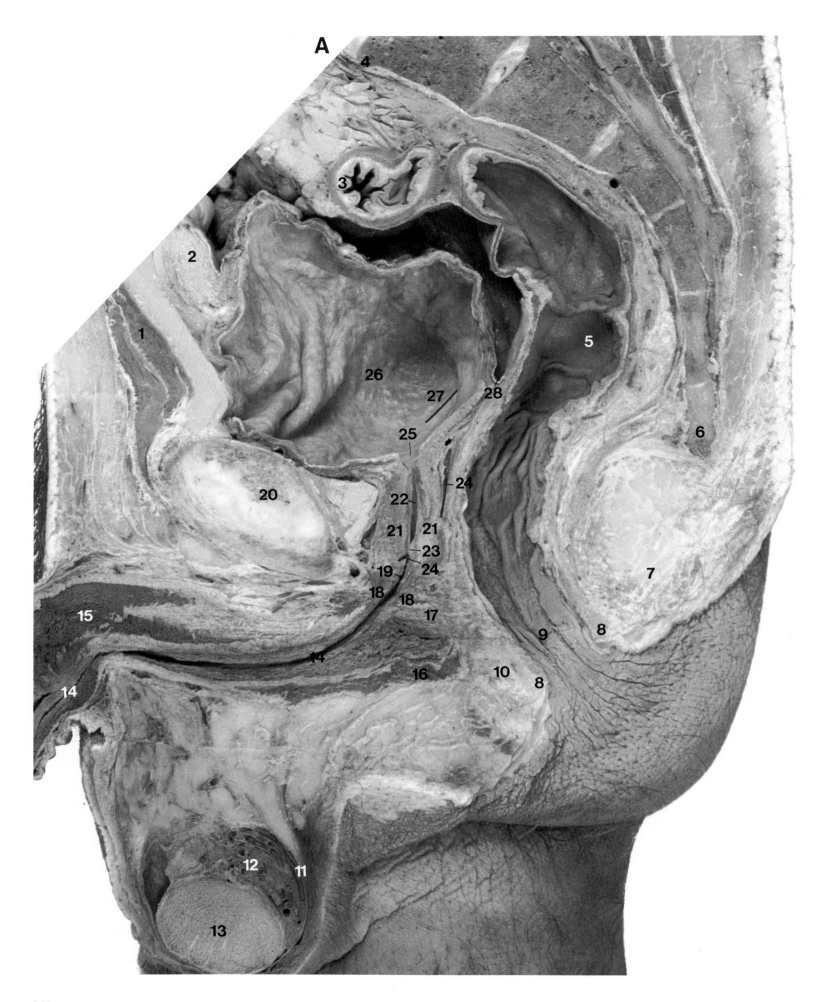

- The various constituents of the spermatic cord come together at the deep inguinal ring, which is in the transversalis fascia *lateral* to the inferior epigastric vessels. The ductus deferens therefore appears to enter the ring by hooking round the lateral side of the vessels.
- The inguinal triangle is the area bounded laterally by the inferior epigastric vessels, medially by the lateral border of rectus abdominis and below by the inguinal ligament. A *direct* inguinal hernia passes forwards through this triangle, *medial* to the inferior epigastric vessels.
- An indirect inguinal hernia passes through the deep inguinal ring *lateral* to the inferior epigastric vessels.
- A femoral hernia passes into the femoral canal through the femoral ring, bounded medially by the lacunar ligament and laterally by the femoral vein (the external iliac vein becomes the femoral vein as it passes beneath the inguinal ligament).

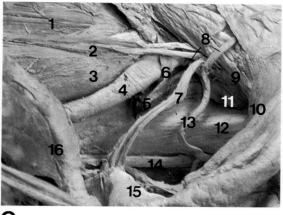

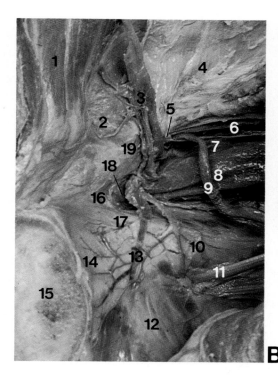

A Right half of a midline sagittal section through the pelvis in the male

(The section has passed through part of the left side of the scrotum and testis)

1 Rectus abdominis
2 Extraperitoneal fat
3 Sigmoid colon
4 Promontory of sacrum
5 Rectum
6 Coccyx
7 Anococcygeal body
8 External anal sphincter
9 Anal canal with anal columns of mucous membrane
10 Perineal body
11 Ductus deferens
12 Epididymis
13 Testis
14 Spongy part of urethra and corpus spongiosum
15 Corpus cavernosum
16 Bulbospongiosus
17 Perineal membrane
18 Sphincter urethrae
19 Membranous part of urethra
20 Pubic symphysis
21 Prostate gland
22 Prostatic part of urethra
23 Seminal colliculus
24 Bristle in ejaculatory duct
25 Internal urethral orifice
26 Bladder
27 Bristle passing up into right ureteral orifice
28 Rectovesical pouch

B Right deep inguinal ring and inguinal triangle, in the male

(As seen when looking into the right half of the pelvis from the left, with the peritoneum removed)

1 Rectus abdominis
2 Conjoint tendon
3 Inferior epigastric vessels
4 Transversalis fascia overlying transversus abdominis
5 Deep inguinal ring
6 Testicular vessels
7 External iliac artery
8 External iliac vein
9 Ductus deferens
10 Superior ramus of pubis
11 Obturator nerve
12 Origin of levator ani from fascia overlying obturator internus
13 Pubic branches of inferior epigastric vessels
14 Body of pubis
15 Pubic symphysis
16 Lacunar ligament
17 Pectineal ligament
18 Femoral ring
19 Inguinal ligament

C Left abnormal obturator artery, in the male, from the right

1 Iliacus
2 Testicular vessels
3 Psoas major
4 External iliac artery
5 External iliac vein (cut end)
6 Deep circumflex iliac vein
7 Ductus deferens
8 Inferior epigastric artery
9 Inguinal ligament
10 Lacunar ligament
11 Femoral ring
12 Superior ramus of pubis and pectineal ligament
13 Abnormal obturator artery
14 Obturator nerve
15 Bladder
16 Right common iliac artery and vein

- The anastomosis between the pubic branches of the inferior epigastric and obturator arteries may be unusually large, forming the vessel known as the abnormal obturator artery, in which case the normal obturator branch from the internal iliac may be absent.
- The abnormal obturator artery *usually* lies at the *lateral* margin of the femoral ring, but rarely it lies at the medial edge of the ring, i.e. at the lateral margin of the lacunar ligament, where it may be at risk if the ligament has to be incised to enlarge the femoral ring in operations to reduce a femoral hernia.

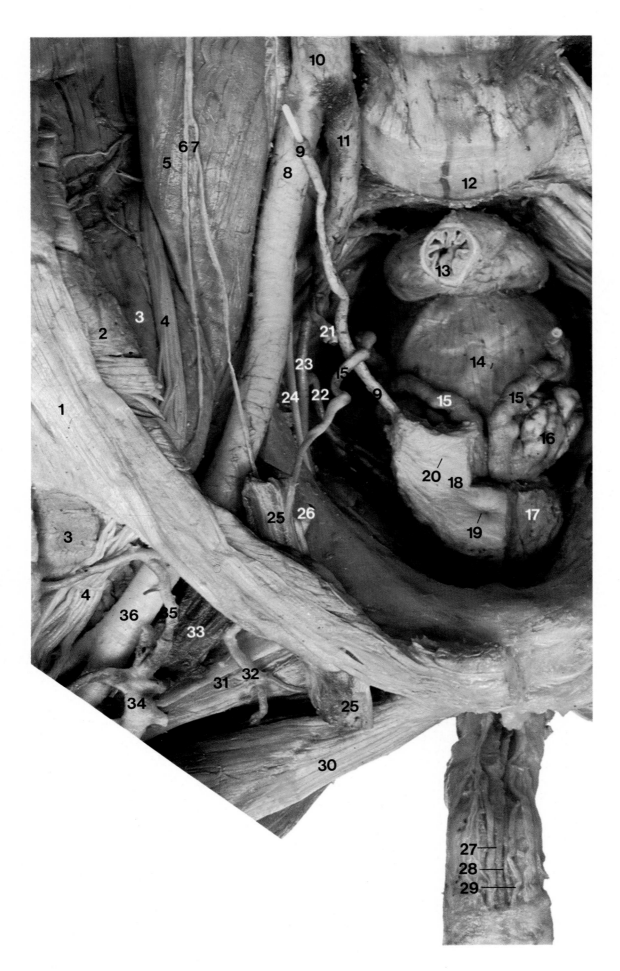

Right inguinal region and pelvis in the male, from above
(Most of the urinary bladder, except for part of the trigone, and pelvic veins have been removed)

 1 External oblique aponeurosis
 2 Internal oblique
 3 Iliacus
 4 Femoral nerve
 5 Psoas major
 6 Femoral ⎫ branch of genito-
 7 Genital ⎬ femoral nerve
 8 External iliac artery
 9 Ureter
10 Common iliac artery
11 Internal iliac artery
12 Fifth lumbar intervertebral disc
13 Sigmoid colon (cut lower end)
14 Rectum
15 Ductus deferens
16 Seminal vesicle
17 Prostate
18 Trigone of bladder
19 Internal urethral orifice
20 Ureteral orifice
21 Superior vesical artery
22 Inferior vesical artery
23 Obturator artery
24 Obturator nerve
25 Spermatic cord
26 Inferior epigastric artery
27 Deep dorsal vein ⎫
28 Dorsal artery ⎬ of penis
29 Dorsal nerve ⎭
30 Adductor longus
31 Pectineus
32 Deep external pudendal artery
33 Femoral vein
34 Great saphenous vein
35 Superficial circumflex iliac vein
36 Femoral artery

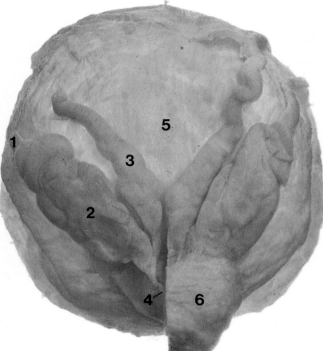

The urinary bladder and prostate gland, from behind

(The bladder has been distended and the left half of the prostate removed)

1 Ureter
2 Seminal vesicle
3 Ductus deferens
4 Left ejaculatory duct
5 Base of bladder
6 Posterior surface of prostate

● The base of the bladder is its posterior surface.
● The base of the prostate is its upper surface, in contact with the neck of the bladder and pierced by the urethra.
● In the male pelvis the ureter is crossed superficially by the ductus deferens. (In the female pelvis the ureter is crossed superficially by the uterine artery.)

Right side of the pelvis in the male, from the left and above

(Most of the urinary bladder and all pelvic veins have been removed)

1 External oblique aponeurosis
2 Internal oblique
3 Transversus abdominis
4 Spermatic cord
5 Ductus deferens
6 Psoas major
7 External iliac vein (cut edge)
8 External iliac artery
9 Genital branch ⎫ of genitofemoral
10 Femoral branch ⎬ nerve
11 Femoral nerve ⎭
12 Psoas minor
13 Ureter
14 Common iliac artery
15 Internal iliac artery
16 Fifth lumbar intervertebral disc
17 Ventral ramus of first sacral nerve and lateral sacral artery
18 Sigmoid colon (cut lower end)
19 Rectum
20 Seminal vesicle
21 Trigone of bladder
22 Internal urethral orifice
23 Ureteral orifice
24 Obturator internus
25 Obturator artery
26 Pubic branch of obturator artery
27 Obturator nerve
28 Inferior vesical artery
29 Superior vesical artery
30 Anterior trunk of internal iliac artery

● The superior gluteal artery is hidden by the internal iliac artery, just above the first sacral nerve.

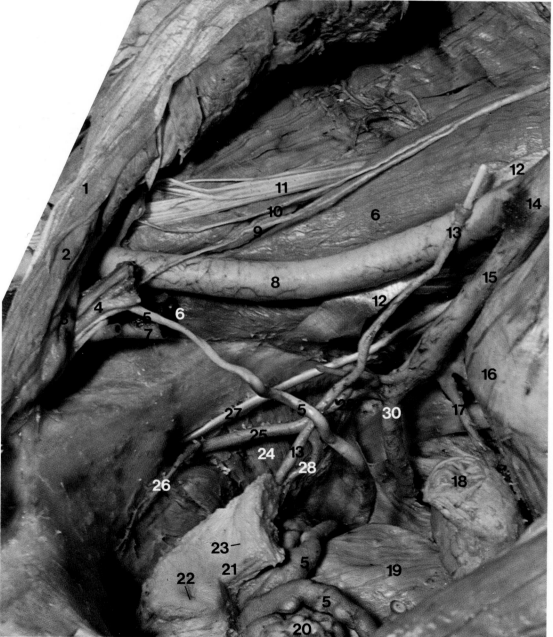

A Left side of the pelvic cavity. Iliac arteries

1 Sacrococcygeal joint
2 Coccygeus and sacrospinous ligament
3 Union of ventral rami of second and third sacral nerves
4 Piriformis
5 Inferior gluteal artery
6 Ventral ramus of first sacral nerve
7 Lateral sacral artery
8 Superior gluteal artery piercing lumbosacral trunk
9 Posterior trunk of internal iliac artery
10 Sacral promontory
11 Internal iliac artery
12 Anterior trunk of internal iliac artery
13 Internal pudendal artery
14 Obturator nerve and artery
15 External iliac artery
16 Inferior epigastric artery
17 Inguinal ligament
18 Lacunar ligament
19 Pubic symphysis
20 Obturator internus
21 Ischial tuberosity

● The internal pudendal and inferior gluteal arteries are the terminal branches of the anterior trunk of the internal iliac artery. The inferior gluteal artery, which passes posteriorly below piriformis into the gluteal region, lies posterior to the internal pudendal.

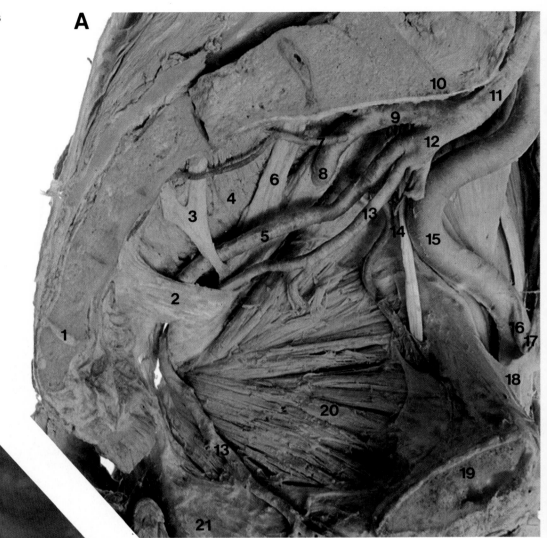

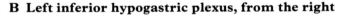

B Left inferior hypogastric plexus, from the right

(After removal of most of the right pelvic wall, but the anterior part of the right levator ani muscle has been preserved)

1 Ventral ramus of first sacral nerve
2 Superior gluteal artery
3 Lumbosacral trunk
4 Arcuate line
5 Fascia overlying obturator internus
6 Left inferior hypogastric plexus
7 Left seminal vesicle
8 Left ductus deferens
9 Rectum
10 Lateral surface of fascia overlying right obturator internus
11 Right levator ani and ischiorectal fossa
12 Right ischiopubic ramus
13 Left coccygeus and nerves to levator ani
14 Ischial spine
15 Left levator ani
16 Pelvic splanchnic nerves (nervi erigentes)
17 Ventral ramus of third sacral nerve
18 Ventral ramus of second sacral nerve
19 Part of left sympathetic trunk

● The pelvic splanchnic nerves are not confined to the pelvis; on the left branches from them pass upwards behind the peritoneum on the posterior abdominal wall to the left colic flexure, descending colon and sigmoid colon.

Left half of the pelvis, internal surface.
Ligaments

1 Sacral promontory
2 Iliac fossa
3 Anterior superior iliac spine
4 Anterior inferior iliac spine and origin of straight head of rectus femoris
5 Inguinal ligament
6 Lacunar ligament
7 Pectineal ligament
8 Pubic symphysis
9 Obturator foramen
10 Obturator membrane
11 Falciform process of sacrotuberous ligament
12 Ischial tuberosity
13 Sacrotuberous ligament
14 Lesser sciatic foramen
15 Ischial spine
16 Sacrospinous ligament
17 Greater sciatic foramen
18 Ventral sacro-iliac ligament

● The sacrospinous and sacrotuberous ligaments convert the greater and lesser sciatic notches into foramina.

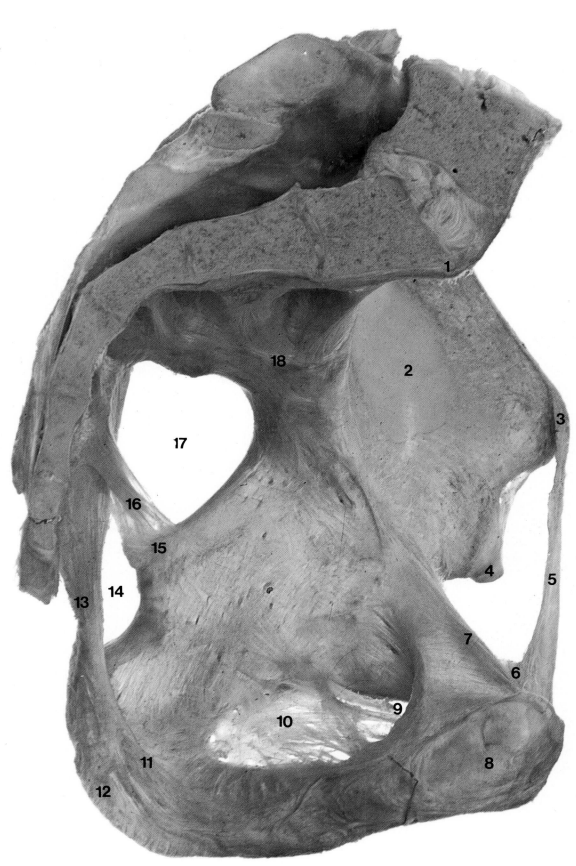

253

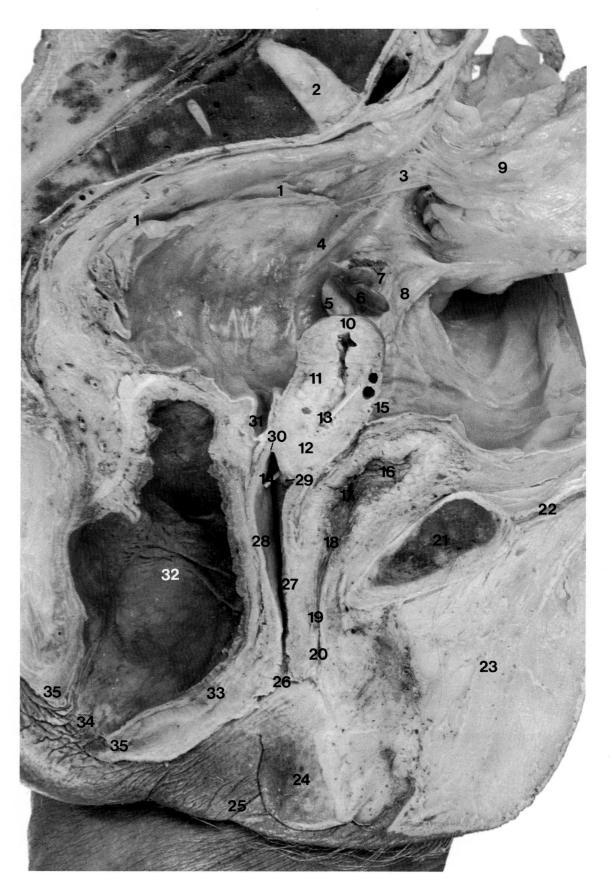

Left half of a midline sagittal section through the pelvis in the female

(The right limb of the sigmoid mesocolon has been detached from the posterior pelvic wall. The lower end of the rectum is dilated, and the bladder, uterus and vagina are contracted)

1 Line of attachment of right limb of sigmoid mesocolon
2 Fifth lumbar intervertebral disc
3 Apex of sigmoid mesocolon
4 Ureter underlying peritoneum
5 Ovary
6 Uterine tube
7 Suspensory ligament of ovary containing ovarian vessels
8 Left limb of sigmoid mesocolon overlying external iliac vessels
9 Sigmoid colon (reflected to left and upwards)
10 Fundus ⎫
11 Body ⎬ of uterus
12 Cervix ⎭
13 Marker in internal os
14 Marker in external os
15 Vesico-uterine pouch
16 Bladder
17 Marker in left ureteral orifice
18 Internal urethral orifice
19 Urethra
20 External urethral orifice
21 Pubic symphysis
22 Rectus abdominis (turned forwards)
23 Fat of mons pubis
24 Labium minor
25 Labium major
26 Vestibule ⎫
27 Anterior wall ⎪
28 Posterior wall ⎬ of vagina
29 Anterior fornix ⎪
30 Posterior fornix ⎭
31 Recto-uterine pouch (of Douglas)
32 Rectum
33 Perineal body
34 Anal canal
35 External anal sphincter

● The apex of the sigmoid mesocolon is a guide to the position of the left ureter which lies under the peritoneum at this point.
● The recto-uterine pouch of peritoneum overlies the posterior fornix of the vagina, but the vesico-uterine pouch does not reach the anterior fornix.

A The uterus and ovaries, from above and in front

1 Recto-uterine pouch (of Douglas)
2 Ligament of ovary
3 Uterine ⎫
4 Tubal ⎬ extremity of ovary
5 Infundibulum ⎫
6 Ampulla ⎬ of uterine tube
7 Isthmus ⎭
8 Round ligament of uterus
9 Fundus of uterus
10 Vesico-uterine pouch
11 Peritoneum overlying bladder
12 Mesosalpinx
13 Posterior surface of broad ligament
14 Mesovarium
15 Suspensory ligament of ovary

● The ovary normally lies against the lateral pelvic wall in front of the ureter and internal iliac artery.

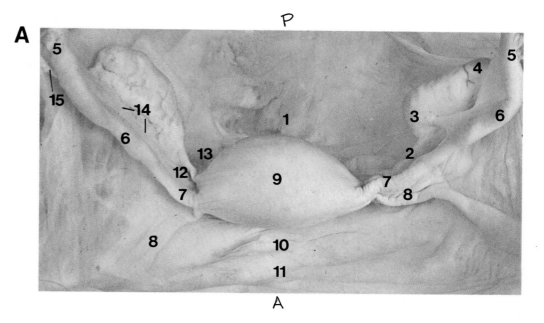

B The bladder, uterus, vagina and rectum, from the right, after removal from the pelvis

(See note below for an explanation of this view)

1 Anterior trunk of internal iliac artery
2 Ureter
3 Ovarian vessels
4 Side of body of uterus
5 Obliterated umbilical artery (medial umbilical ligament)
6 Bladder
7 Superior vesical artery
8 Obliterated urachus (median umbilical ligament)
9 Vagina
10 Levator ani
11 Rectum
12 Superior rectal artery
13 Internal pudendal artery
14 Vaginal artery
15 Obturator artery
16 Vaginal venous plexus
17 Inferior vesical artery
18 Uterine venous plexus
19 Uterine artery
20 Lateral fornix of vagina and cervix of uterus
21 Inferior gluteal artery

● With the removal of the viscera from the pelvis, the structures that are normally situated retroperitoneally are displayed from the lateral side. The peritoneum has been stripped upwards off the viscera. In the absence of the lateral and posterior pelvic walls, the obturator and inferior gluteal branches of the internal iliac artery are inevitably cut and their proximal ends displaced from their normal course.

● The origins of the branches of the internal iliac artery are variable, and here the superior vesical branch arises from the uterine artery, and the vaginal branch from the internal pudendal. There is a separate inferior vesical branch; in the female the vaginal artery usually takes the place of this vessel. The middle rectal artery is absent, as it usually is in the female (in the male it supplies the prostate).

● In the female pelvis the ureter is crossed superficially by the uterine artery and then lies in the lower and medial part of the connective tissue between the two layers of peritoneum that form the broad ligament.

● The transverse cervical ligaments (of Mackenrodt; cardinal ligaments) are important in anchoring the uterine cervix and vaginal fornices in their normal position. They pass from the lateral side of the cervix and fornices to the lateral pelvic walls, becoming continuous with the connective tissue surrounding the branches of the internal iliac artery, and have therefore been removed in dissections such as B.

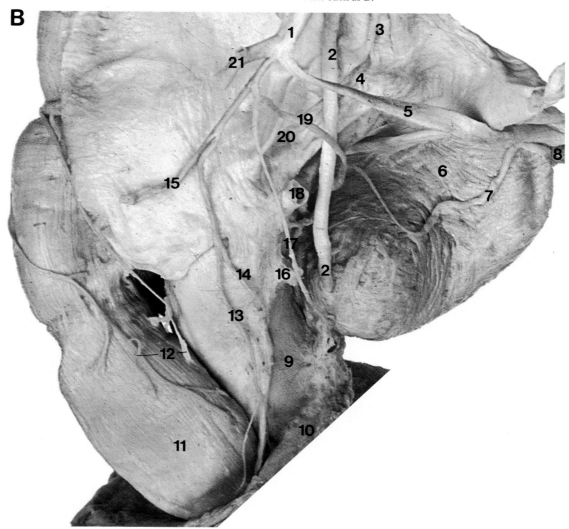

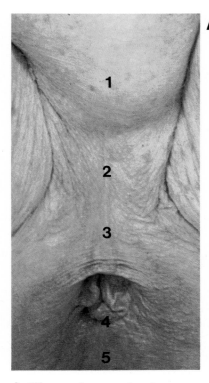

B Ischiorectal fossae and perineum in the male, from below

(On the right the perineal membrane and urogenital diaphragm have been removed)

1 Perineal branch of posterior cutaneous nerve of thigh
2 Adductor magnus
3 Gracilis
4 Adductor longus
5 Posterior scrotal vessels and nerves
6 Corpus cavernosum of penis
7 Corpus spongiosum of penis
8 Bulbospongiosus overlying bulb of penis
9 Ischiocavernosus overlying crus of penis

10 Superficial transverse perineal muscle overlying posterior border of perineal membrane
11 Inferior rectal vessels and nerve in ischiorectal fossa
12 Perforating cutaneous nerve
13 Gluteus maximus
14 Anococcygeal body
15 Margin of anus
16 Sacrotuberous ligament
17 Perineal nerve
18 Internal pudendal artery
19 Perineal artery
20 Artery to bulb
21 Dorsal nerve and artery of penis
22 Levator ani

C Root of the penis, from in front and below

1 Pubic tubercle
2 Pubic crest
3 Pubic symphysis
4 Suspensory ligament
5 Deep dorsal vein
6 Dorsal artery
7 Dorsal nerve
8 Corpus cavernosum
9 Corpus spongiosum
10 Urethra
11 Perineal membrane
12 Ischiopubic ramus
13 Obturator membrane

● In the male the subpubic arch (below the pubic symphysis between the inferior pubic rami) makes an angle measuring about 50 to 60°, but in the female it more nearly approaches a right angle.

A The perineum, in the male from below (with the scrotum pulled upwards)

1 Scrotum overlying left testis
2 Raphe overlying bulb of penis
3 Perineal body
4 Margin of anus
5 Anococcygeal body

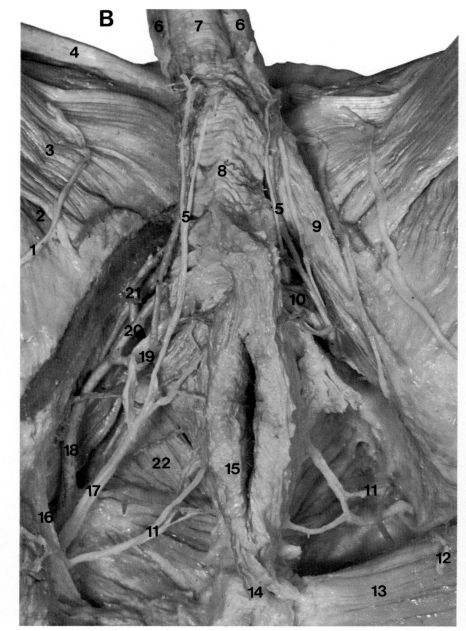

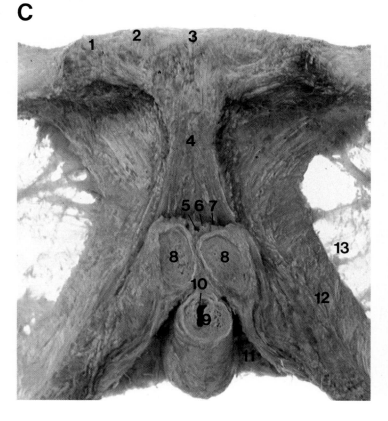

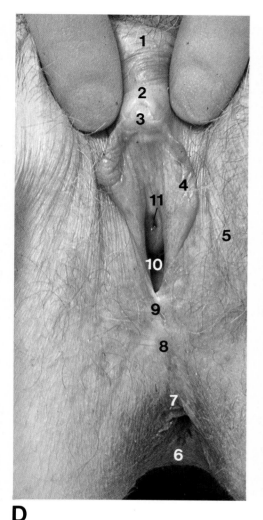

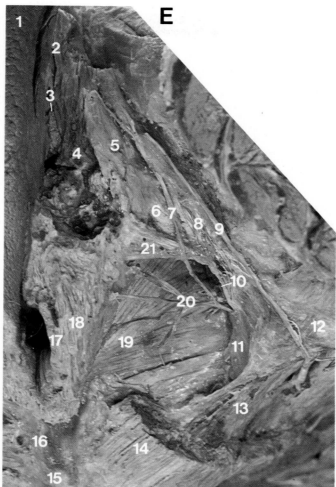

E

D

● The pudendal cleft is the region between the two labia majora into which the vagina and urethra open.
● The vestibule is the cleft between the labia minora. The lesser vestibular glands open on the inner surface of these labia.

● In B the pudendal canal on the lateral wall of the ischiorectal fossa has been opened to display the internal pudendal artery and the terminal branches of the pudendal nerve (perineal nerve and dorsal nerve of penis). The canal is shown intact in the female in F.
● The inferior rectal nerve and vessels cross the fossa transversely.

F

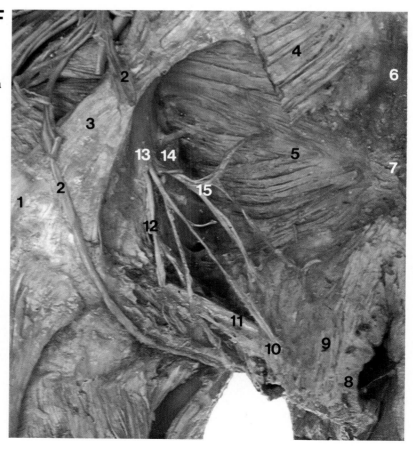

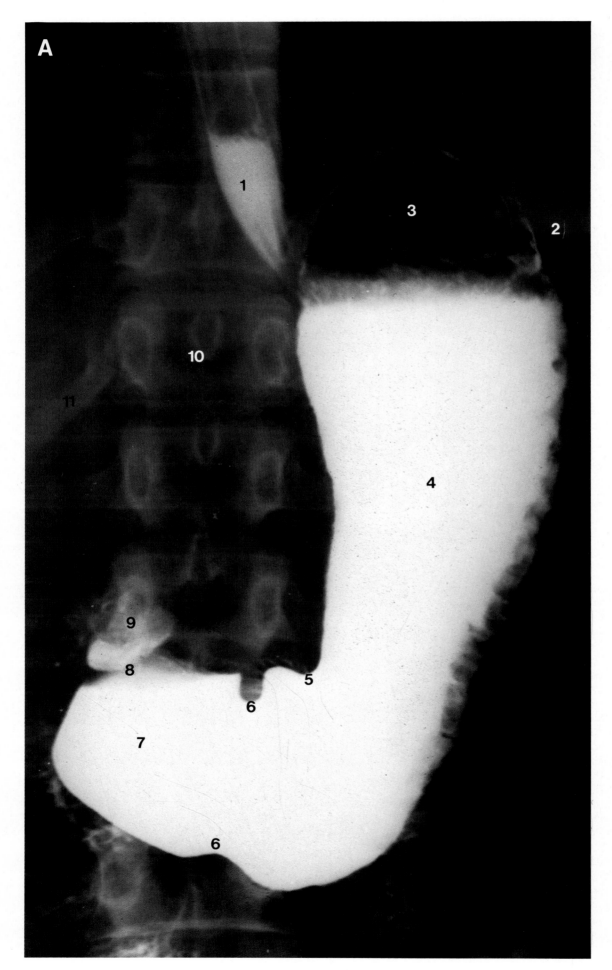

A Radiograph of the stomach in the female, a few minutes after drinking a barium meal

1 Lower end of oesophagus
2 Lower margin of shadow of left breast
3 Fundus
4 Body
5 Angular notch
6 Peristaltic wave
7 Pyloric antrum
8 Pylorus
9 Superior (first) part of duodenum (duodenal cap)
10 Twelfth thoracic vertebra
11 Twelfth rib

● A small amount of barium has entered the descending (second) part of the duodenum.

B Radiograph of the small intestine, three hours after a barium meal

1 Superior (first)
2 Descending (second) ⎤ part of
3 Horizontal (third)   ⎥ duodenum
4 Ascending (fourth) ⎦
5 Pylorus
6 Pyloric antrum
7 Body of stomach
8 Coils of jejunum and ileum

● The junction of the descending and horizontal parts of the duodenum is obscured by an overlying loop of bowel. The duodenojejunal flexure is behind the lower part of the stomach.

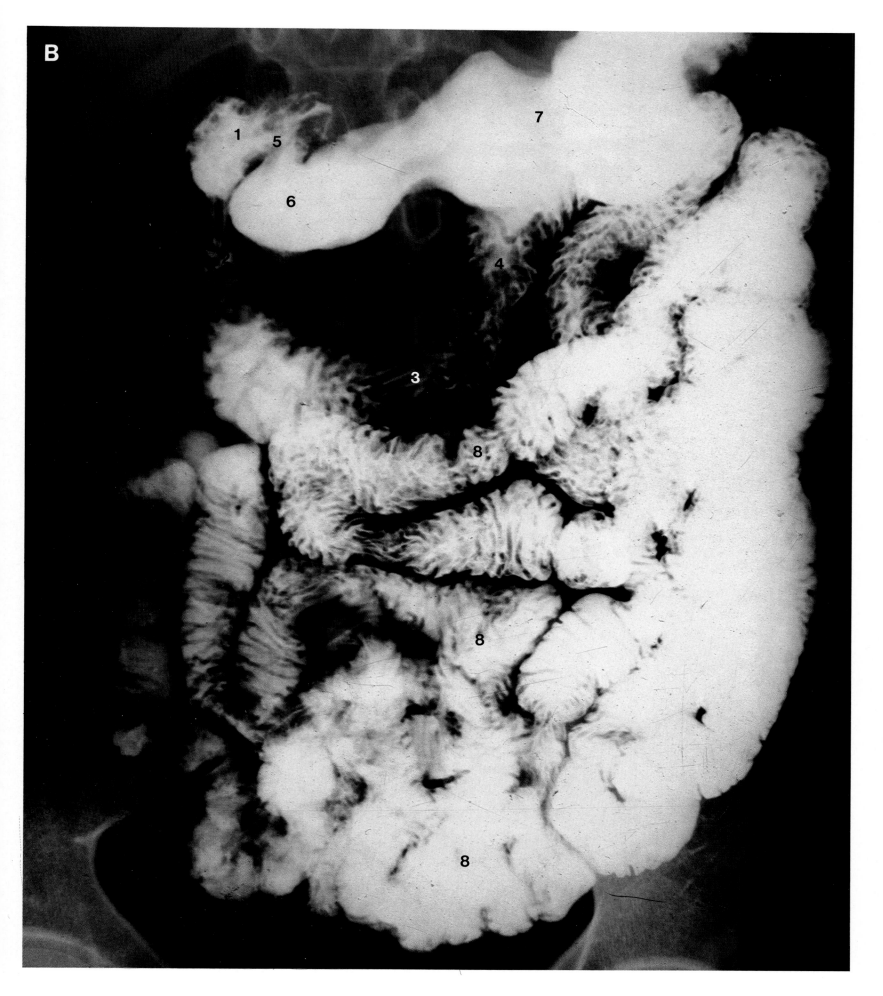

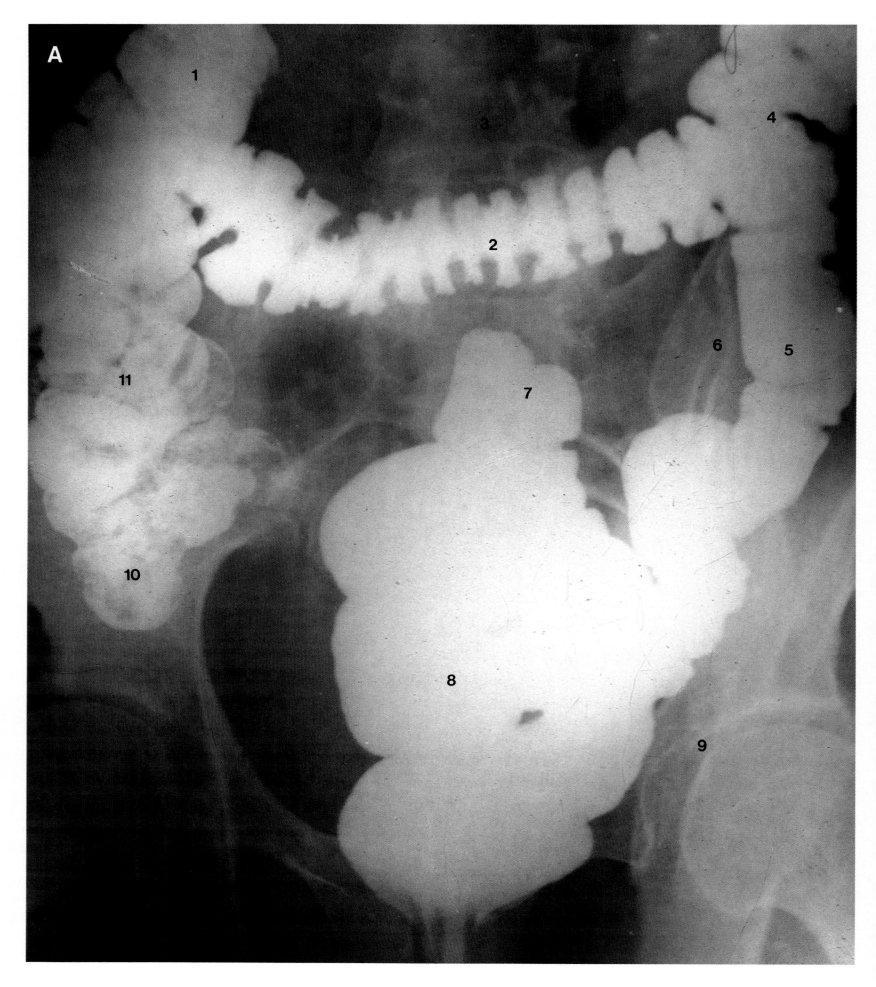

A Radiograph of the large intestine after a barium enema

1 Right colic flexure
2 Transverse colon
3 Fourth lumbar vertebra
4 Left colic flexure
5 Descending colon
6 Sacro-iliac joint
7 Sigmoid colon
8 Rectum
9 Hip joint
10 Caecum
11 Ascending colon

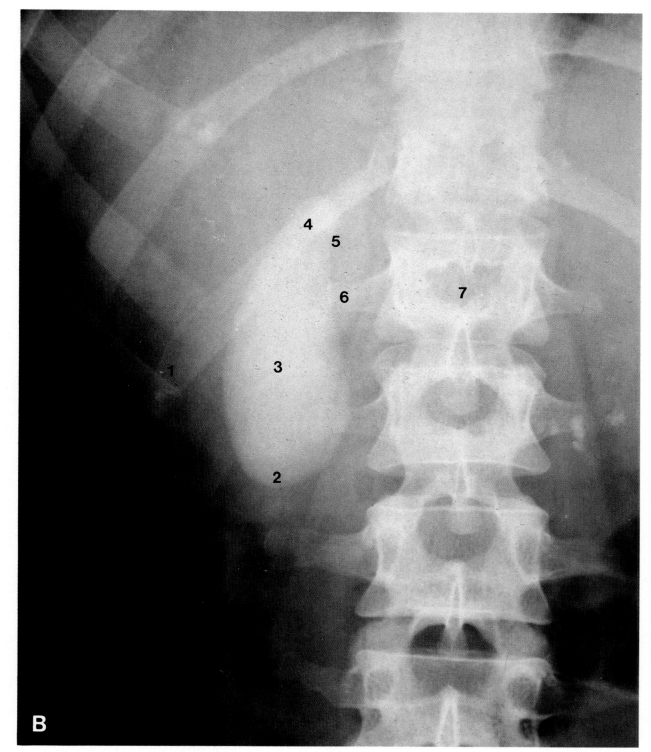

B Radiograph of the gall bladder (cholecystogram), one hour after the intravenous injection of contrast medium

1 Right twelfth rib
2 Fundus ⎫
3 Body ⎬ of gall bladder
4 Neck ⎭
5 Cystic duct
6 Bile duct
7 First lumbar vertebra

● Radiologically the gall bladder is frequently seen in the angle between the twelfth rib and the upper lumbar vertebrae.

261

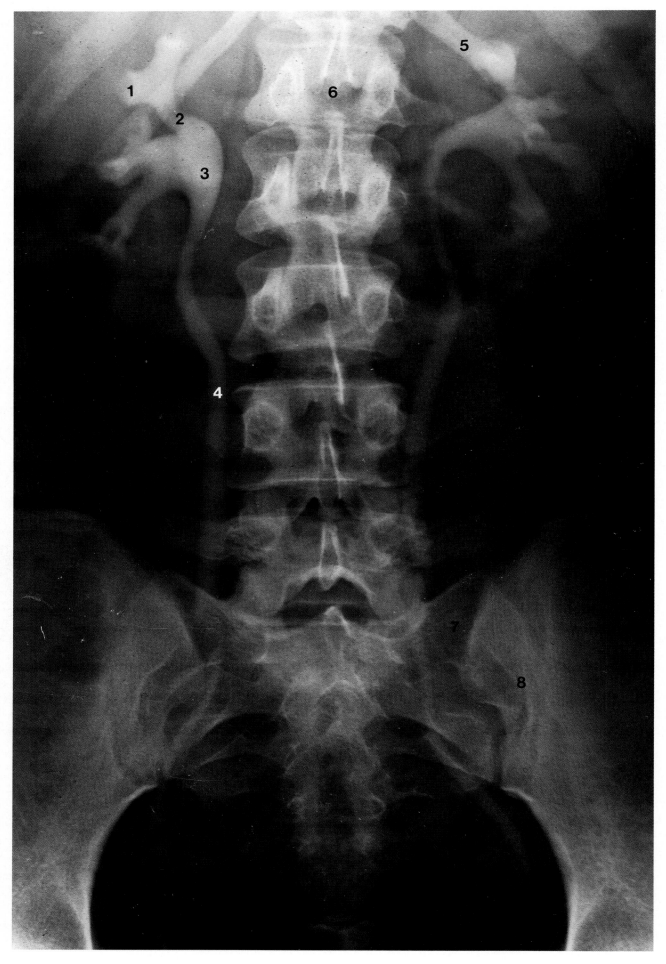

Radiograph of the kidneys and ureter (pyelogram), ten minutes after the intravenous injection of contrast medium

1 Minor calyx
2 Major calyx
3 Pelvis of kidney
4 Ureter
5 Twelfth rib
6 First lumbar vertebra
7 Lateral part of sacrum
8 Sacro-iliac joint

● Radiologically the ureters normally lie near the tips of the transverse processes of the lumbar vertebrae.

Lower Limb

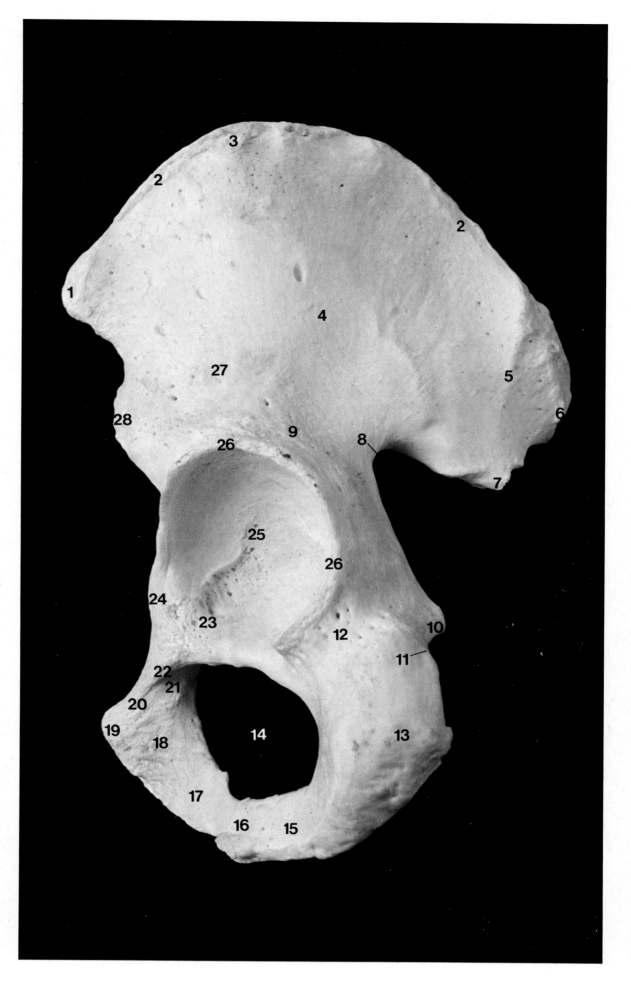

Left hip bone, lateral surface
1 Anterior superior iliac spine
2 Iliac crest
3 Tubercle of iliac crest
4 Anterior gluteal line
5 Posterior gluteal line
6 Posterior superior iliac spine
7 Posterior inferior iliac spine
8 Greater sciatic notch
9 Body of ilium
10 Ischial spine
11 Lesser sciatic notch
12 Body of ischium
13 Ischial tuberosity
14 Obturator foramen
15 Ramus of ischium
16 Junction of 15 and 17
17 Inferior ramus of pubis
18 Body of pubis
19 Pubic tubercle
20 Superior ramus of pubis
21 Obturator groove
22 Obturator crest
23 Acetabular notch
24 Iliopubic eminence
25 Acetabulum
26 Rim of acetabulum
27 Inferior gluteal line
28 Anterior inferior iliac spine

● The hip (innominate) bone is formed by the union of the ilium, ischium and pubis.
● It bears on its lateral surface the cup-shaped acetabulum, to which the ilium, ischium and pubis each contribute a part (see page 290).
● The two hip bones articulate in the midline anteriorly at the pubic symphysis; posteriorly they are separated by the sacrum, forming the sacro-iliac joints. The two hip bones with the sacrum and coccyx constitute the pelvis.
● The ischiopubic ramus is formed by the union of the ramus of the ischium with the inferior ramus of the pubis.

Left hip bone, lateral surface. Attachments

(Epiphysial line, dotted; capsule attachment, interrupted line)

1 External oblique
2 Tensor fasciae latae
3 Gluteus minimus
4 Gluteus medius
5 Gluteus maximus
6 Piriformis
7 Ischiofemoral ligament
8 Superior gemellus
9 Semimembranosus
10 Semitendinosus and long head of biceps
11 Quadratus femoris
12 Adductor magnus
13 Obturator externus
14 Gracilis
15 Adductor brevis
16 Adductor longus
17 Transverse ligament
18 Reflected head of rectus femoris
19 Iliofemoral ligament
20 Straight head of rectus femoris
21 Sartorius
22 Inguinal ligament

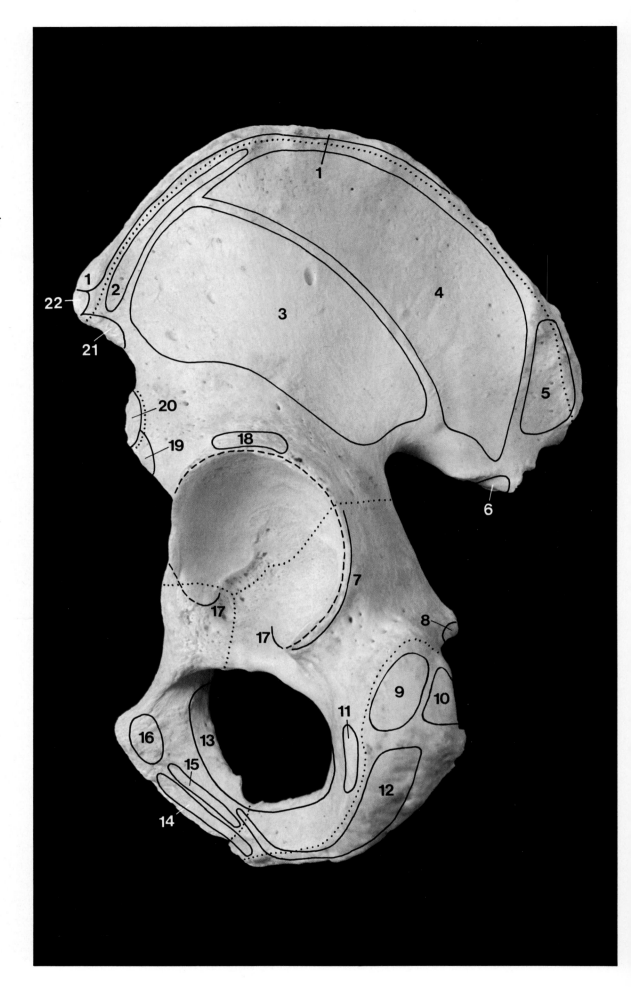

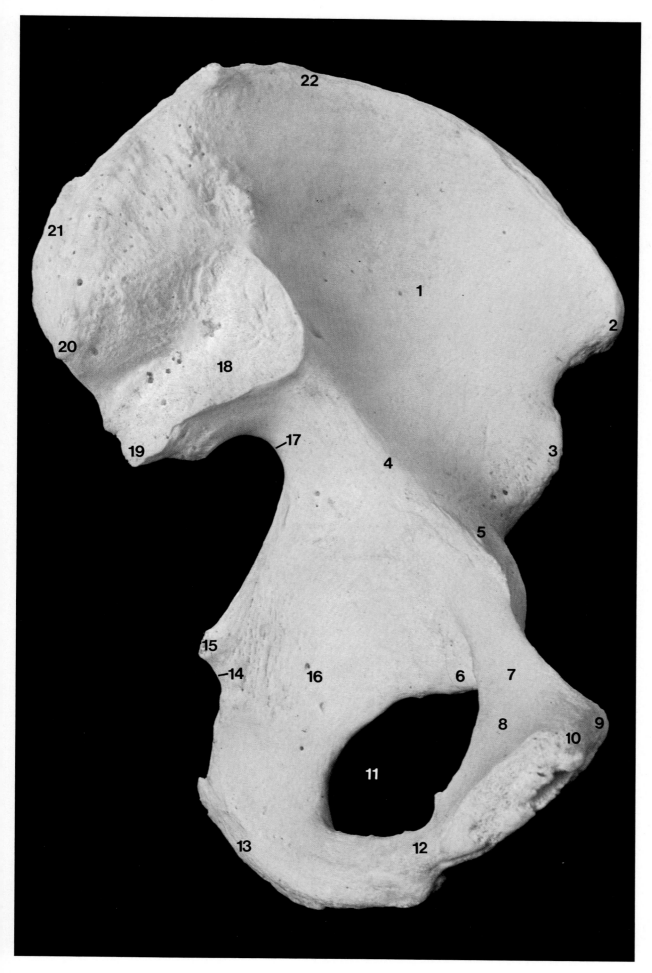

Left hip bone, medial surface

1 Iliac fossa
2 Anterior superior iliac spine
3 Anterior inferior iliac spine
4 Arcuate line
5 Iliopubic eminence
6 Obturator groove
7 Superior ramus of pubis
8 Body of pubis
9 Pubic tubercle
10 Pubic crest
11 Obturator foramen
12 Ischiopubic ramus
13 Ischial tuberosity
14 Lesser sciatic notch
15 Ischial spine
16 Body of ischium
17 Greater sciatic notch
18 Auricular surface
19 Posterior inferior iliac spine
20 Posterior superior iliac spine
21 Iliac tuberosity
22 Iliac crest

● The auricular surface of the ilium is the articular surface for the sacro-iliac joint.

Left hip bone, medial surface. Attachments
(Epiphysial line, dotted; capsule attachment, interrupted line)

1 Erector spinae
2 Interosseous ligament
3 Iliolumbar ligament
4 Quadratus lumborum
5 Transversus abdominis
6 Iliacus
7 Inguinal ligament
8 Sartorius
9 Straight head of rectus femoris
10 Psoas minor
11 Levator ani
12 Pubic symphysis
13 Obturator internus
14 Sphincter urethrae
15 Superficial transverse perineal and ischiocavernosus
16 Falciform process of sacro-tuberous ligament
17 Sacrotuberous ligament
18 Inferior gemellus
19 Coccygeus and sacrospinous ligament

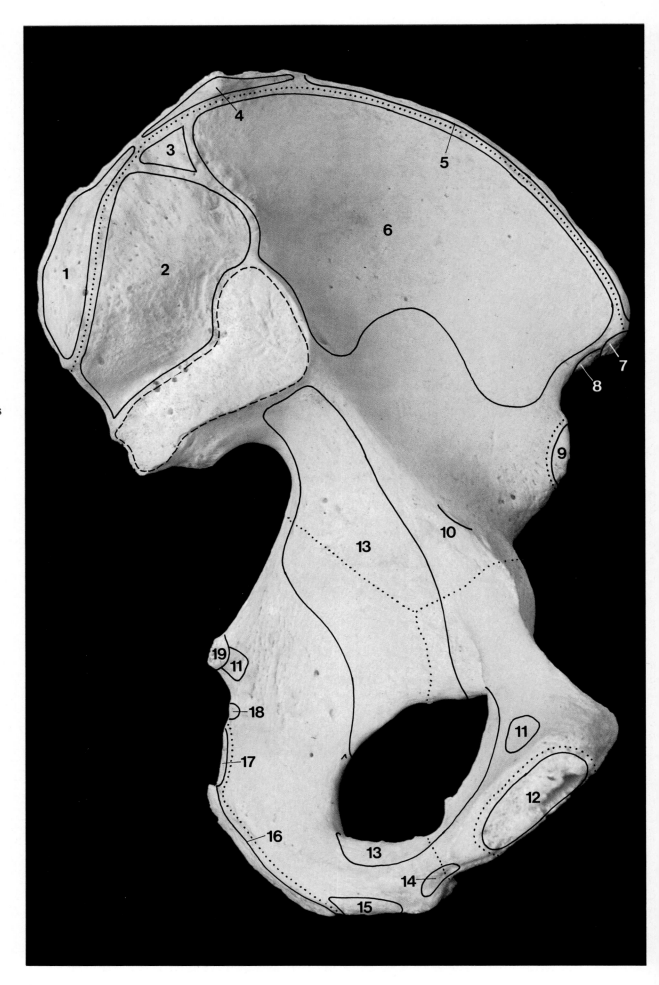

266

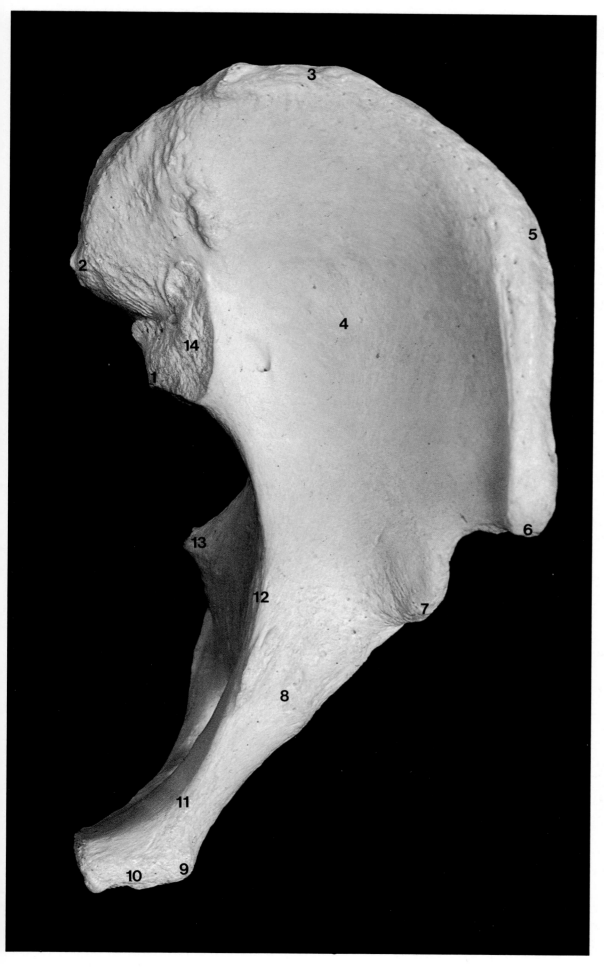

Left hip bone, from above
1 Posterior inferior iliac spine
2 Posterior superior iliac spine
3 Iliac crest
4 Iliac fossa
5 Tubercle of iliac crest
6 Anterior superior iliac spine
7 Anterior inferior iliac spine
8 Iliopubic eminence
9 Pubic tubercle
10 Pubic crest
11 Pecten of pubis (pectineal line)
12 Arcuate line
13 Ischial spine
14 Auricular surface

● The arcuate line of the ilium and the pecten and crest of the pubis form part of the brim of the pelvis (the rest of the brim being formed by the promontory and upper surface of the lateral part of the sacrum – see page 79).

● The pecten of the pubis is more commonly called the pectineal line.

Left hip bone, from above. Attachments

(Epiphysial line, dotted; capsule attachment, interrupted line)

1 Interosseous sacro-iliac ligament
2 Iliolumbar ligament
3 Quadratus lumborum
4 Iliacus
5 Transversus abdominis
6 Internal oblique
7 External oblique
8 Inguinal ligament
9 Straight head of rectus femoris
10 Iliofemoral ligament
11 Psoas minor
12 Pectineal ligament
13 Pectineus
14 Lacunar ligament
15 Anterior wall of rectus sheath
16 Pyramidalis
17 Lateral head of rectus abdominis
18 Conjoint tendon
19 Medial head of rectus abdominis

● The inguinal ligament is formed by the lower border of the aponeurosis of the external oblique muscle, and extends from the anterior superior iliac spine to the pubic tubercle.

● The lacunar ligament (sometimes called the pectineal part of the inguinal ligament) is the part of the inguinal ligament that extends backwards from the medial end of the inguinal ligament to the pecten of the pubis.

● The pectineal ligament is the lateral extension of the lacunar ligament along the pecten. It is not classified as a part of the inguinal ligament, and must not be confused with the alternative name for the lacunar ligament, i.e. with the pectineal part of the inguinal ligament.

● The conjoint tendon is formed by the aponeuroses of the internal oblique and transversus muscles, and is attached to the pubic crest and the adjoining part of the pecten, blending medially with the anterior wall of the rectus sheath.

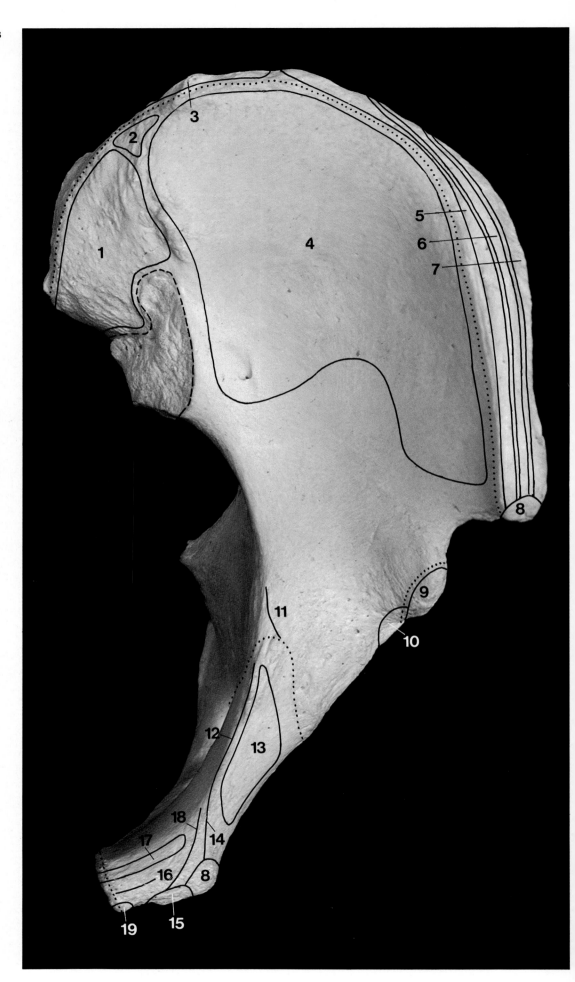

A **Left hip bone. Ischial tuberosity, from behind and below**
 1 Ischial spine
 2 Lesser sciatic notch
 3 Upper part of tuberosity
 4 Transverse ridge
 5 Lower part of tuberosity
 6 Longitudinal ridge
 7 Ischiopubic ramus
 8 Obturator groove
 9 Acetabular notch
10 Rim of acetabulum
11 Acetabulum

B **Left hip bone, from the front**
 1 Tubercle of iliac crest
 2 Anterior superior iliac spine
 3 Anterior inferior iliac spine
 4 Rim of acetabulum
 5 Acetabular notch
 6 Ischial tuberosity
 7 Ischiopubic ramus
 8 Obturator foramen
 9 Body of pubis
10 Pubic crest
11 Pubic tubercle
12 Obturator groove
13 Obturator crest
14 Pecten of pubis (pectineal line)
15 Iliopubic eminence
16 Iliac fossa

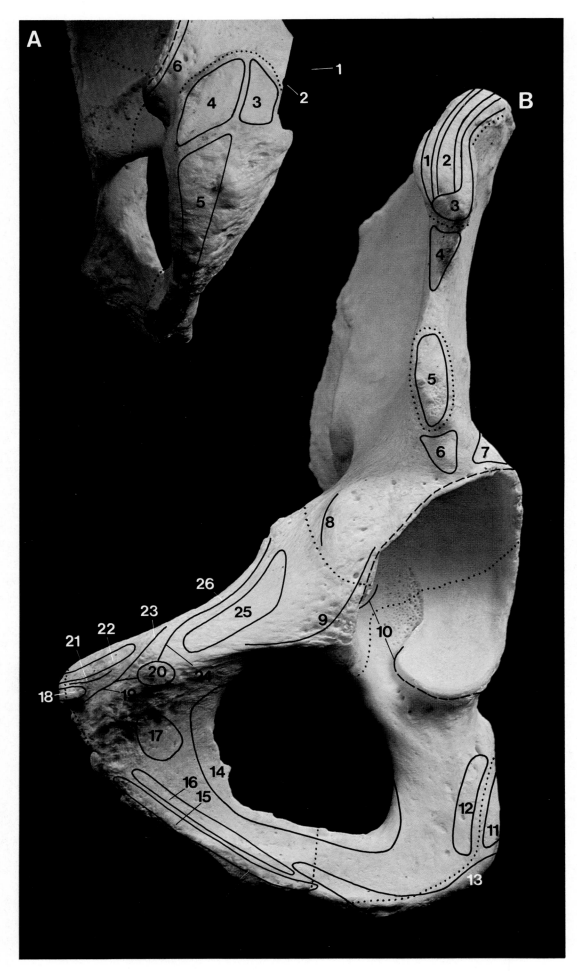

A Left hip bone. Ischial tuberosity, from behind and below. Attachments
(Epiphysial line, dotted; capsule attachment, interrupted line)

1 Superior gemellus
2 Inferior gemellus
3 Semitendinosus and long head of biceps
4 Semimembranosus
5 Adductor magnus
6 Ischiofemoral ligament

● The area on the ischial tuberosity medial to the adductor magnus attachment is covered by fibrofatty tissue and the ischial bursa underlying gluteus maximus.

B Left hip bone, from the front. Attachments
(Epiphysial line, dotted; capsule attachment, interrupted line)

1 Transversus abdominis
2 Internal oblique
3 External oblique and inguinal ligament
4 Sartorius
5 Straight head of rectus femoris
6 Iliofemoral ligament
7 Reflected head of rectus femoris
8 Psoas minor
9 Pubofemoral ligament
10 Transverse ligament
11 Semimembranosus
12 Quadratus femoris
13 Adductor magnus
14 Obturator externus
15 Gracilis
16 Adductor brevis
17 Adductor longus
18 Medial head of rectus abdominis
19 Rectus sheath
20 Inguinal ligament
21 Pyramidalis
22 Lateral head of rectus abdominis
23 Conjoint tendon
24 Lacunar ligament
25 Pectineus
26 Pectineal ligament

Left femur, upper end, A from the front, B from the medial side

1 Head
2 Neck
3 Greater trochanter
4 Intertrochanteric line
5 Lesser trochanter
6 Shaft
7 Facet of head
8 Spiral line
9 Pectineal line
10 Quadrate tubercle on intertrochanteric crest
11 Trochanteric fossa

● The intertrochanteric *line* is at the junction of the neck and shaft on the anterior surface; the intertrochanteric *crest* is in a similar position on the posterior surface.

● The neck makes an angle with the shaft of about 125°.

● The pectineal line of the femur must not be confused with the pectineal line (pecten) of the pubis (page 267), nor with the spiral line of the femur which is usually more prominent than the pectineal line

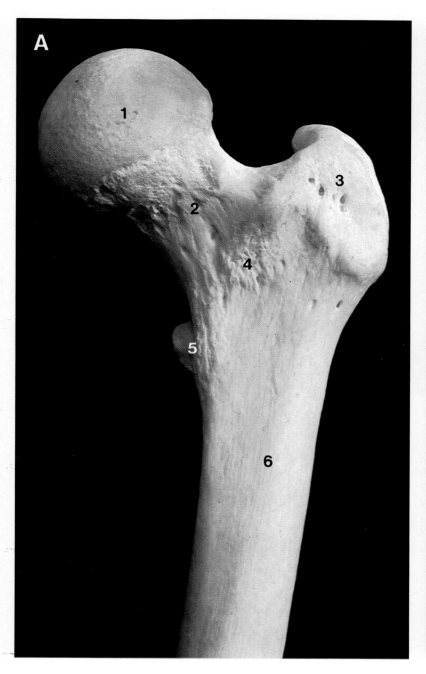
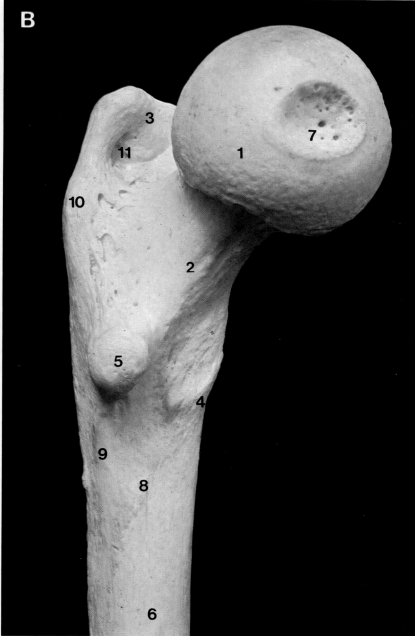

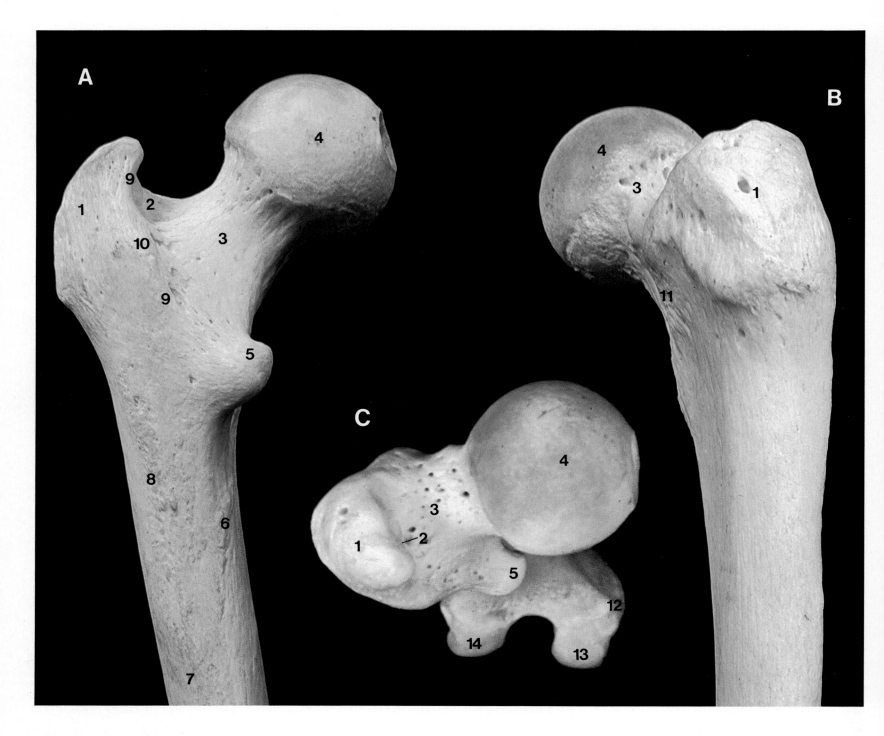

Left femur, upper end, A from behind, B from the lateral side, C from above

1 Greater trochanter
2 Trochanteric fossa
3 Neck
4 Head
5 Lesser trochanter
6 Spiral line
7 Linea aspera
8 Gluteal tuberosity
9 Intertrochanteric crest
10 Quadrate tubercle
11 Intertrochanteric line
12 Adductor tubercle ⎤
13 Medial condyle ⎬ at lower end
14 Lateral condyle ⎦

● The neck of the femur passes forwards as well as upwards and medially, making an angle of about 15° with the transverse axis of the lower end (the angle of femoral torsion).
● The lesser trochanter projects backwards and medially.

272

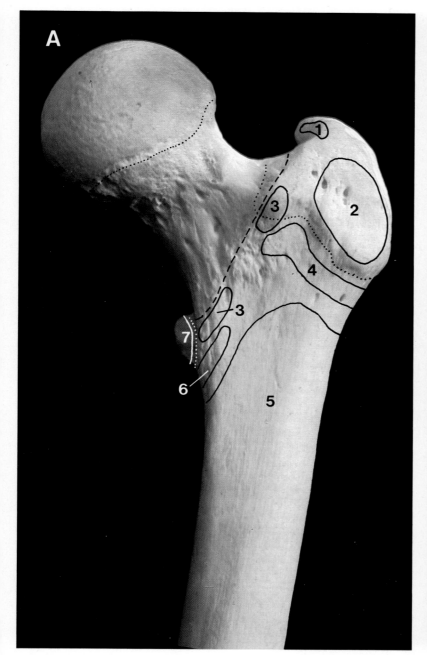

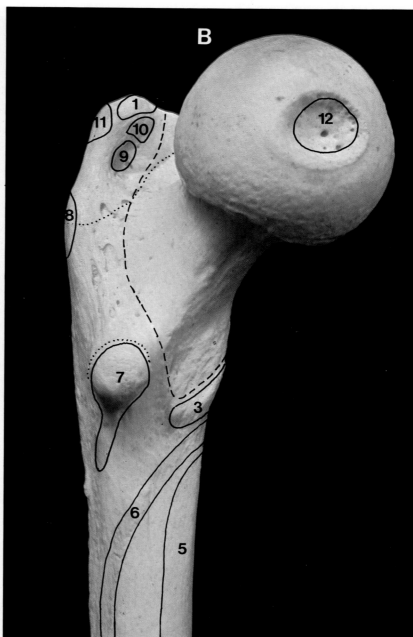

Left femur, upper end, A from the front, B from the medial side. Attachments

(Epiphysial line, dotted; capsule attachment, interrupted line)

1 Piriformis
2 Gluteus minimus
3 Iliofemoral ligament
4 Vastus lateralis
5 Vastus intermedius
6 Vastus medialis
7 Psoas major and iliacus
8 Quadratus femoris
9 Obturator externus
10 Obturator internus
11 Gluteus medius
12 Ligament of head of femur

● The iliofemoral ligament has the shape of an inverted Y, with the stem attached to the anterior inferior iliac spine of the hip bone, and the limbs attached to the upper (lateral) and lower (medial) ends of the intertrochanteric line, blending with the capsule of the hip joint.
● The tendon of psoas major is attached to the lesser trochanter; many of the muscle fibres of iliacus are inserted into the psoas tendon but some reach the femur below the trochanter.

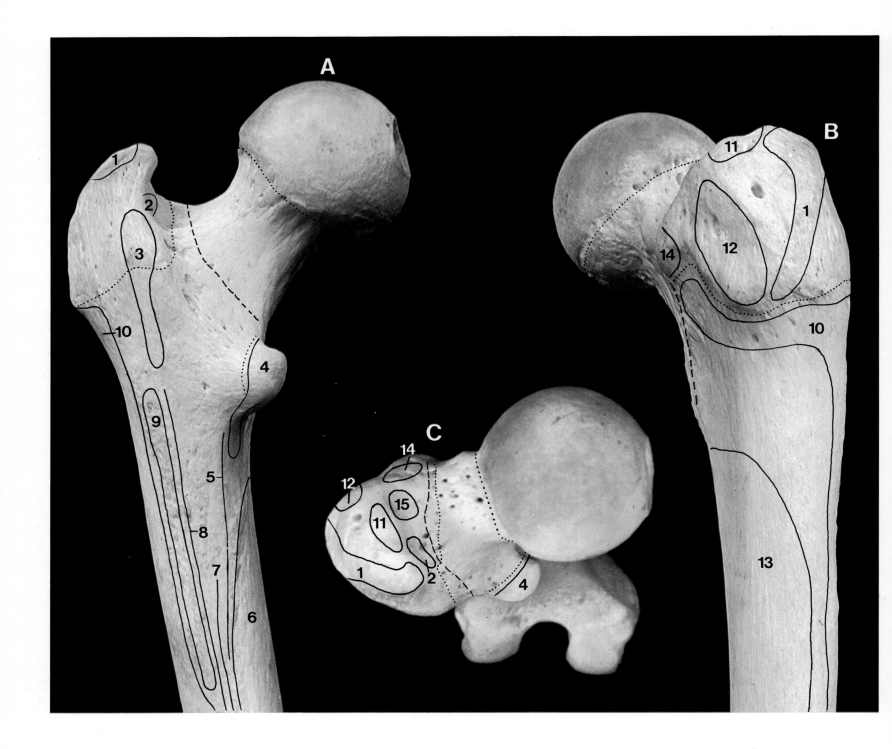

Left femur, upper end, A from behind, B from the lateral side, C from above. Attachments

(Epiphysial line, dotted; capsule attachment, interrupted line)

1 Gluteus medius
2 Obturator externus
3 Quadratus femoris
4 Psoas major and iliacus
5 Pectineus
6 Vastus medialis
7 Adductor brevis
8 Adductor magnus
9 Gluteus maximus
10 Vastus lateralis
11 Piriformis
12 Gluteus minimus
13 Vastus intermedius
14 Iliofemoral ligament
15 Obturator internus

● On the front of the femur the capsule of the hip joint is attached to the intertrochanteric line, but at the back the capsule is attached to the neck of the femur and does not extend as far laterally as the intertrochanteric crest.

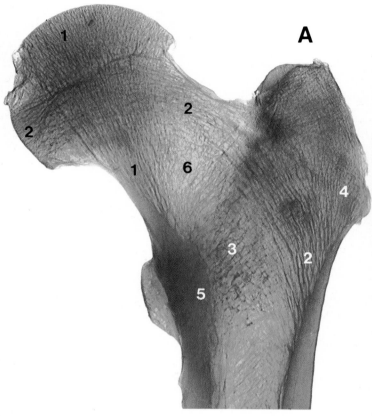

A Left femur, upper end. Posterior half of cleared bisected specimen, from the front, showing major groups of trabeculae

1 From medial ⎫
2 From lateral ⎬ surface of shaft to head

3 From medial ⎫
4 From lateral ⎬ surface of shaft to greater trochanter

5 Calcar femorale
6 Triangular area of few trabeculae

● The calcar femorale is a dense concentration of trabeculae passing from the region of the lesser trochanter to the under surface of the neck.

B Left femur, shaft, from behind

1 Gluteal tuberosity
2 Lesser trochanter
3 Pectineal line
4 Linea aspera
5 Medial supracondylar line
6 Lateral supracondylar line

● The rough linea aspera often shows distinct medial and lateral lips; the lateral lip continues upwards as the gluteal tuberosity.

C Left femur, shaft, from behind. Attachments

1 Vastus lateralis
2 Quadratus femoris
3 Gluteus maximus
4 Adductor magnus
5 Psoas and iliacus
6 Pectineus
7 Adductor brevis
8 Vastus medialis
9 Adductor longus
10 Short head of biceps
11 Vastus intermedius

● For diagrammatic clarity the muscle attachments to the linea aspera have been slightly separated.

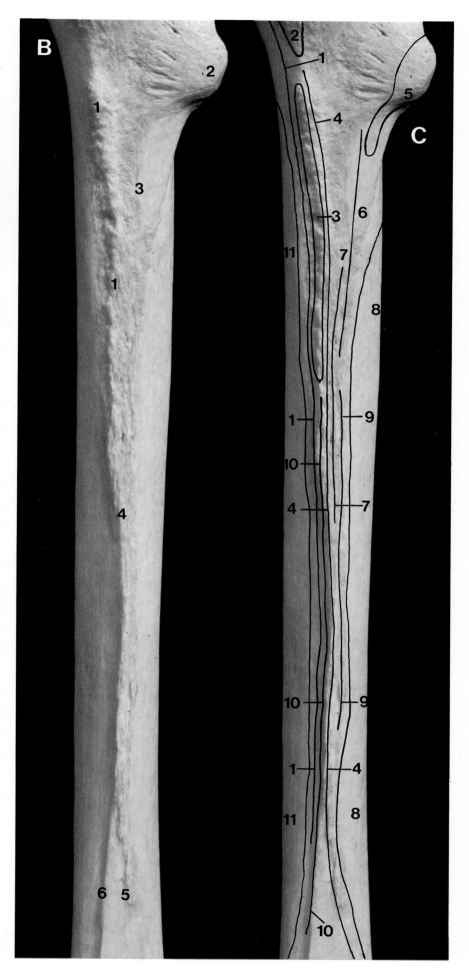

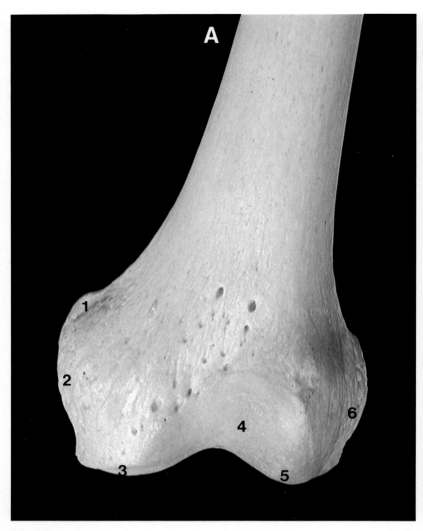

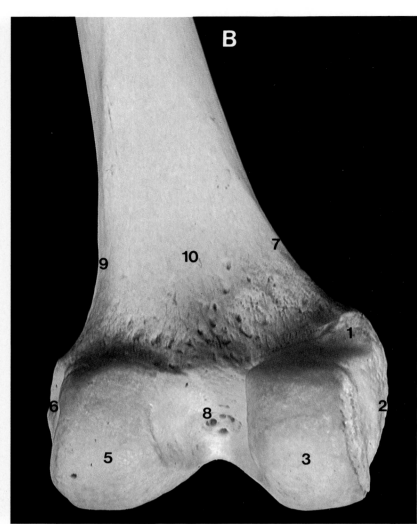

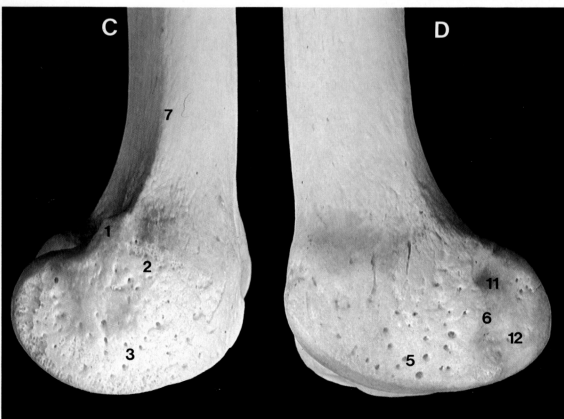

Left femur, lower end, A from the front, B from behind, C from the medial side, D from the lateral side

1 Adductor tubercle
2 Medial epicondyle
3 Medial condyle
4 Patellar surface
5 Lateral condyle
6 Lateral epicondyle
7 Medial supracondylar line
8 Intercondylar fossa
9 Lateral supracondylar line
10 Popliteal surface
11 Impression for lateral head of gastrocnemius
12 Groove for popliteus tendon

● The condyles bear the articular surfaces for the tibia, and project backwards; the epicondyles are the most prominent points on the (non-articular) sides of the condyles.

● The lower ends of the condyles lie in the same horizontal plane in order to rest squarely on the condyles of the tibia at the knee joint. The shaft therefore passes obliquely outwards and upwards from the knee towards the hip.

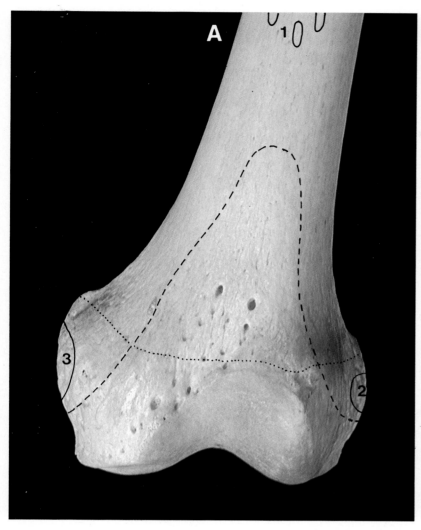

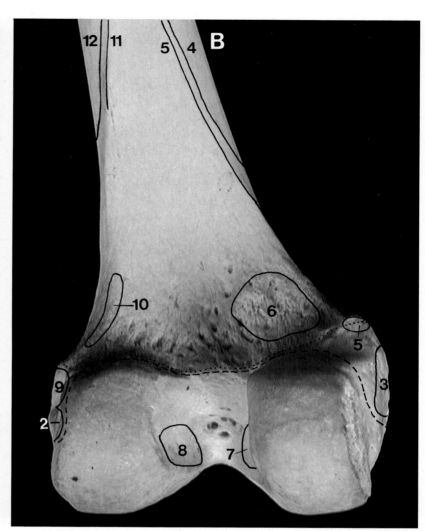

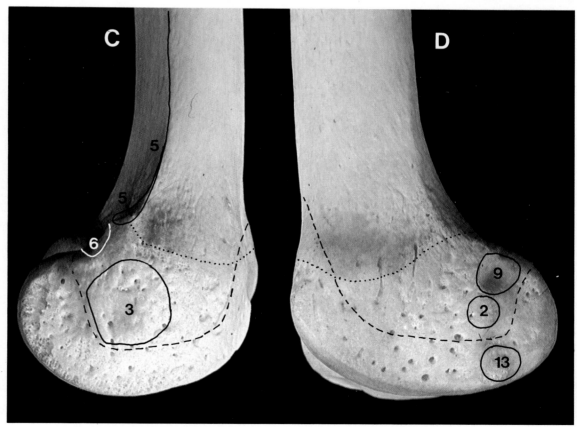

Left femur, lower end, A from the front, B from behind, C from the medial side, D from the lateral side. Attachments

(Epiphysial line, dotted; capsule attachment, interrupted line)

 1 Articularis genu
 2 Fibular collateral ligament
 3 Tibial collateral ligament
 4 Vastus medialis
 5 Adductor magnus
 6 Medial head of gastrocnemius
 7 Posterior cruciate ligament
 8 Anterior cruciate ligament
 9 Lateral head of gastrocnemius
10 Plantaris
11 Short head of biceps
12 Vastus intermedius
13 Popliteus

● The medial head of gastrocnemius arises from the popliteal surface of the femur above the medial condyle and from the adjacent part of the capsule; the lateral head arises from an impression on the lateral surface of the lateral condyle above the lateral epicondyle (not from the popliteal surface of the femur) and from the adjacent part of the capsule.

277

Left patella, A anterior surface, B articular (posterior) surface

1 Base
2 Apex
3 Facet for lateral condyle of femur
4 Vertical ridge
5 Facet for medial condyle of femur

● The lateral part of the articular surface is larger than the medial.
● The articular surface does not extend on to the apex.

Left patella, C anterior surface, D articular (posterior) surface. Attachments

1 Vastus intermedius ⎤
2 Rectus femoris ⎥ parts of quadriceps tendon
3 Vastus medialis ⎥
4 Vastus lateralis ⎦
5 Facets for femur in flexion
6 Facets for femur in extension
7 Area for medial condyle in extreme flexion
8 Area for infrapatellar fat pad
9 Patellar ligament

Left femur, E from below, articulated with the patella in the extended position, F from below and behind, articulated with the patella in the flexed position

1 Medial condyle
2 Lateral condyle

● The most medial facet of the patella only comes into contact with the medial condyle in extreme flexion.

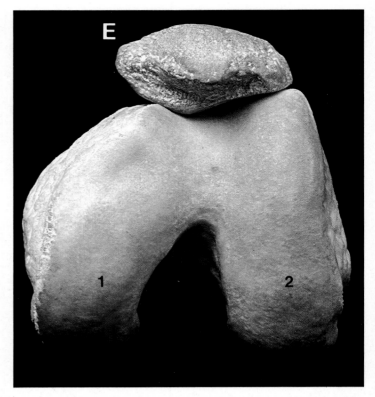

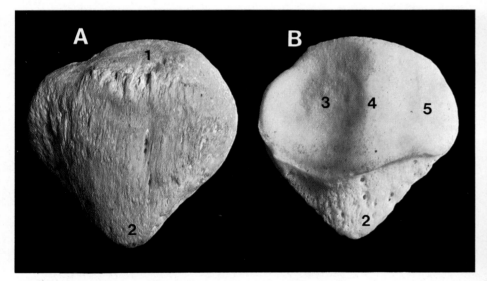

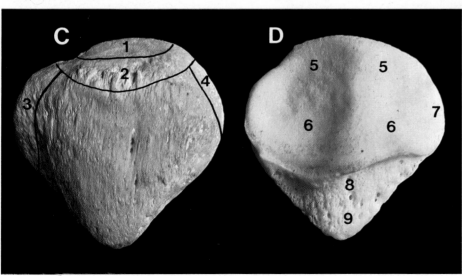

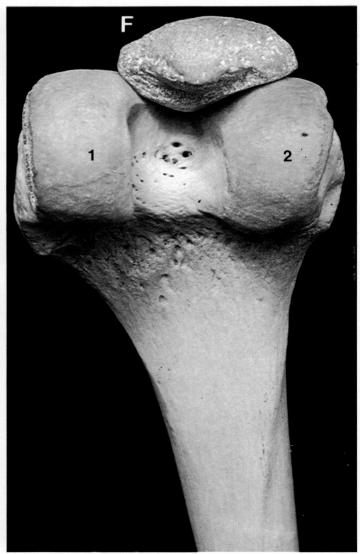

Left tibia, upper end, A from the front, B from behind

1 Tubercles of intercondylar eminence
2 Lateral condyle
3 Impression for iliotibial tract
4 Tuberosity
5 Lateral surface
6 Interosseous border
7 Anterior border
8 Medial surface
9 Medial border
10 Medial condyle
11 Groove for semimembranosus
12 Posterior surface
13 Soleal line
14 Vertical line
15 Articular facet for fibula

● The shaft of the tibia has three borders – anterior, medial and interosseous – and three surfaces – medial, lateral and posterior.

● Much of the anterior border forms a slightly curved crest commonly known as the shin. Most of the smooth medial surface is subcutaneous. The posterior surface contains the soleal and vertical lines.

● The tuberosity is at the upper end of the anterior border.

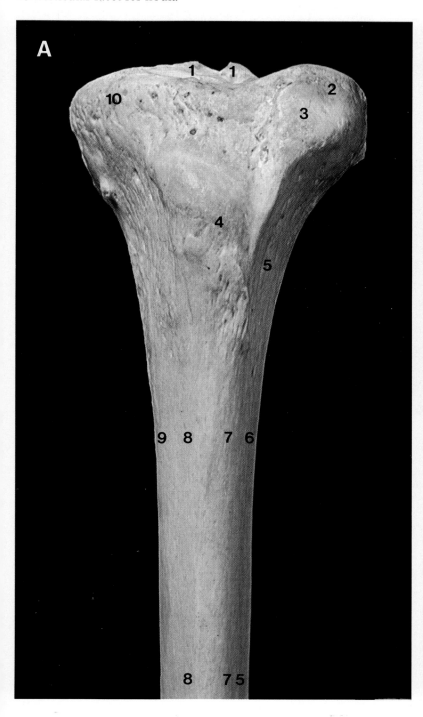

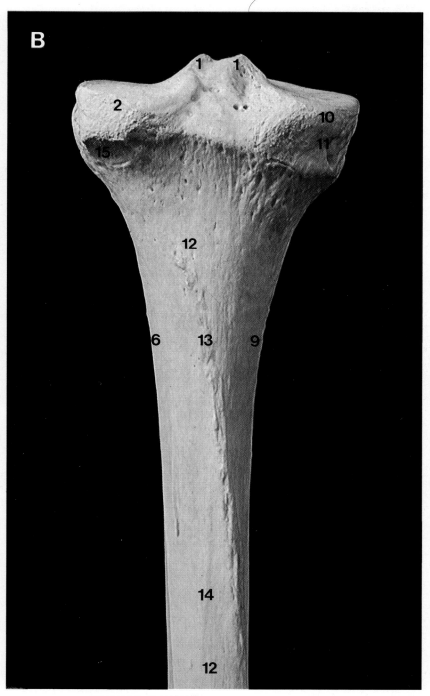

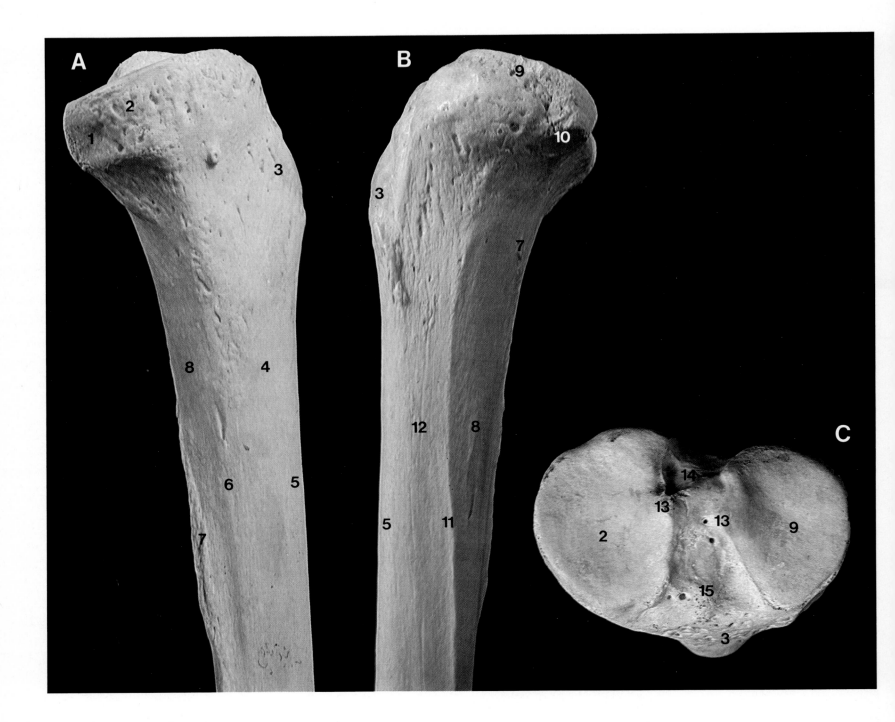

Left tibia, upper end, A from the medial side, B from the lateral side, C from above

1 Groove for semimembranosus
2 Medial condyle
3 Tuberosity
4 Medial surface
5 Anterior border
6 Medial border
7 Soleal line
8 Posterior surface
9 Lateral condyle
10 Articular facet for fibula
11 Interosseous border
12 Lateral surface
13 Tubercles of intercondylar eminence
14 Posterior intercondylar area
15 Anterior intercondylar area

● The medial condyle is larger than the lateral condyle.
● The articular facet for the fibula is on the postero-inferior aspect of the lateral condyle.

Left tibia, upper end, A from the front, B from behind. Attachments
(Epiphysial line, dotted; capsule attachment, interrupted line)

1 Iliotibial tract
2 Tibialis anterior
3 Patellar ligament
4 Sartorius
5 Gracilis
6 Semitendinosus
7 Tibial collateral ligament
8 Semimembranosus
9 Vastus medialis
10 Popliteus
11 Soleus
12 Flexor digitorum longus
13 Tibialis posterior
14 Posterior cruciate ligament

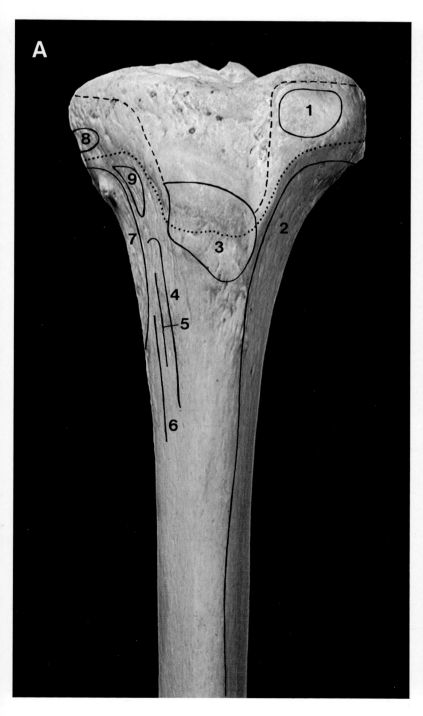

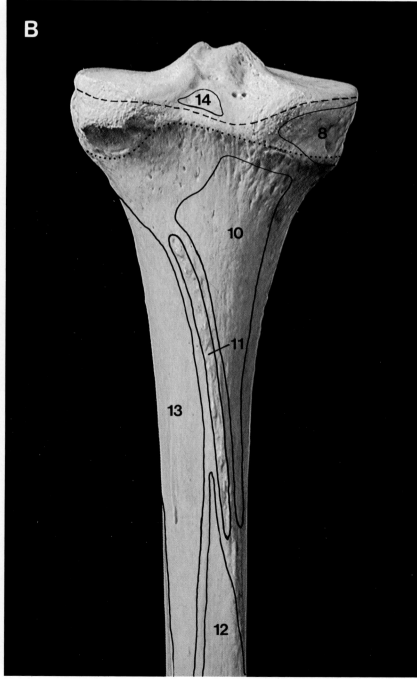

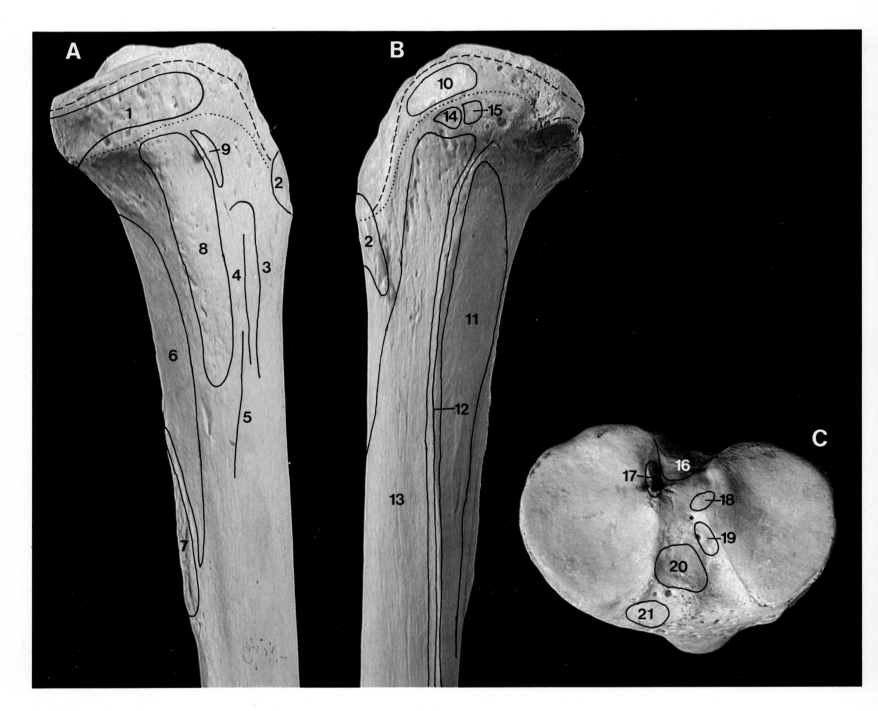

Left tibia, upper end, A from the medial side, B from the lateral side, C from above
Attachments
(Epiphysial line, dotted; capsule attachment, interrupted line)

1 Semimembranosus
2 Patellar ligament
3 Sartorius
4 Gracilis
5 Semitendinosus
6 Popliteus
7 Soleus
8 Tibial collateral ligament
9 Vastus medialis
10 Iliotibial tract
11 Tibialis posterior
12 Interosseous membrane
13 Tibialis anterior
14 Extensor digitorum longus
15 Peroneus longus
16 Posterior cruciate ligament
17 Posterior horn of medial meniscus
18 Posterior horn of lateral meniscus
19 Anterior horn of lateral meniscus
20 Anterior cruciate ligament
21 Anterior horn of medial meniscus

● Although arising mainly from the fibula (see page 285), extensor digitorum longus and peroneus longus have a small attachment to the tibia above tibialis anterior.
● The horns of the lateral meniscus are attached close to one another on either side of the intercondylar eminence, but the horns of the medial meniscus are more widely separated (see page 309).

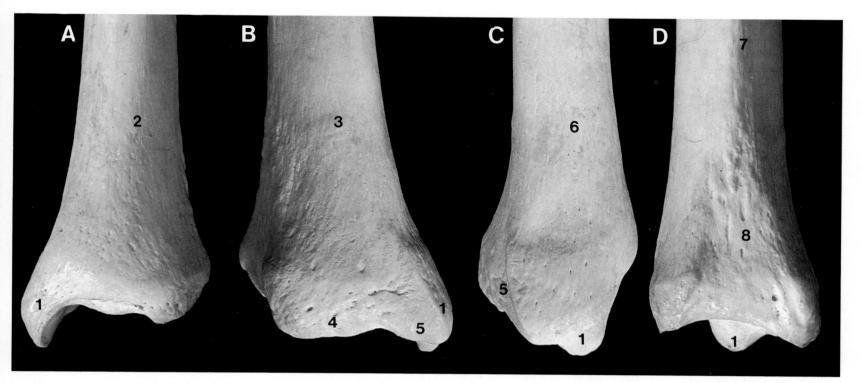

Left tibia, lower end, A from the front, B from behind, C from the medial side, D from the lateral side

1 Medial malleolus
2 Anterior surface
3 Posterior surface
4 Groove for flexor hallucis longus
5 Groove for tibialis posterior
6 Medial surface
7 Interosseous border
8 Fibular notch

● The lower end of the tibia has five surfaces – anterior, posterior, medial, lateral and inferior (for the inferior surface see page 286).
● The medial surface is continuous below with the medial surface of the medial malleolus (the lateral malleolus is the lower end of the fibula).
● The fibular notch is triangular and constitutes the lateral surface of the lower end.

Left tibia, lower end, E from the front, F from behind, G from the medial side, H from the lateral side. Attachments
(Epiphysial line, dotted; capsule attachment, interrupted line)

1 Medial collateral ligament
2 Interosseous membrane
3 Interosseous ligament
4 Posterior tibiofibular ligament
5 Inferior transverse ligament

● The medial collateral ligament is commonly known as the deltoid ligament.
● The lowest fibres of the posterior tibiofibular ligament (attached most medially to the tibia) are known as the inferior transverse ligament.

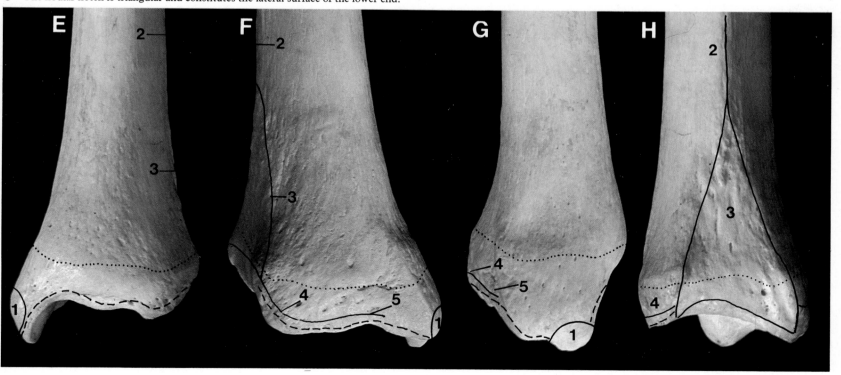

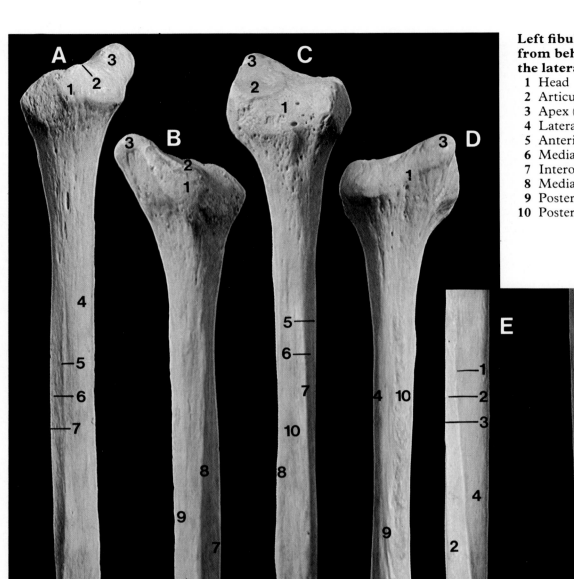

Left fibula, upper end, A from the front, B from behind, C from the medial side, D from the lateral side
  1 Head
  2 Articular facet on upper surface
  3 Apex (styloid process)
  4 Lateral surface
  5 Anterior border
  6 Medial surface
  7 Interosseous border
  8 Medial crest
  9 Posterior border
  10 Posterior surface

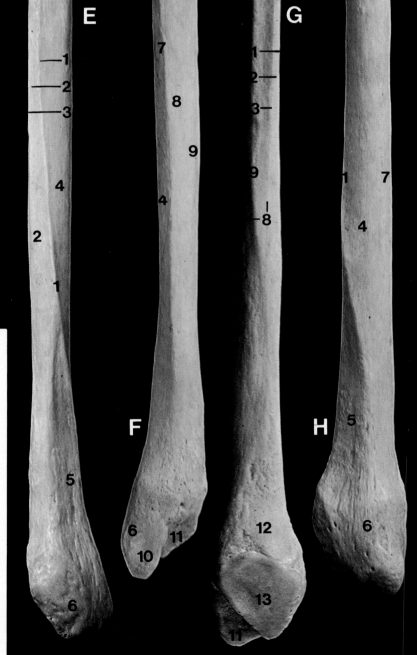

Left fibula, lower end, E from the front, F from behind, G from the medial side, H from the lateral side

  1 Anterior border
  2 Medial surface
  3 Interosseous border
  4 Lateral surface
  5 Triangular subcutaneous area
  6 Lateral malleolus
  7 Posterior border
  8 Posterior surface
  9 Medial crest
  10 Groove for peroneus brevis
  11 Malleolar fossa
  12 Surface for interosseous ligament
  13 Articular surface of lateral malleolus

● The fibula has three borders – anterior, interosseous and posterior – and three surfaces – medial, lateral and posterior.

● At first sight much of the shaft appears to have four borders and four surfaces, but this is because the posterior surface is divided into two parts (medial and lateral) by the medial crest.

● At the lower end the lateral surface comes to face posteriorly, so leaving the triangular subcutaneous area above the lateral malleolus.

● The anterior border is easily identified by following it upwards from the apex of the triangular subcutaneous area; the interosseous border is usually two or three millimetres behind the anterior border (although in the upper part of the shaft these two borders may fuse into one).

● The malleolar fossa is posterior to the articular surface.

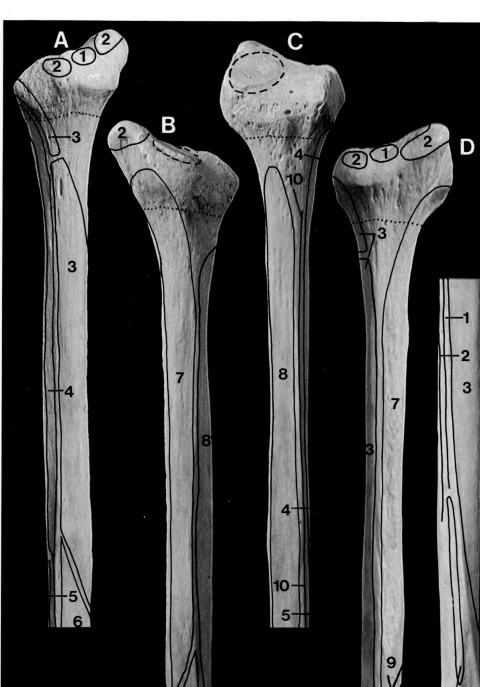

285

Left fibula, upper end, A from the front, B from behind, C from the medial side, D from the lateral side. Attachments

(Epiphysial line, dotted; capsule attachment, interrupted line)

1 Fibular collateral ligament
2 Biceps
3 Peroneus longus
4 Extensor digitorum longus
5 Extensor hallucis longus
6 Peroneus brevis
7 Soleus
8 Tibialis posterior
9 Flexor hallucis longus
10 Interosseous membrane

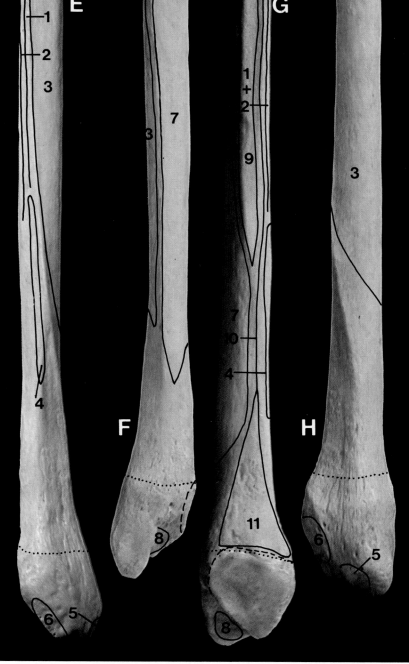

Left fibula, lower end, E from the front, F from behind, G from the medial side, H from the lateral side. Attachments

(Epiphysial line, dotted; capsule attachment, interrupted line)

1 Extensor digitorum longus
2 Extensor hallucis longus
3 Peroneus brevis
4 Peroneus tertius
5 Calcaneofibular ligament
6 Anterior talofibular ligament
7 Flexor hallucis longus
8 Posterior talofibular ligament
9 Tibialis posterior
10 Interosseous membrane
11 Interosseous ligament

● The medial surface (between the anterior and interosseous borders) gives origin to extensor muscles (digitorum longus and hallucis longus, and peroneus tertius).
● The lateral surface (between the anterior and posterior borders) gives origin to peroneus longus and brevis.
● The posterior surface (between the interosseous and posterior borders) gives origin to flexor muscles (soleus and flexor hallucis longus lateral to the medial crest; tibialis posterior medial to the medial crest).
● The gap at the upper end of the peroneus longus attachment is for the common peroneal nerve.

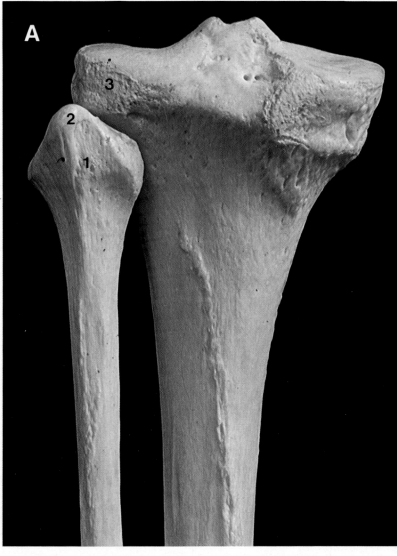

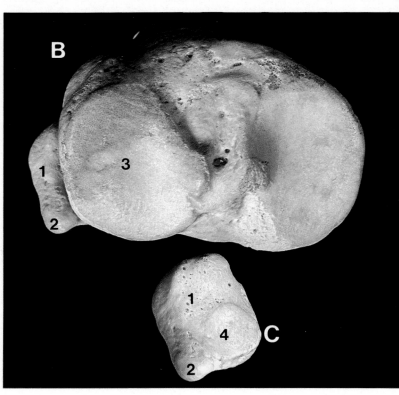

Articulation of left tibia and fibula, A upper ends from behind, B upper ends from above, C upper end of fibula from above, D lower ends of tibia and fibula from behind, E lower ends from below

1 Head of fibula
2 Apex of head (styloid process)
3 Lateral condyle of tibia
4 Articular facet
5 Lateral malleolus
6 Malleolar fossa
7 Inferior surface of tibia
8 Medial malleolus

● The superior tibiofibular joint is synovial, with the tibial facet of the joint on the posterolateral and lower aspect of the lateral condyle. The facet on the fibula is towards the posterior and medial part of the upper surface of the head.

● The inferior tibiofibular joint is fibrous.

● The lateral malleolus extends lower than the medial malleolus. The articular surfaces of the malleoli together with the inferior surface of the tibia embrace the talus to form the ankle (talocrural) joint.

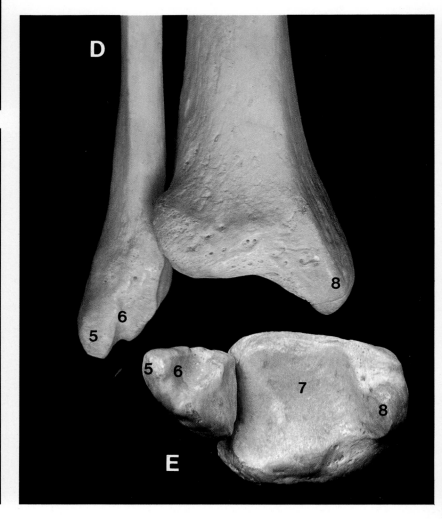

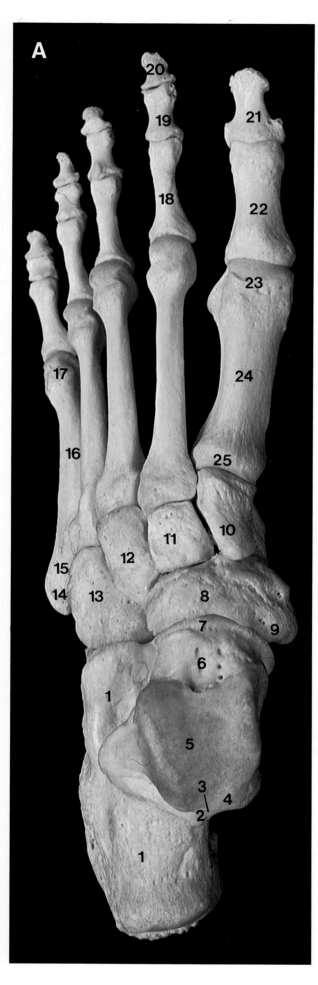

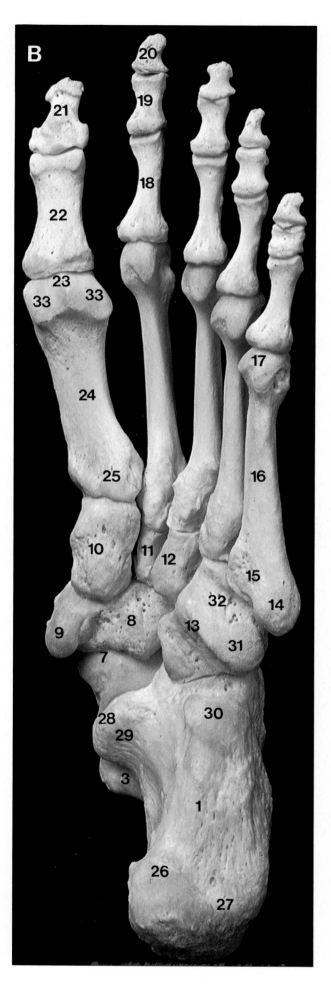

Bones of the left foot, A from above (dorsum), B from below (plantar surface)

1 Calcaneus
2 Lateral tubercle of talus
3 Groove on talus for flexor hallucis longus
4 Medial tubercle of talus
5 Trochlear surface of body of talus
6 Neck of talus
7 Head of talus
8 Navicular
9 Tuberosity of navicular
10 Medial cuneiform
11 Intermediate cuneiform
12 Lateral cuneiform
13 Cuboid
14 Tuberosity of base of fifth metatarsal
15 Base of fifth metatarsal
16 Shaft of fifth metatarsal
17 Head of fifth metatarsal
18 Proximal phalanx of second toe
19 Middle phalanx of second toe
20 Distal phalanx of second toe
21 Distal phalanx of great toe
22 Proximal phalanx of great toe
23 Head of first metatarsal
24 Shaft of first metatarsal
25 Base of first metatarsal
26 Medial process of calcaneus
27 Lateral process of calcaneus
28 Sustentaculum tali of calcaneus
29 Groove on calcaneus for flexor hallucis longus
30 Anterior tubercle of calcaneus
31 Tuberosity of cuboid
32 Groove on cuboid for peroneus longus
33 Grooves for sesamoid bones in flexor hallucis brevis tendons

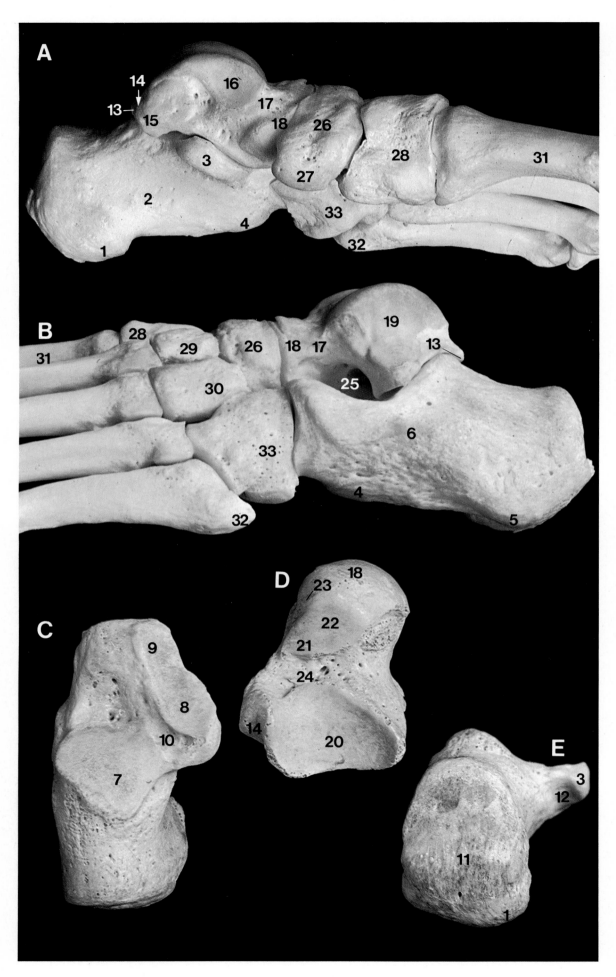

Bones of the left foot, A from the medial side, B from the lateral side, C calcaneus from above, D talus from below, E calcaneus from behind

1 Medial process ⎫
2 Medial surface ⎪
3 Sustentaculum tali ⎪
4 Anterior tubercle ⎪
5 Lateral process ⎪
6 Peroneal trochlea ⎬ of calcaneus
7 Posterior ⎱ talal ⎱ ⎪
8 Middle ⎬ articular ⎪
9 Anterior ⎰ surface ⎪
10 Sulcus ⎪
11 Posterior surface ⎪
12 Groove for flexor ⎪
   hallucis longus ⎭

13 Lateral tubercle ⎫
14 Groove for flexor ⎪
   hallucis longus ⎪
15 Medial tubercle ⎪
16 Medial malleolar surface ⎪
17 Neck ⎪
18 Head ⎪
19 Lateral malleolar surface ⎬ of talus
20 Posterior ⎱ calcanean ⎪
21 Middle ⎬ articular ⎪
22 Anterior ⎰ surface ⎪
23 Surface for plantar ⎪
   calcaneonavicular ⎪
   ligament ⎪
24 Sulcus ⎭

25 Tarsal sinus
26 Navicular
27 Tuberosity of navicular
28 Medial ⎫
29 Intermediate ⎬ cuneiform
30 Lateral ⎭
31 First metatarsal
32 Tuberosity of base of fifth
   metatarsal
33 Cuboid

288

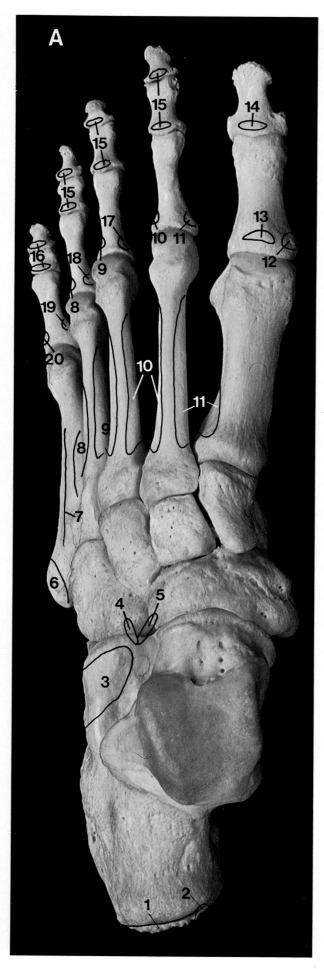

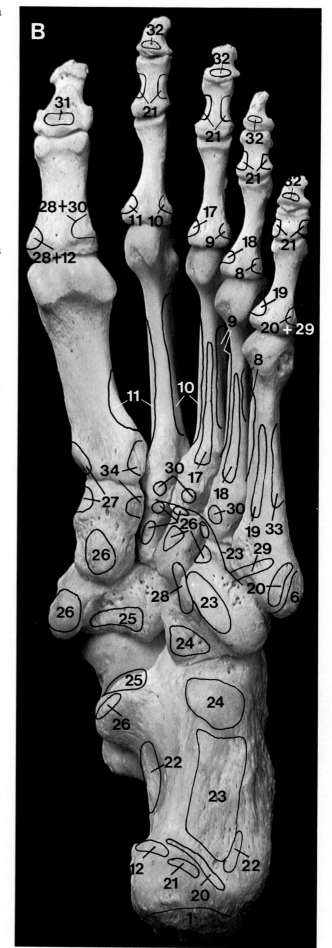

Bones of the left foot, A from above, B from below. Attachments

(Joint capsules and minor ligaments have been omitted)

1 Tendo calcaneus (Achilles' tendon)
2 Plantaris
3 Extensor digitorum brevis
4 Calcaneocuboid part of bifurcate ligament
5 Calcaneonavicular part of bifurcate ligament
6 Peroneus brevis
7 Peroneus tertius
8 Fourth ⎫
9 Third ⎬ dorsal interosseous
10 Second ⎪
11 First ⎭
12 Abductor hallucis
13 Extensor hallucis brevis
14 Extensor hallucis longus
15 Extensor digitorum longus and brevis
16 Extensor digitorum longus
17 First ⎫
18 Second ⎬ plantar interosseous
19 Third ⎭
20 Abductor digiti minimi
21 Flexor digitorum brevis
22 Flexor accessorius
23 Long plantar ligament
24 Short plantar ligament
25 Plantar calcaneonavicular ligament
26 Tibialis posterior
27 Tibialis anterior
28 Flexor hallucis brevis
29 Flexor digiti minimi brevis
30 Adductor hallucis
31 Flexor hallucis longus
32 Flexor digitorum longus
33 Opponens digiti minimi (part of 29)
34 Peroneus longus

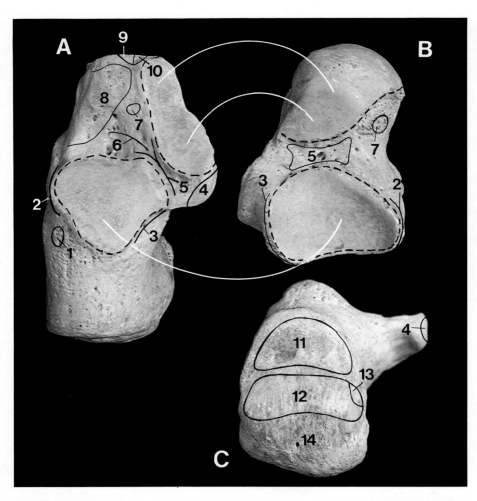

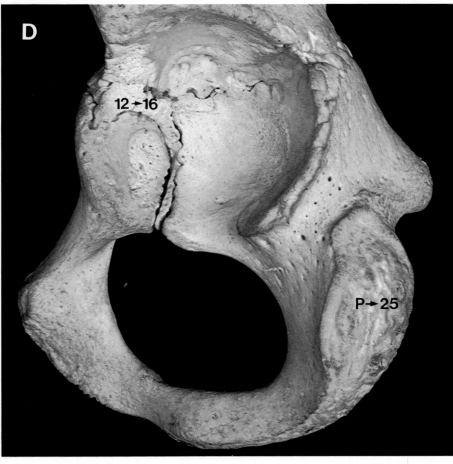

Left calcaneus, A from above, C from behind, and B left talus, from below. Attachments

(Capsule, interrupted line; curved lines indicate corresponding articular surfaces)

1 Calcaneofibular ligament
2 Lateral ⎫
3 Medial ⎬ talocalcanean ligament
4 Tibiocalcanean part of deltoid ligament
5 Interosseous talocalcanean ligament
6 Inferior extensor retinaculum
7 Cervical ligament
8 Extensor digitorum brevis
9 Calcaneocuboid ⎫
10 Calcaneonavicular ⎬ parts of bifurcate ligament
11 Area for bursa
12 Tendo calcaneus (Achilles' tendon)
13 Plantaris
14 Area for fibrofatty tissue

● The interosseous talocalcanean ligament is formed by thickening of the adjacent capsules of the talocalcanean and talocalcaneonavicular joints.

Secondary centres of ossification of left lower limb bones

(Figures in years, commencement of ossification → fusion; B, ninth intrauterine month; P, puberty)

D Lower lateral surface of hip bone, E upper and F lower end of femur, G upper and H lower end of tibia, J upper and K lower end of fibula, L calcaneus, M metatarsal and phalanges of second toe, N metatarsal and phalanges of great toe

● See note on page 106.
● In the hip bone one or more secondary centres appear in the Y-shaped cartilage between ilium, ischium and pubis. Other centres (not illustrated) are usually present for the iliac crest, anterior inferior iliac spine, and (possibly) the pubic tubercle and pubic crest (all P → 25).
● The patella (not illustrated) begins to ossify from one or more centres between the third to sixth year.
● The calcaneus is the only tarsal bone to have a secondary centre.
● All the phalanges, and the first metatarsal, have a secondary centre at their proximal ends; the other metatarsals have one at their distal ends.

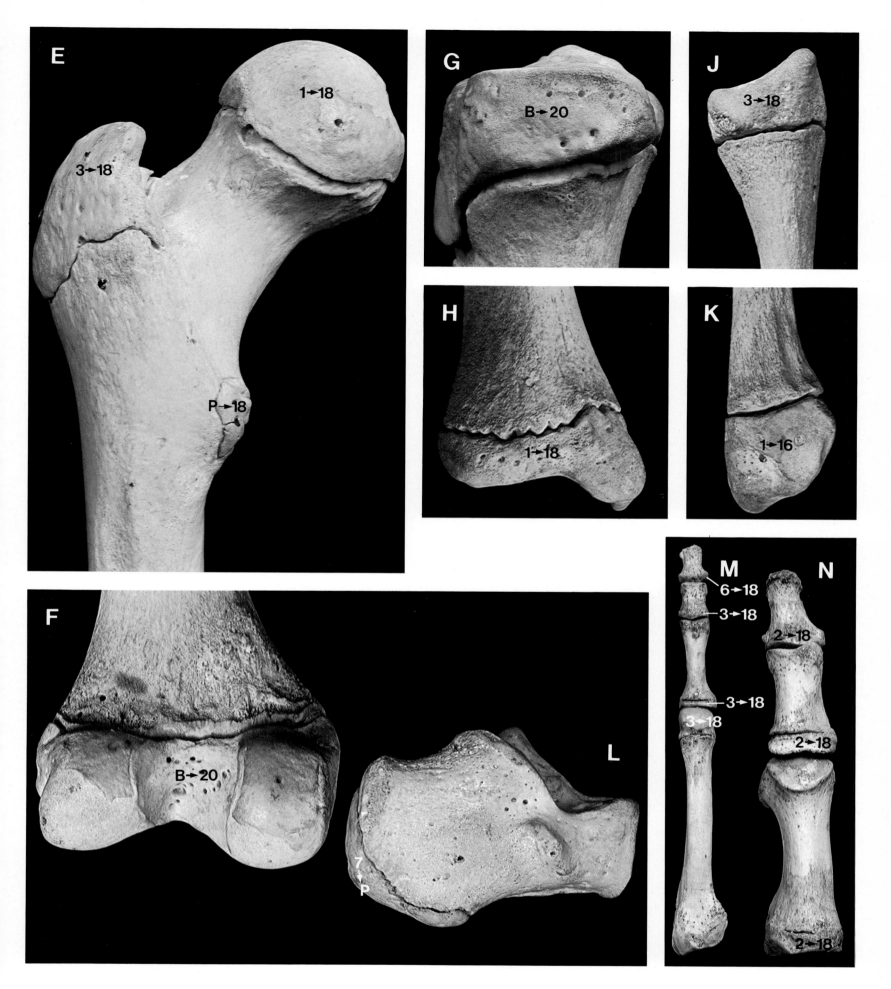

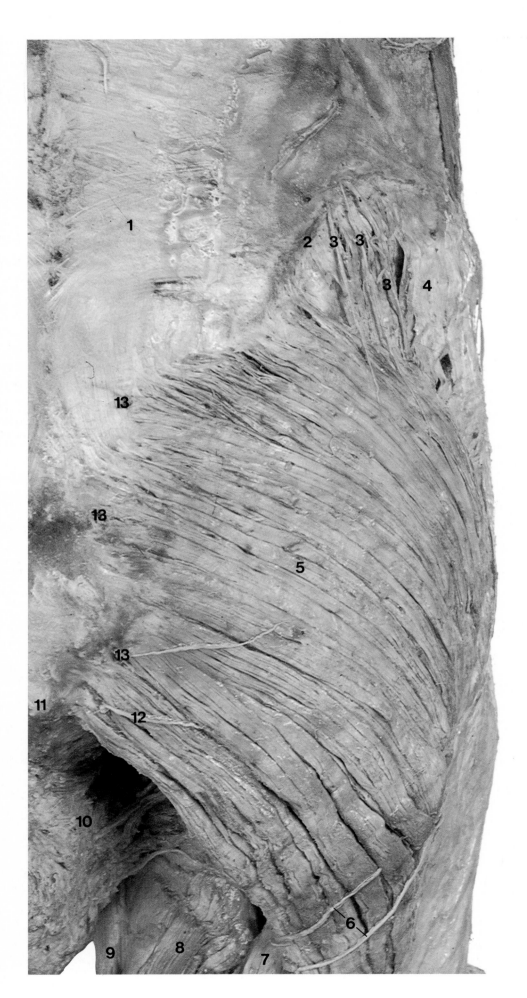

Right gluteal region. Superficial nerves
1 Posterior layer of lumbar fascia overlying erector
   spinae
2 Iliac crest
3 Cutaneous branches of dorsal rami of first three
   lumbar nerves
4 Gluteal fascia overlying gluteus medius
5 Gluteus maximus
6 Gluteal branches of posterior cutaneous nerve of
   thigh
7 Semitendinosus
8 Adductor magnus
9 Gracilis
10 Ischiorectal fossa and levator ani
11 Coccyx
12 Perforating cutaneous nerve
13 Gluteal branches of dorsal rami of first three sacral
   nerves

● The first three lumbar nerves and the first three sacral nerves
supply skin over the gluteal region (by the lateral branches of their
dorsal rami) but the intervening fourth and fifth lumbar nerves do
not have a cutaneous distribution in this region.

A Right gluteal region.
Branches of the sacral plexus
(Most of gluteus maximus, piriformis and the superior gemellus have been removed, together with the blood vessels)
1 Gluteus maximus
2 Piriformis
3 Branches of superior and inferior gluteal nerves
4 Gluteus minimus
5 Gluteus medius
6 Greater trochanter
7 Obturator internus
8 Inferior gemellus
9 Obturator externus
10 Quadratus femoris
11 Adductor magnus
12 Common peroneal part of sciatic nerve
13 Tibial part of sciatic nerve
14 Posterior cutaneous nerve of thigh
15 Ischial tuberosity
16 Long head of biceps
17 Semitendinosus
18 Sacrotuberous ligament
19 Nerve to quadratus femoris (superficial to marker)
20 Nerve to obturator internus (superficial to marker)
21 Pudendal nerve
● The lower edge of the piriformis muscle is here penetrated by the common peroneal part of the sciatic nerve and by numerous filaments forming the inferior gluteal nerve (supplying gluteus maximus). The lowest part of piriformis here gives off a tendon that joins that of obturator internus.

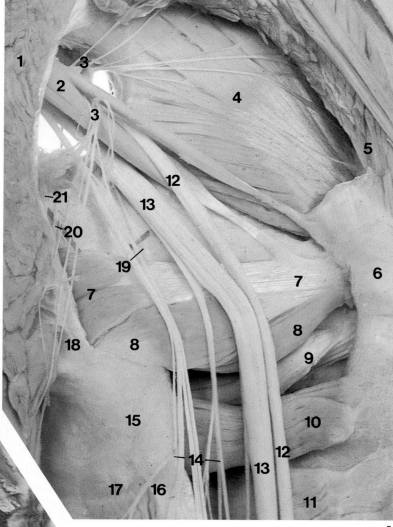

A

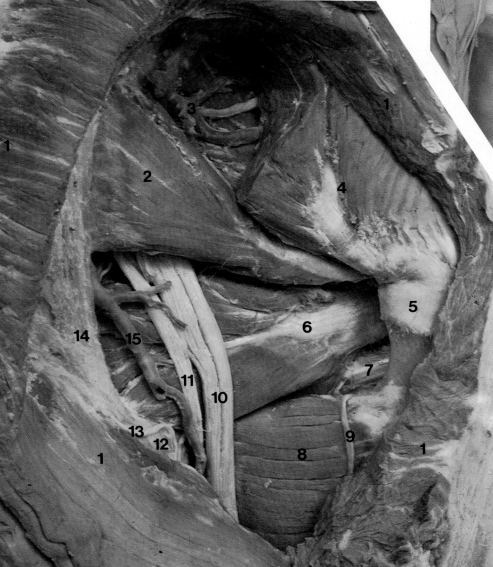

B

B Right gluteal region with the central part of gluteus maximus removed
1 Gluteus maximus
2 Piriformis
3 Superior gluteal nerve and vessels overlying gluteus minimus
4 Gluteus medius
5 Greater trochanter of femur
6 Obturator internus and gemelli
7 Obturator externus
8 Quadratus femoris
9 Ascending branch of medial circumflex femoral artery
10 Sciatic nerve
11 Posterior cutaneous nerve of thigh
12 Ischial tuberosity
13 Perforating cutaneous nerve
14 Sacrotuberous ligament
15 Inferior gluteal artery
● Of the numerous structures that pass out of the greater sciatic foramen, only the superior gluteal nerve and vessels do so *above* the piriformis.

293

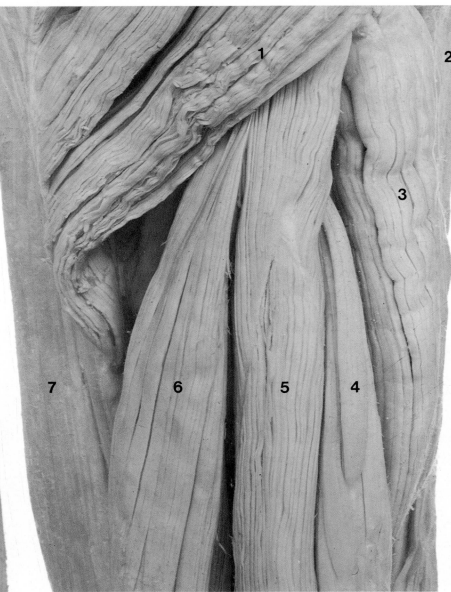

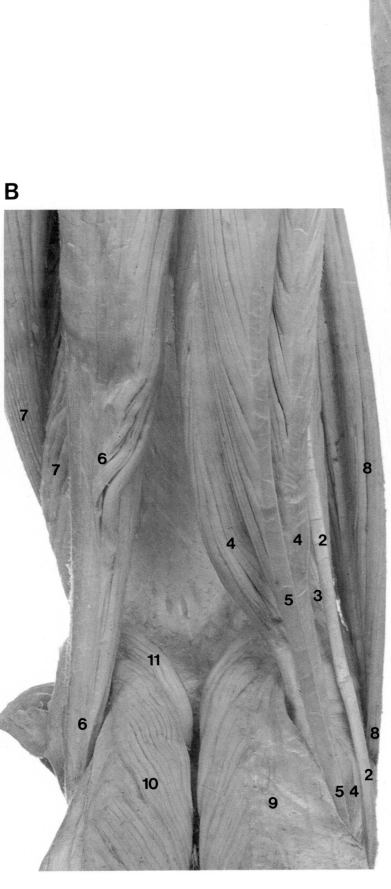

Back of the left thigh. Muscles, A in the upper part, B in the lower part and bordering the popliteal fossa

  1 Gluteus maximus
  2 Gracilis
  3 Adductor magnus
  4 Semimembranosus
  5 Semitendinosus
  6 Biceps
  7 Vastus lateralis
  8 Sartorius
  9 Medial ⎫
  10 Lateral ⎬ head of gastrocnemius
  11 Plantaris

● The long head of biceps (the part seen in illustration A), semimembranosus and semitendinosus are commonly called the hamstrings. The short head of biceps, which is under cover of the long head and arises from the back of the femur, not from the ischial tuberosity, is not classified as a hamstring. The true hamstrings span both the hip and the knee joints.

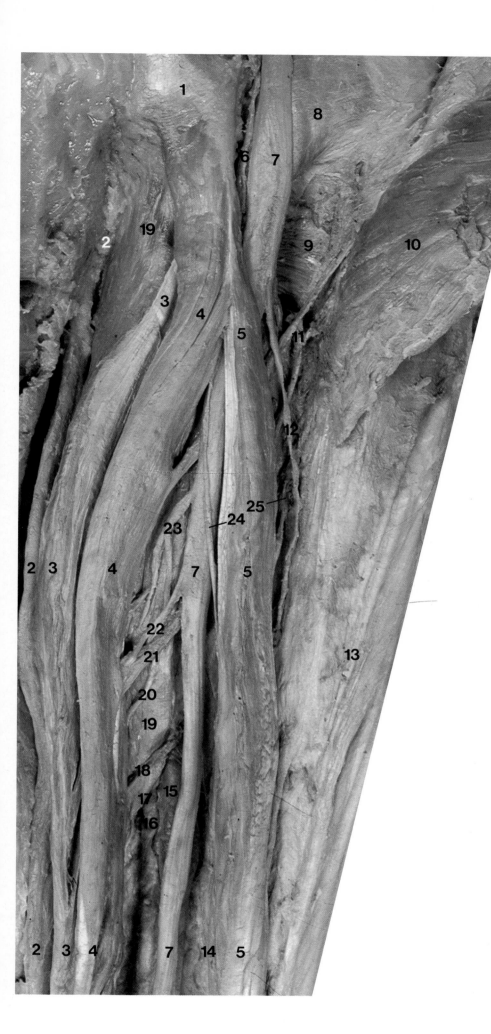

Back of the right thigh. Hamstrings and muscular branches of the sciatic nerve

(Gluteus maximus has been reflected laterally and the hamstrings separated)

1 Ischial tuberosity
2 Gracilis
3 Semimembranosus
4 Semitendinosus
5 Long head of biceps
6 Anastomotic branch of inferior gluteal artery
7 Sciatic nerve
8 Quadratus femoris
9 Upper part of adductor magnus ('adductor minimus')
10 Gluteus maximus
11 First perforating artery
12 Nerve to short head of biceps
13 Iliotibial tract overlying vastus lateralis
14 Short head of biceps
15 Popliteal vein
16 Popliteal artery
17 Opening in adductor magnus
18 Fourth perforating artery
19 Adductor magnus
20 Nerve to semimembranosus
21 Third perforating artery
22 Nerve to semitendinosus
23 Nerve to semimembranosus and adductor magnus
24 Nerve to long head of biceps
25 Second perforating artery

● The only muscular branch to arise from the *lateral* side of the sciatic nerve (i.e. from the common peroneal part) is the nerve to the *short* head of biceps. All the other muscular branches arise from the medial side of the nerve (i.e. from the tibial part).

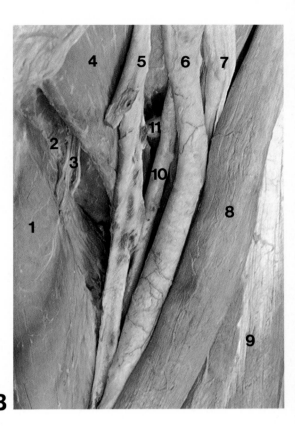

B Left femoral vessels and profunda femoris artery
(From the same specimen as in A, with the femoral artery displaced laterally)

1 Adductor longus
2 Adductor brevis
3 Branches of anterior branch of obturator nerve
4 Pectineus
5 Femoral vein
6 Femoral artery
7 Femoral nerve
8 Sartorius
9 Rectus femoris
10 Profunda femoris artery
11 Medial circumflex femoral artery

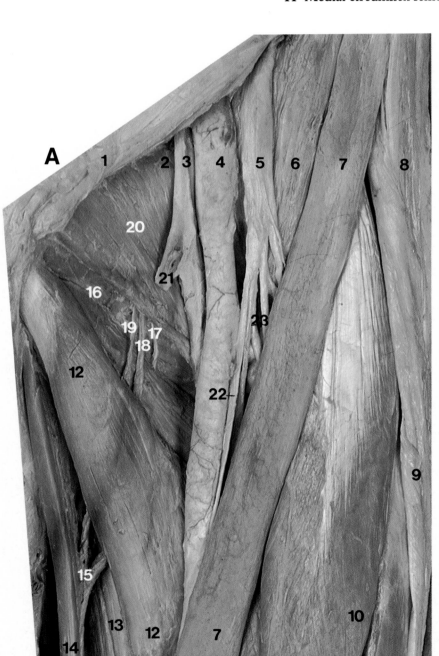

A Left femoral triangle
(The superficial vessels, cutaneous branches of the femoral nerve and the anterior part of the fascia lata have been removed)

1 Inguinal ligament
2 Position of femoral canal
3 Femoral vein
4 Femoral artery
5 Femoral nerve
6 Iliacus
7 Sartorius
8 Fascia lata overlying tensor fasciae latae
9 Iliotibial tract overlying vastus lateralis
10 Rectus femoris
11 Vastus medialis
12 Adductor longus
13 Adductor magnus
14 Gracilis
15 Nerve and vessels to gracilis
16 Adductor brevis
17 Nerve to adductor brevis ⎫ from anterior
18 Nerve to adductor longus ⎬ branch of
19 Nerve to gracilis ⎭ obturator nerve
20 Pectineus
21 Great saphenous vein
22 Saphenous nerve
23 Muscular branches of femoral nerve overlying lateral circumflex femoral vessels

● For superficial dissection of this region see page 207.
● The boundaries of the femoral triangle are the inguinal ligament, the *medial* border of sartorius and the *medial* border of adductor longus.
● The adjacent borders of pectineus and adductor longus are usually in contact with one another, but if they are not (as in this specimen) the anterior branch of the obturator nerve and its muscular branches are visible in the floor of the triangle lying in front of adductor brevis.
● The femoral canal is the medial compartment of the femoral sheath (removed) which contains in its middle compartment the femoral vein, and in the lateral compartment the femoral artery. The femoral nerve is *lateral* to the sheath, not within it.

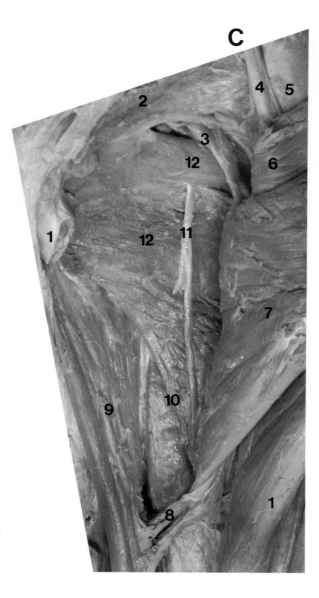

C Posterior branch of the left obturator nerve

(Adductor longus, adductor brevis and pectineus have been detached from their origins and reflected laterally)

1 Adductor longus
2 Superior ramus of pubis
3 Anterior branch of obturator nerve
4 Femoral vein
5 Femoral artery
6 Pectineus
7 Adductor brevis
8 Nerve and vessels to gracilis
9 Gracilis
10 Adductor magnus
11 Posterior branch of obturator nerve
12 Obturator externus

● The obturator nerve divides into its anterior and posterior branches when in the obturator foramen. The anterior branch emerges anterior to obturator externus, while the posterior branch pierces the muscle.

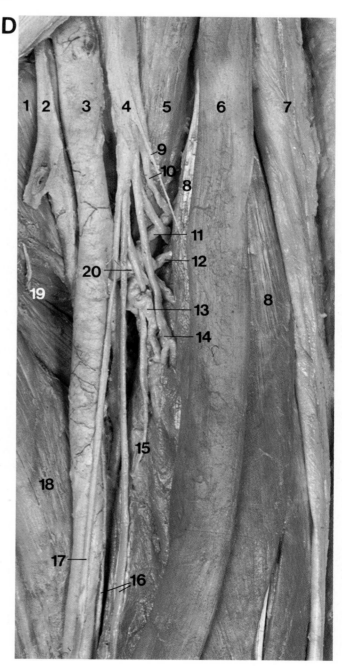

D Left femoral nerve and branches

(From the same specimen as in A, with sartorius and rectus femoris displaced laterally)

1 Pectineus	11 Ascending	branch of lateral
2 Femoral vein	12 Transverse	circumflex femoral
3 Femoral artery	13 Descending	artery
4 Femoral nerve	14 Nerve to vastus lateralis	
5 Iliacus	15 Vastus intermedius and nerve	
6 Sartorius	16 Vastus medialis and nerves	
7 Tensor fasciae latae	17 Saphenous nerve	
8 Rectus femoris	18 Adductor longus	
9 Nerve to sartorius	19 Adductor brevis and nerve	
10 Nerve to rectus femoris	20 Profunda femoris artery	

● The femoral artery (with the vein behind it) passes down the thigh in front of adductor longus and adductor magnus in the adductor canal, and enters the back of the thigh through the opening in adductor magnus (pages 295 and 299) to become the popliteal artery.
● The profunda femoris artery passes down the thigh behind adductor longus, and ends by piercing adductor magnus as the fourth perforating artery (page 295).

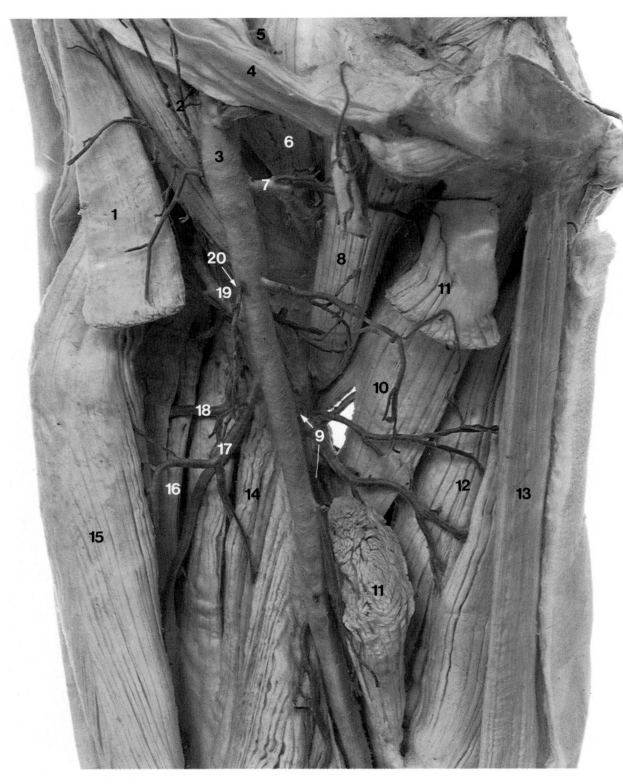

Right femoral artery and branches, with parts of adjacent muscles removed

(Some muscular branches are not named)

1 Sartorius
2 Superficial circumflex iliac vessels overlying iliacus
3 Femoral artery
4 Inguinal ligament
5 Inferior epigastric artery
6 Psoas major
7 Medial circumflex femoral artery
8 Pectineus
9 Profunda femoris artery
10 Adductor brevis
11 Adductor longus
12 Adductor magnus
13 Gracilis
14 Vastus intermedius
15 Rectus femoris (displaced laterally)
16 Vastus lateralis
17 Descending ⎱ branch of
18 Transverse ⎰ lateral circumflex
19 Ascending ⎰ femoral artery
20 Lateral circumflex femoral artery

● In this specimen the medial circumflex femoral artery is a branch of the femoral artery (a frequent occurrence), and not from the profunda artery which is the standard parent vessel.

● The medial circumflex femoral artery passes backwards between the tendon of psoas and pectineus to take part in the cruciate anastomosis on the back of the thigh.

Lower left thigh, from the front and medial side. Vastus medialis and the lower end of the adductor canal

(Sartorius and gracilis have been displaced medially)

1 Gracilis
2 Adductor magnus
3 Sartorius
4 Femoral artery
5 Saphenous nerve
6 Opening in adductor magnus
7 · Vastus medialis and nerve
8 Rectus femoris
9 Iliotibial tract
10 Quadriceps tendon
11 Patella
12 Medial patellar retinaculum
13 Lowest (horizontal) fibres of vastus medialis
14 Saphenous branch of descending genicular artery

● The saphenous nerve is lateral to the femoral artery in the femoral triangle but medial to it in the lower end of the adductor canal, and becomes superficial by passing between sartorius and gracilis at the medial side of the knee.

● The lowest fibres of vastus medialis pass *horizontally* to the patella and are of the utmost importance for obtaining complete extension of the knee joint.

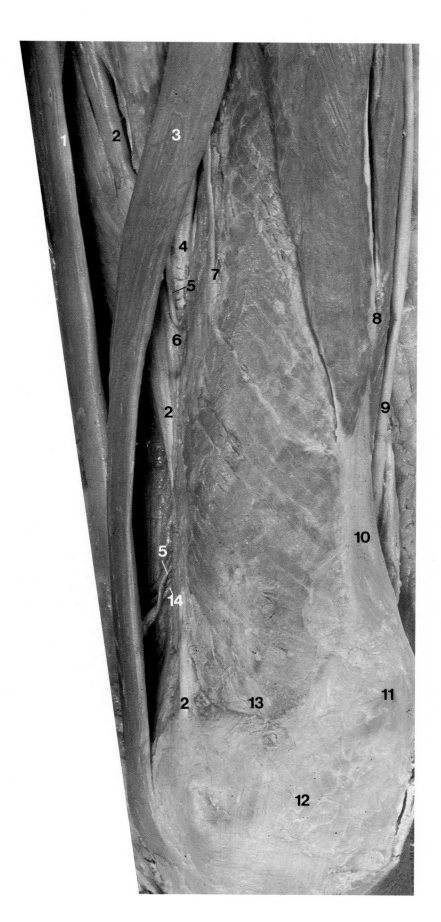

**Right hip joint in the male, A from the front,
B from behind**

 1 Anterior inferior iliac spine
 2 Inguinal ligament
 3 Superficial inguinal ring and spermatic cord
 4 Iliopubic eminence
 5 Obturator canal
 6 Obturator externus
 7 Pubofemoral ligament
 8 Iliofemoral ligament
 9 Lesser trochanter
10 Intertrochanteric line and capsule attachment
11 Greater trochanter
12 Ischiofemoral ligament
13 Zona orbicularis
14 Intertrochanteric crest
15 Ischial tuberosity
16 Lesser sciatic notch and surface for obturator
     internus
17 Ischial spine

● The iliofemoral ligament has the shape of an inverted Y. It and
the interosseous sacro-iliac ligament are the two strongest ligaments
in the body.

● Some of the fibres of the ischiofemoral ligament help to form the
zona orbicularis – circular fibres of the capsule that form a collar
round the neck of the femur.

● Posteriorly the capsule is attached to the neck of the femur, not
to the intertrochanteric crest. (Anteriorly it is attached to the
intertrochanteric line).

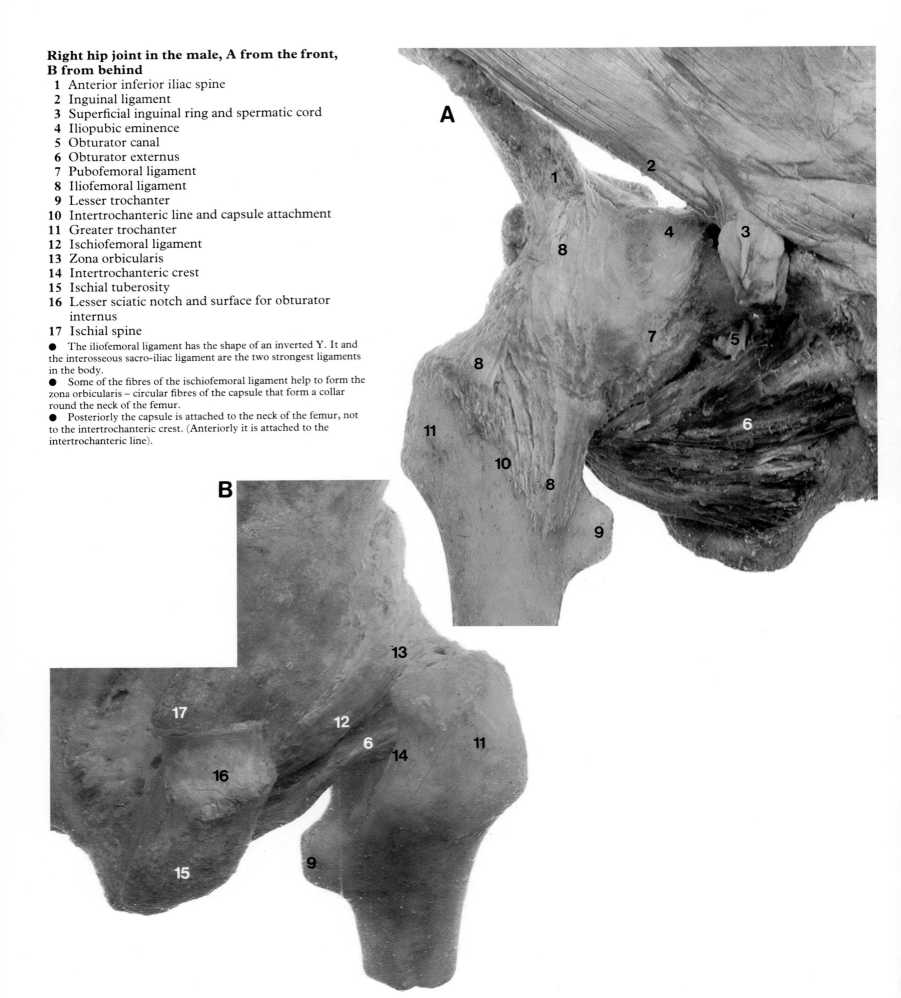

● The vertebropelvic ligaments are the iliolumbar, sacrotuberous and ·
sacrospinous ligaments.
● The dorsal sacro-iliac ligaments cover the interosseous sacro-iliac
ligament.

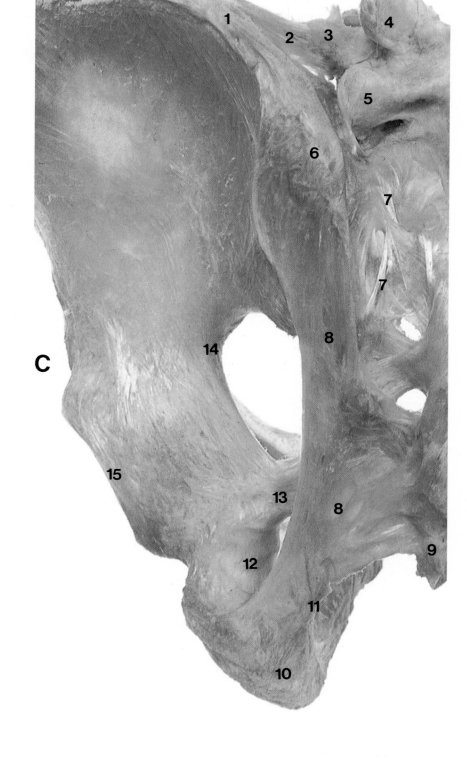

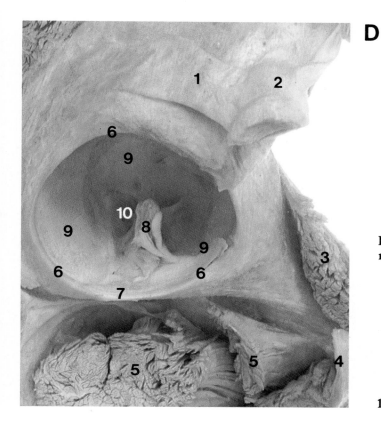

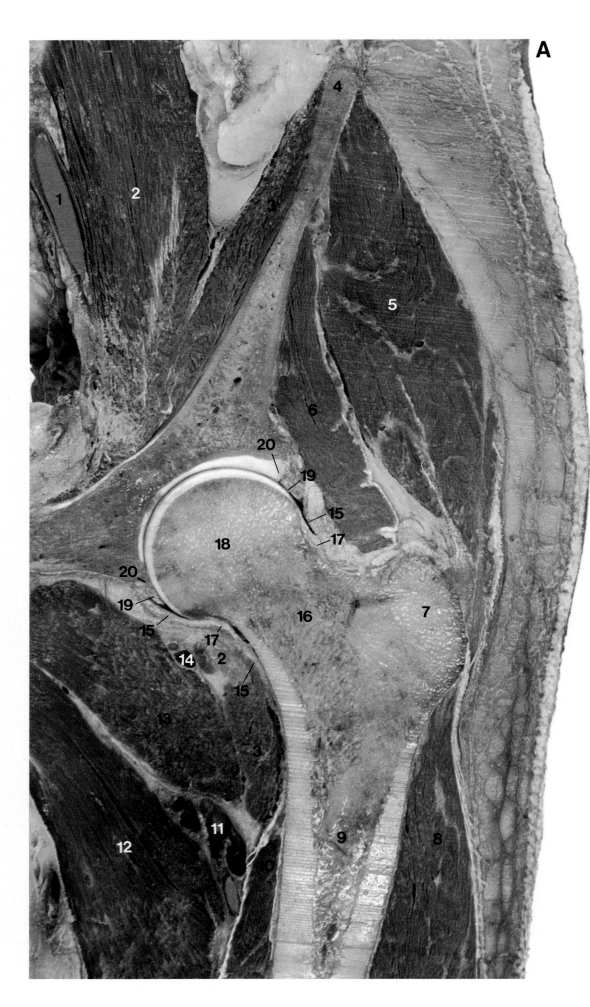

A Left hip joint. Coronal section, from the front

1 External iliac artery
2 Psoas major
3 Iliacus
4 Iliac crest
5 Gluteus medius
6 Gluteus minimus
7 Greater trochanter
8 Vastus lateralis
9 Shaft of femur
10 Vastus medialis
11 Profunda femoris vessels
12 Adductor longus
13 Pectineus
14 Medial circumflex femoral vessels
15 Capsule of hip joint
16 Neck of femur
17 Zona orbicularis of capsule
18 Head of femur
19 Acetabular labrum
20 Rim of acetabulum

● In this section the convergence of gluteus medius and minimus on to the greater trochanter is well illustrated. In walking these muscles prevent the pelvis from falling to the opposite side when the opposite leg is off the ground, i.e. they are acting more as preventers of adduction than as abductors.

B Radiograph of the left hip joint, from the front in the female

1 Transverse process of fifth lumbar vertebra
2 Sacro-iliac joint
3 Anterior superior iliac spine
4 Rim of acetabulum
5 Head ⎫
6 Neck ⎬ of femur
7 Greater trochanter ⎪
8 Lesser trochanter ⎭
9 Ischial tuberosity
10 Pectineal line
11 Pubic tubercle
12 Pubic symphysis
13 Shadow of pudendal cleft
14 First coccygeal vertebra
15 Calcified lymph nodes
16 Ischial spine

B

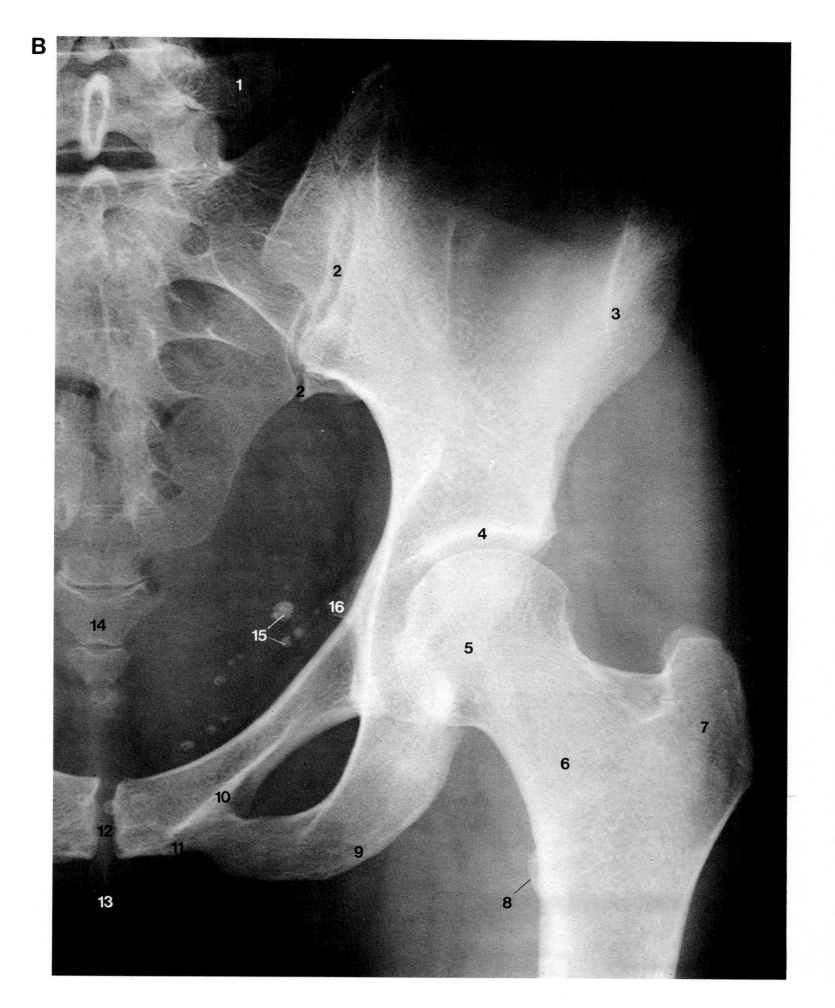

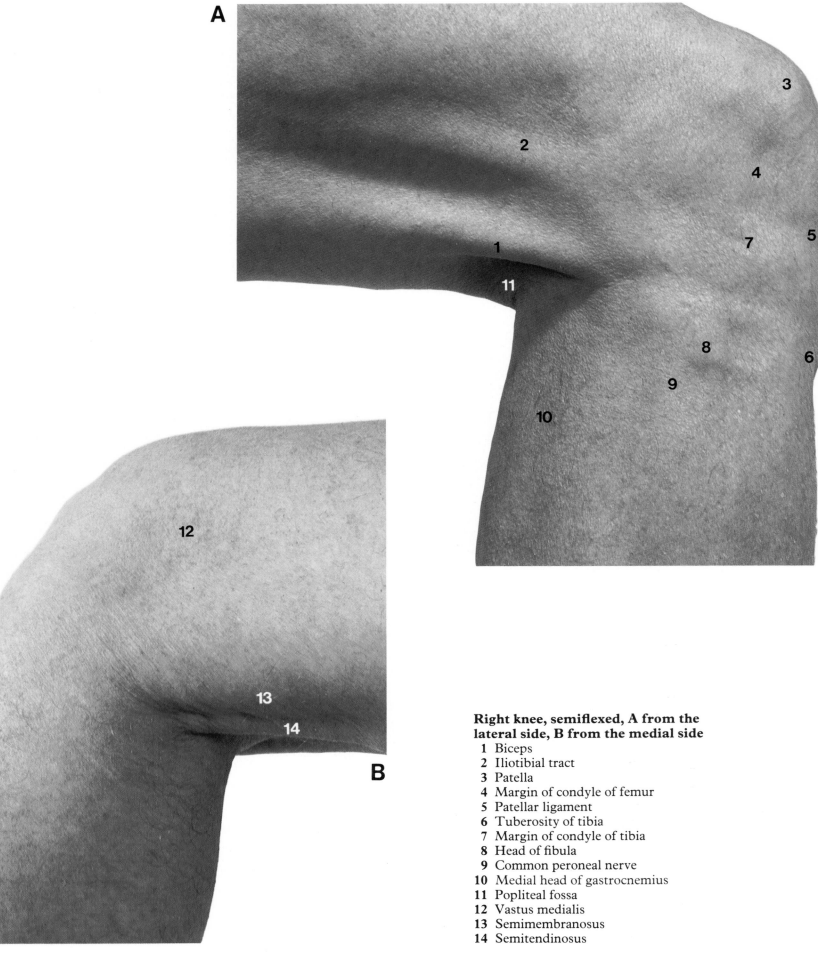

Right knee, semiflexed, A from the lateral side, B from the medial side

1 Biceps
2 Iliotibial tract
3 Patella
4 Margin of condyle of femur
5 Patellar ligament
6 Tuberosity of tibia
7 Margin of condyle of tibia
8 Head of fibula
9 Common peroneal nerve
10 Medial head of gastrocnemius
11 Popliteal fossa
12 Vastus medialis
13 Semimembranosus
14 Semitendinosus

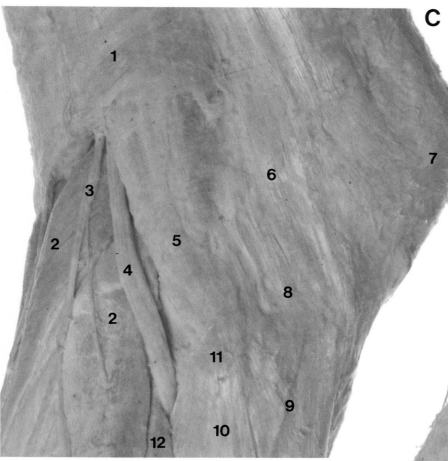

C Right knee, from the lateral side. Iliotibial tract and common peroneal nerve

1 Fascia lata
2 Lateral head of gastrocnemius
3 Lateral cutaneous nerve of calf
4 Common peroneal nerve
5 Biceps
6 Iliotibial tract
7 Patella
8 Attachment of iliotibial tract to tibia
9 Deep fascia overlying extensor muscles
10 Deep fascia overlying peroneus longus
11 Head of fibula
12 Soleus

● The iliotibial tract is the thickened lateral part of the fascia lata. At its upper part the tensor fasciae latae and most of gluteus maximus are inserted into it; its lower end is attached to the lateral condyle of the tibia.

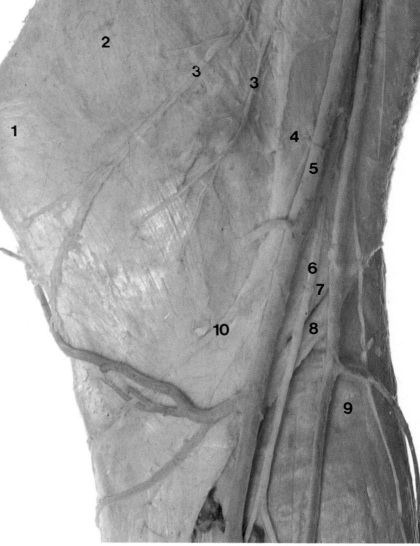

D Right knee, from the medial side. Superficial vessels and nerves

1 Patella
2 Vastus medialis
3 Cutaneous branches of femoral nerve
4 Sartorius
5 Great saphenous vein
6 Saphenous nerve
7 Gracilis
8 Semitendinosus
9 Medial head of gastrocnemius
10 Infrapatellar branch of saphenous nerve

● At the level of the knee joint the great saphenous vein lies one handsbreadth behind the medial border of the patella.
● The saphenous nerve becomes superficial behind the lower end of sartorius.

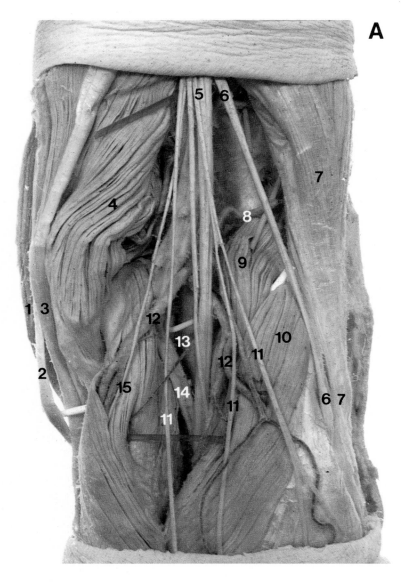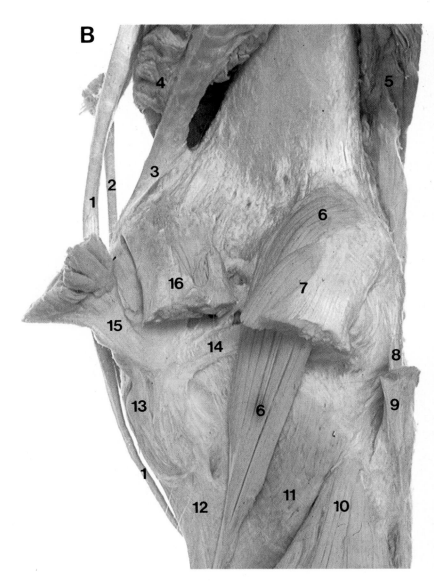

A Right popliteal fossa

1 Sartorius
2 Gracilis (displaced backwards by white marker)
3 Semitendinosus
4 Semimembranosus
5 Tibial nerve
6 Common peroneal nerve
7 Biceps
8 Superior lateral genicular artery (passing over blue marker)
9 Plantaris (superficial to white marker)
10 Lateral head of gastrocnemius
11 Branches of sural nerve
12 Sural arteries
13 Popliteal artery
14 Popliteal vein (displaced medially by blue marker)
15 Medial head of gastrocnemius (displaced medially by red marker) and branch from tibial nerve

● The upper red marker passes between the tibial nerve and the underlying popliteal vein.
● The uppermost blue marker is crossed by a muscular branch of the popliteal artery.
● The sural nerve has divided at an unusually high level into several branches. The peroneal communicating branch of the common peroneal nerve is not present.
● The principal structures in the middle of the fossa – the tibial nerve, popliteal vein and popliteal artery – lie in that order from superficial to deep. The deep position of the artery makes palpation of its pulsation difficult.

● The small saphenous vein (here removed) normally drains into the popliteal vein by piercing the deep fascia that forms the roof of the fossa.
● The most lateral branch of the sural nerve may here take the place of the lateral cutaneous nerve of the calf which normally arises from the common peroneal nerve.

B Right knee joint from behind. Semimembranosus attachment and fibrous expansions

1 Semitendinosus
2 Gracilis
3 Adductor magnus
4 Vastus medialis
5 Vastus lateralis
6 Plantaris
7 Lateral head of gastrocnemius
8 Fibular collateral ligament
9 Biceps
10 Soleus
11 Popliteus
12 Fascia overlying popliteus
13 Expansion to tibia
14 Oblique popliteal ligament
15 Semimembranosus
16 Medial head of gastrocnemius

● The semimembranosus tendon gives three main slips or expansions: to the tibia behind the tibial collateral ligament, to join the fascia over popliteus, and to form the oblique popliteal ligament.

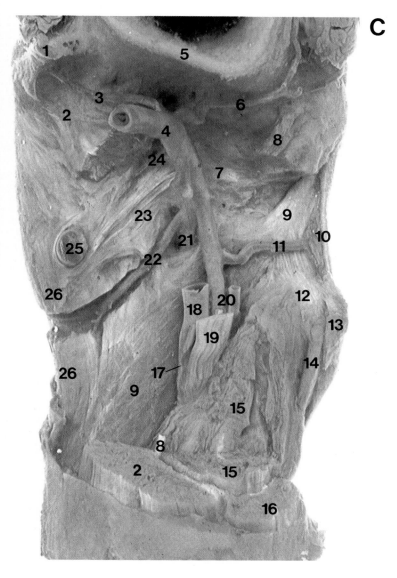

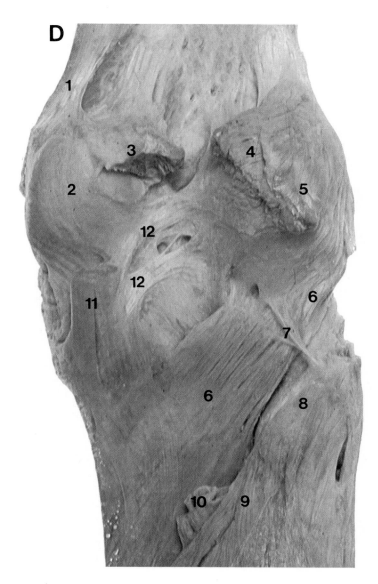

C Right popliteal fossa with the knee joint flexed. Deep dissection of popliteal artery (with unusually high division) and genicular vessels

1 Adductor magnus
2 Medial head of gastrocnemius
3 Superior medial genicular artery
4 Popliteal artery
5 Popliteal surface of femur in section
6 Superior lateral genicular artery
7 Capsule of knee joint
8 Plantaris
9 Popliteus
10 Fibular collateral ligament
11 Inferior lateral genicular artery
12 Head of fibula
13 Biceps
14 Common peroneal nerve
15 Soleus
16 Lateral head of gastrocnemius
17 Nerve to popliteus
18 Popliteal vein
19 Tibial nerve
20 Posterior tibial artery and vein
21 Anterior tibial artery
22 Inferior medial genicular artery
23 Oblique popliteal ligament

24 Middle genicular artery
25 Semimembranosus
26 Tibial collateral ligament

● The popliteal artery normally divides into anterior and posterior tibial vessels at the lower border of popliteus, but in this specimen the division is unusually high and the anterior tibial artery passes deep to popliteus.

D Right knee joint, from behind. Capsule and popliteal ligaments

1 Adductor magnus
2 Capsule overlying medial condyle of femur
3 Medial head of gastrocnemius
4 Plantaris
5 Lateral head of gastrocnemius
6 Popliteus
7 Arcuate popliteal ligament
8 Head of fibula
9 Soleus
10 Popliteal vessels and tibial nerve
11 Semimembranosus
12 Oblique popliteal ligament

● The oblique popliteal ligament is derived from the semimembranosus tendon and reinforces the central posterior part of the joint capsule; it is pierced by the middle genicular artery which passes through the capsule to supply the cruciate ligaments.

● The arcuate popliteal ligament arches over the popliteus as it emerges from the capsule.

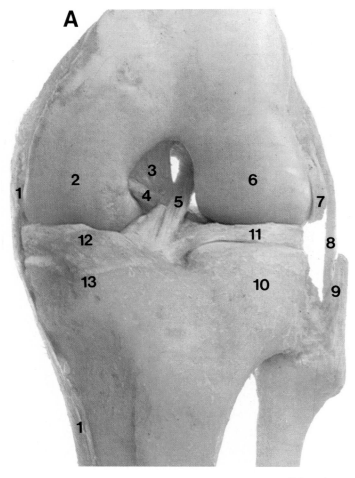

A

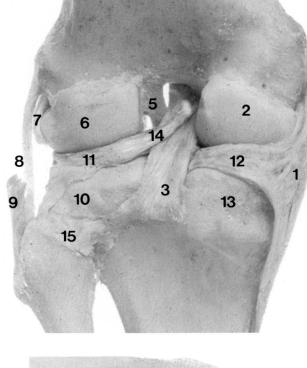

B

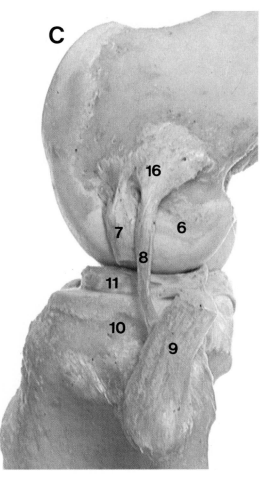

C

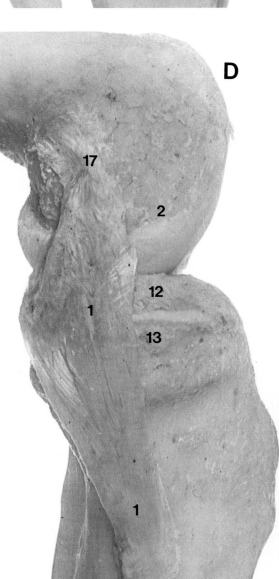

D

**Ligaments of the left knee joint, A
from the front, B from behind, C from
the lateral side, D from the medial
side**

1 Tibial collateral ligament
2 Medial condyle of femur
3 Posterior cruciate ligament
4 Anterior meniscofemoral ligament
5 Anterior cruciate ligament
6 Lateral condyle of femur
7 Popliteus
8 Fibular collateral ligament
9 Biceps
10 Lateral condyle of tibia
11 Lateral meniscus
12 Medial meniscus
13 Medial condyle of tibia
14 Posterior meniscofemoral ligament
15 Capsule of superior tibiofibular joint
16 Lateral ⎫
17 Medial ⎬ epicondyle of femur

● The transverse ligament, connecting the medial
and lateral menisci anteriorly, is not present in this
specimen (see opposite page).
● The tibial collateral (medial) ligament is a broad
band about 12cm long.
● The fibular collateral (lateral) ligament is a
rounded cord about 5cm long.
● The medial meniscus is attached to the tibial
collateral ligament but the lateral meniscus is *not*
attached to the fibular collateral ligament.
● The posterior and anterior meniscofemoral
ligaments are both derived from the lateral meniscus
and are named from their relationship to the posterior
cruciate ligament.

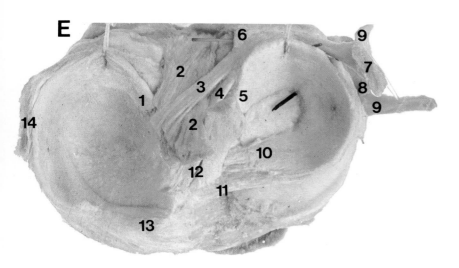

E Left knee joint, with the femur removed, from above
1 Posterior horn of medial meniscus
2 Posterior cruciate ligament
3 Posterior ⎱ meniscofemoral
4 Anterior ⎰ ligament
5 Posterior horn of lateral meniscus
6 Popliteal attachment to lateral meniscus (with underlying bristle)
7 Popliteus tendon
8 Fibular collateral ligament
9 Biceps tendon
10 Anterior horn of lateral meniscus
11 Transverse ligament

12 Anterior cruciate ligament
13 Anterior horn of medial meniscus
14 Tibial collateral ligament attached to medial meniscus

● The anterior cruciate ligament is attached to the intercondylar area of the tibia some distance behind the anterior margin of the upper surface of the bone, but the attachment of the posterior cruciate ligament overlaps the posterior margin on to the posterior surface.

● The cruciate ligaments are named from their attachments to the tibia. The anterior cruciate passes upwards, backwards and laterally to be attached to the medial side of the lateral condyle of the femur; the posterior cruciate passes upwards, forwards and medially to be attached to the lateral surface of the medial condyle of the femur.

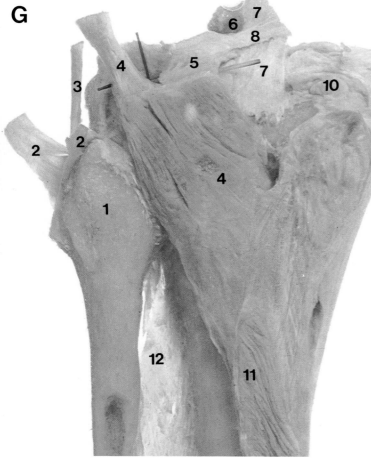

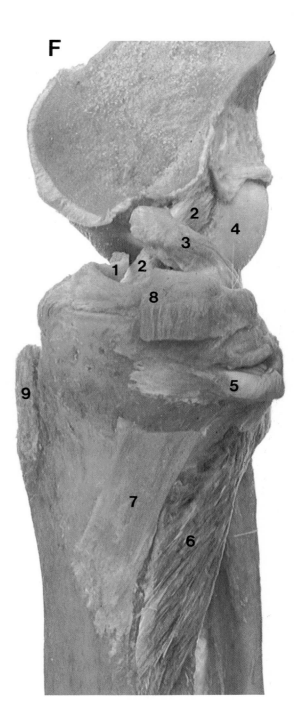

G Left knee joint, from behind with the femur removed
1 Head of fibula
2 Biceps
3 Fibular collateral ligament
4 Popliteus
5 Attachment of lateral meniscus to popliteus
6 Anterior cruciate ligament
7 Posterior cruciate ligament
8 Posterior meniscofemoral ligament
9 Medial meniscus attached to tibial collateral ligament
10 Semimembranosus
11 Soleus
12 Interosseous membrane

F Right knee joint, with the medial femoral condyle removed, from the medial side
1 Transverse ligament (displaced backwards)
2 Anterior cruciate ligament
3 Posterior cruciate ligament
4 Lateral condyle of femur
5 Semimembranosus
6 Popliteus
7 Tibial collateral ligament
8 Medial meniscus and attachment of tibial collateral ligament
9 Patellar ligament

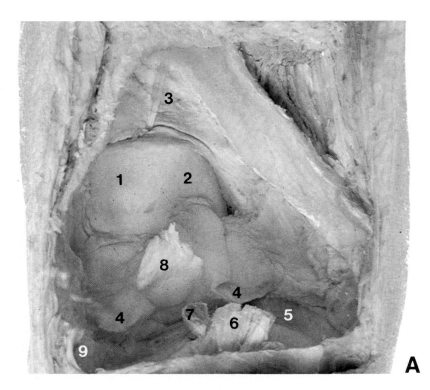

A Left knee joint, opened from behind with the femur removed

1 Lateral ⎫
2 Medial ⎭ articular surface of patella
3 Suprapatellar bursa (supported by glass rod)
4 Alar fold
5 Medial meniscus
6 Posterior ⎫
7 Anterior ⎭ cruciate ligament
8 Infrapatellar fold (ligamentum mucosum)
9 Lateral meniscus

● Below the patella the synovial membrane is projected backwards by the infrapatellar fat pad, so forming the two alar folds which have posterior free borders, and the central infrapatellar fold which is attached to the front of the intercondylar area of the femur.

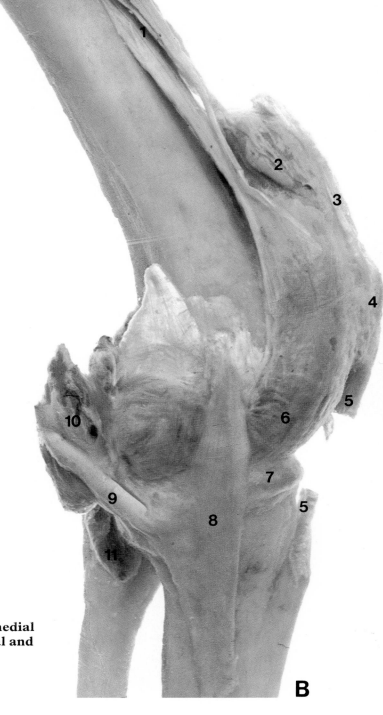

B Left knee joint, from the medial side, with injection of synovial and bursal cavities

1 Articularis genu
2 Suprapatellar bursa
3 Quadriceps tendon
4 Patella
5 Patellar ligament
6 Capsule
7 Medial meniscus
8 Tibial collateral ligament
9 Semimembranosus
10 Semimembranosus bursa
11 Bursa of popliteal tendon

● The normal knee joint (the largest of all synovial joints) contains less than 1 ml of synovial fluid; the joint illustrated contains about 80 ml of injected resin which has distended the synovial cavity.

● The suprapatellar bursa always communicates with the joint cavity. The bursa around the popliteus tendon usually does so. The semimembranosus bursa may do so.

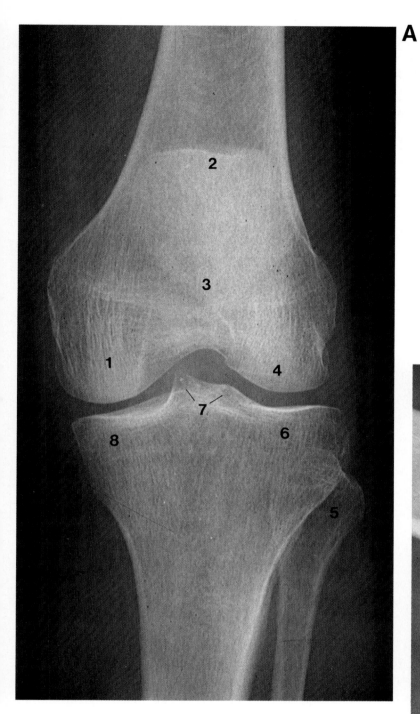
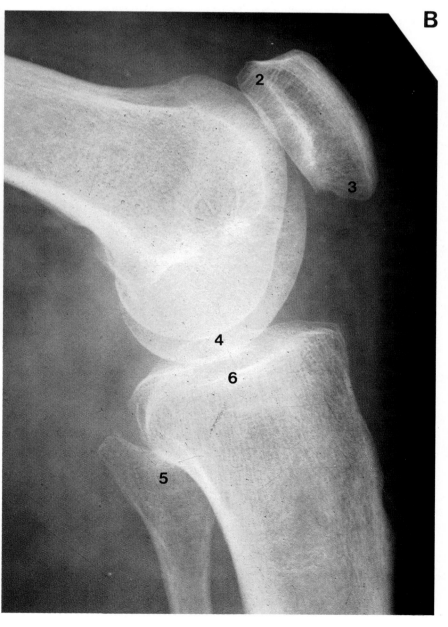

**Radiographs of the knee, A from behind,
B from the lateral side, in partial flexion**
1 Medial condyle of femur
2 Base ⎱
3 Apex ⎰ of patella
4 Lateral condyle of femur
5 Head of fibula
6 Lateral condyle of tibia
7 Tubercles of intercondylar eminence
8 Medial condyle of tibia

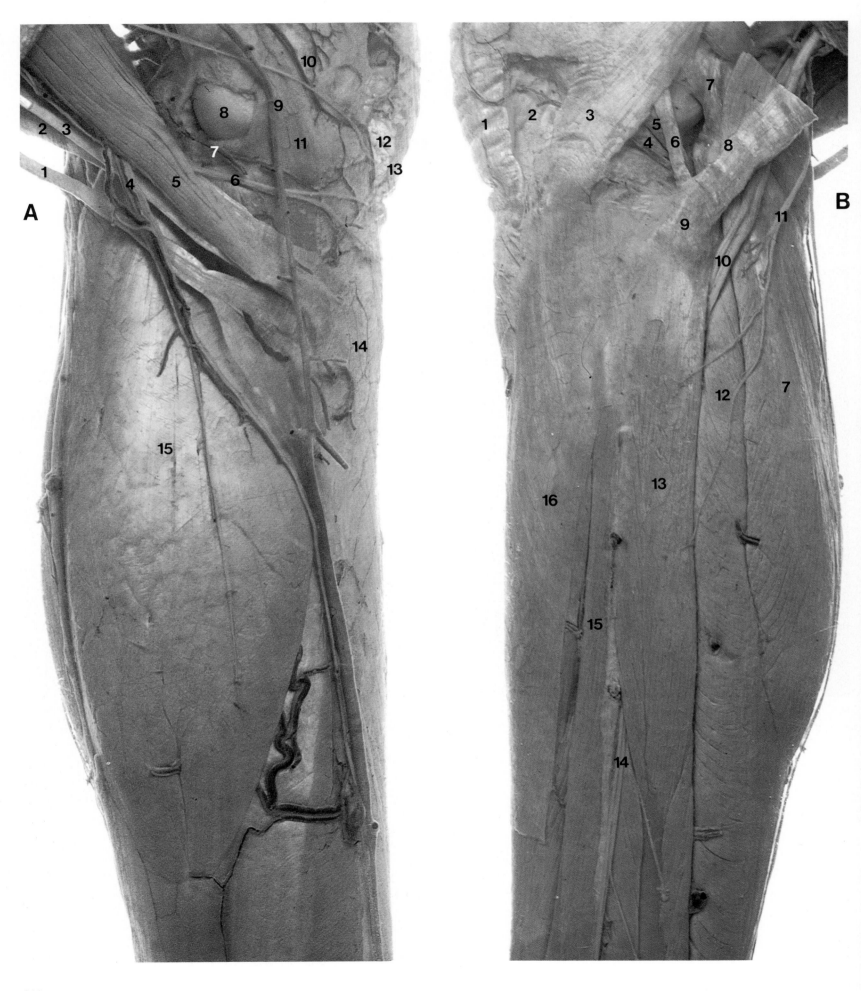

**A Left knee and leg, from the medial side.
Tendons, vessels and nerves**
  1 Semitendinosus
  2 Semimembranosus
  3 Gracilis
  4 Saphenous nerve and artery
  5 Sartorius
  6 Infrapatellar branch of saphenous nerve
  7 Branch of saphenous artery overlying medial meniscus
  8 Medial condyle of femur (part of capsule removed)
  9 Great saphenous vein
 10 Branches of superior medial genicular artery
 11 Tibial collateral ligament
 12 Infrapatellar fat pad
 13 Patellar ligament
 14 Medial surface of tibia
 15 Medial head of gastrocnemius
● In this specimen the great saphenous vein at the level of the knee is unusually small.

**B Left knee and leg, from the lateral side.
Muscles and nerves**
  1 Patellar ligament
  2 Infrapatellar fat pad
  3 Iliotibial tract
  4 Lateral meniscus
  5 Popliteus
  6 Fibular collateral ligament
  7 Lateral head of gastrocnemius
  8 Biceps
  9 Head of fibula
 10 Common peroneal nerve
 11 Lateral cutaneous nerve of calf
 12 Soleus
 13 Peroneus longus
 14 Superficial peroneal nerve
 15 Extensor digitorum longus
 16 Fascia overlying tibialis anterior

C Middle of the calf of the left leg. Superficial vessels and nerves
  1 Lateral head of gastrocnemius
  2 Lateral cutaneous nerve of calf
  3 Small saphenous vein
  4 Medial head of gastrocnemius
  5 Sural nerve
  6 Aponeurotic part of tendo calcaneus
  7 Soleus
  8 Peroneus longus
  9 Deep fascia
● The medial head of gastrocnemius extends to a lower level than the lateral head.

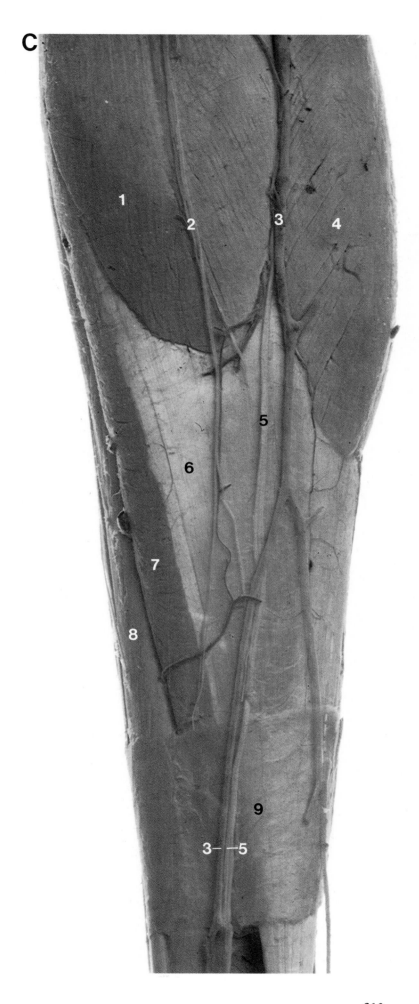

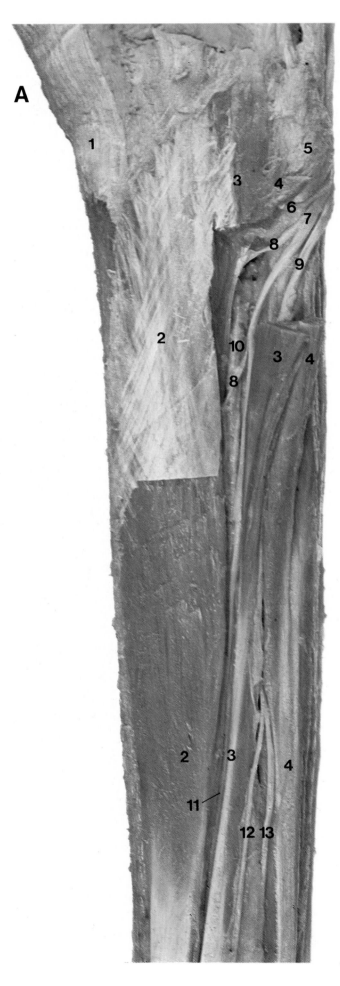

A Left leg, from the front and lateral side. Extensor muscles and branches of common peroneal nerve

1 Tuberosity of tibia and patellar ligament
2 Tibialis anterior and overlying fascia
3 Extensor digitorum longus
4 Peroneus longus
5 Head of fibula
6 Recurrent branch of common peroneal nerve
7 Deep peroneal nerve
8 Branch to tibialis anterior
9 Superficial peroneal nerve
10 Anterior tibial artery overlying interosseous membrane
11 Extensor hallucis longus
12 Medial ⎫ branch of superficial
13 Lateral ⎭ peroneal nerve

● The upper ends of peroneus longus and extensor digitorum longus have been partly removed and displaced backwards.

● The common peroneal nerve divides into its superficial and deep parts immediately below the lateral side of the head of the fibula where it is in contact with the bone under cover of peroneus longus.

B Left ankle, from the front and lateral side. Tendons, vessels and nerves

1 Medial malleolus
2 Tibialis anterior
3 Extensor hallucis longus
4 Anterior tibial vessels
5 Deep peroneal nerve
6 Extensor digitorum longus
7 Medial branch of superficial peroneal nerve
8 Lateral malleolus

● On the front of the ankle the *extensor hallucis* longus tendon is immediately adjacent to the *tibialis anterior* tendon. Behind the medial malleolus (page 320) it is the *flexor digitorum* longus tendon that lies immediately adjacent to the *tibialis posterior* tendon.

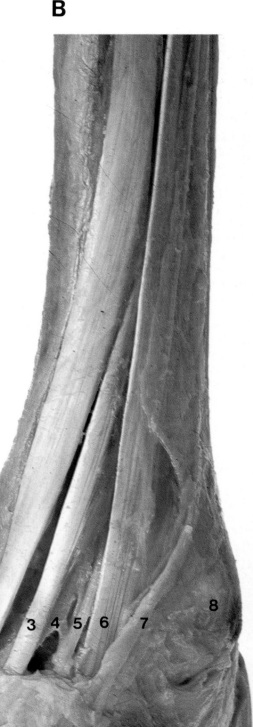

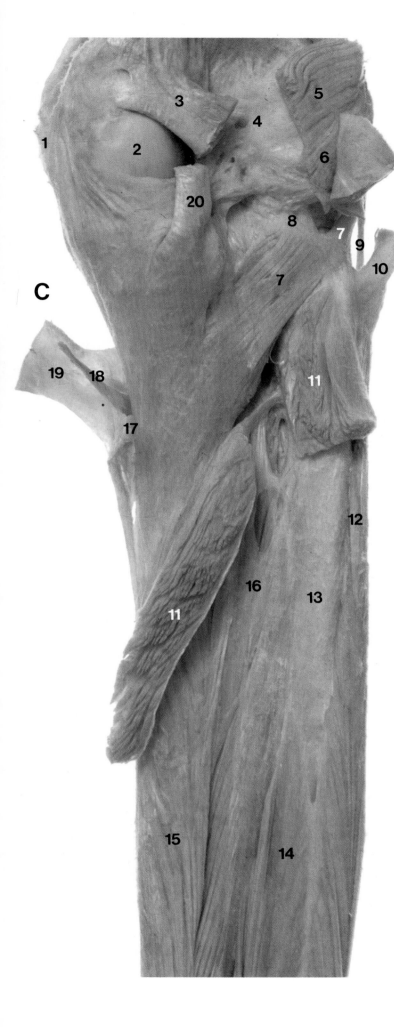

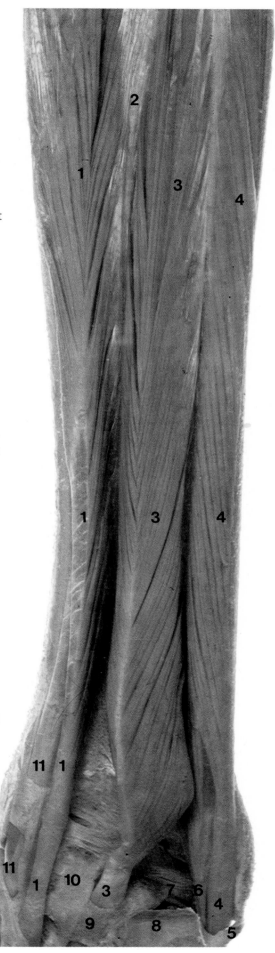

C Right popliteal fossa and upper calf. Deep dissection of muscles

1 Tibial collateral ligament
2 Medial condyle of femur
3 Medial head of gastrocnemius
4 Capsule of knee joint
5 Plantaris
6 Lateral head of gastrocnemius
7 Popliteus
8 Attachment of popliteus to lateral meniscus
9 Fibular collateral ligament
10 Biceps
11 Soleus
12 Peroneus longus
13 Posterior surface of fibula (soleus removed)
14 Flexor hallucis longus
15 Flexor digitorum longus
16 Tibialis posterior
17 Semitendinosus
18 Gracilis
19 Sartorius
20 Semimembranosus

● Tibialis posterior is the deepest muscle of the calf.
● Flexor hallucis longus, although passing to the great toe on the *medial* side of the foot, arises from the fibula on the *lateral* side of the leg.

D Calf of the right leg. Deep muscles

1 Flexor digitorum longus
2 Fascia overlying tibialis posterior
3 Flexor hallucis longus
4 Peroneus longus
5 Superior peroneal retinaculum
6 Peroneus brevis
7 Posterior talofibular ligament
8 Tendo calcaneus (Achilles' tendon)
9 Part of flexor retinaculum
10 Position of posterior tibial vessels and tibial nerve
11 Tibialis posterior

315

A

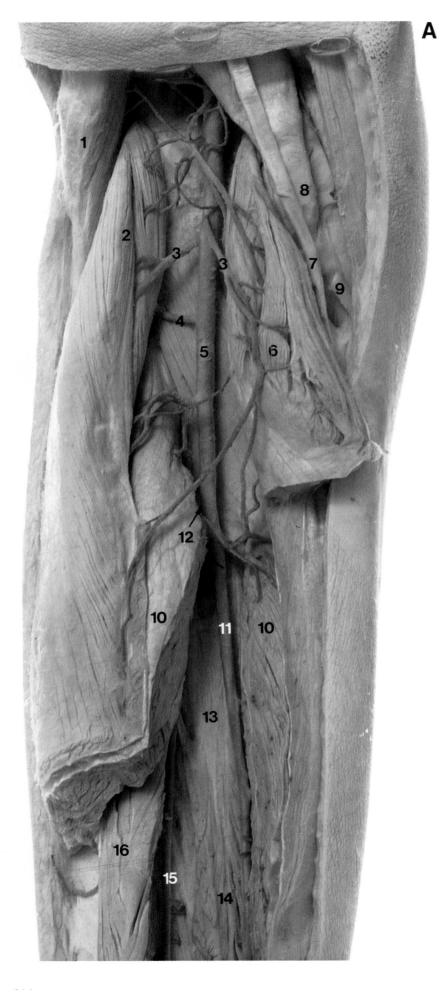

B

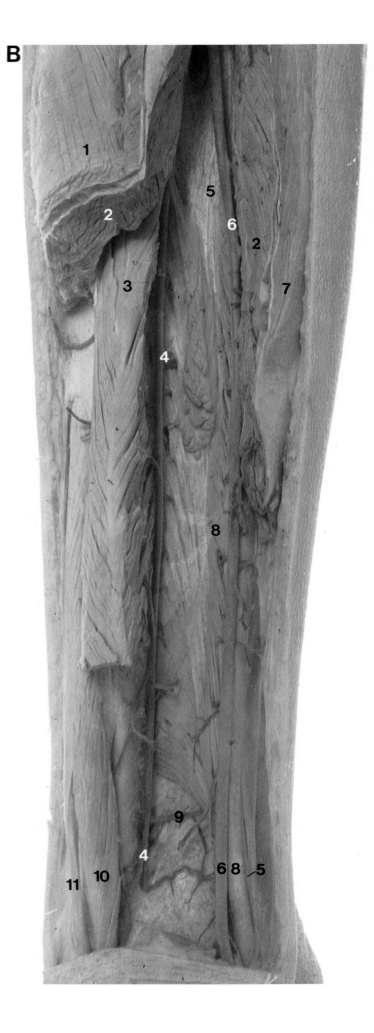

A Left popliteal fossa and calf. Popliteal artery and branches

1 Biceps
2 Lateral head of gastrocnemius
3 Sural arteries
4 Inferior lateral genicular artery overlying popliteus
5 Popliteal artery
6 Medial head of gastrocnemius
7 Semitendinosus
8 Semimembranosus
9 Gracilis
10 Soleus
11 Posterior tibial artery
12 Anterior tibial artery
13 Tibialis posterior
14 Flexor digitorum longus
15 Peroneal artery
16 Flexor hallucis longus

● The arrow indicates the origin (hidden by the overlying soleus) of the peroneal artery; it arises from the posterior tibial below the lower border of popliteus.
● The popliteal artery ends at the lower border of popliteus by dividing into the anterior and posterior tibial vessels. The anterior tibial artery passes forwards above tibialis posterior into the extensor compartment.

B Calf of the left leg. Deep dissection of arteries

1 Lateral head of gastrocnemius
2 Soleus
3 Flexor hallucis longus
4 Peroneal artery
5 Tibialis posterior
6 Posterior tibial artery
7 Medial head of gastrocnemius
8 Flexor digitorum longus
9 Communicating branch
10 Peroneus brevis
11 Peroneus longus

● The peroneal artery passes down the medial crest of the fibula between flexor hallucis longus and tibialis posterior. It ends by dividing into a number of lateral calcanean branches.
● The posterior tibial artery passes down the medial side of the calf on tibialis posterior and flexor digitorum longus, to lie behind the digitorum tendon behind the medial malleolus where it ends by dividing into the medial and lateral plantar arteries.

C Left popliteal fossa and calf, from the right and behind

(With the soleus bisected in the midline and displaced to each side to show the branches of the tibial nerve. The knee joint has been injected with resin and the capsule removed. Most of gastrocnemius and all veins have also been removed)

1 Common peroneal nerve
2 Sural nerve (double origin)
3 Tibial nerve
4 Popliteal artery
5 Semimembranosus
6 Semitendinosus
7 Gracilis (displaced laterally at upper end)
8 Sartorius
9 Medial head of gastrocnemius
10 Popliteus
11 Plantaris
12 Soleus
13 Flexor digitorum longus
14 Nerve to flexor hallucis longus
15 Flexor hallucis longus
16 Peroneal artery
17 Fascia over tibialis posterior
18 Posterior tibial artery
19 Nerve to deep surface of soleus
20 Nerve to tibialis posterior
21 Nerve to superficial surface of soleus
22 Nerve to popliteus
23 Nerve to lateral head of gastrocnemius
24 Nerve to medial head of gastrocnemius

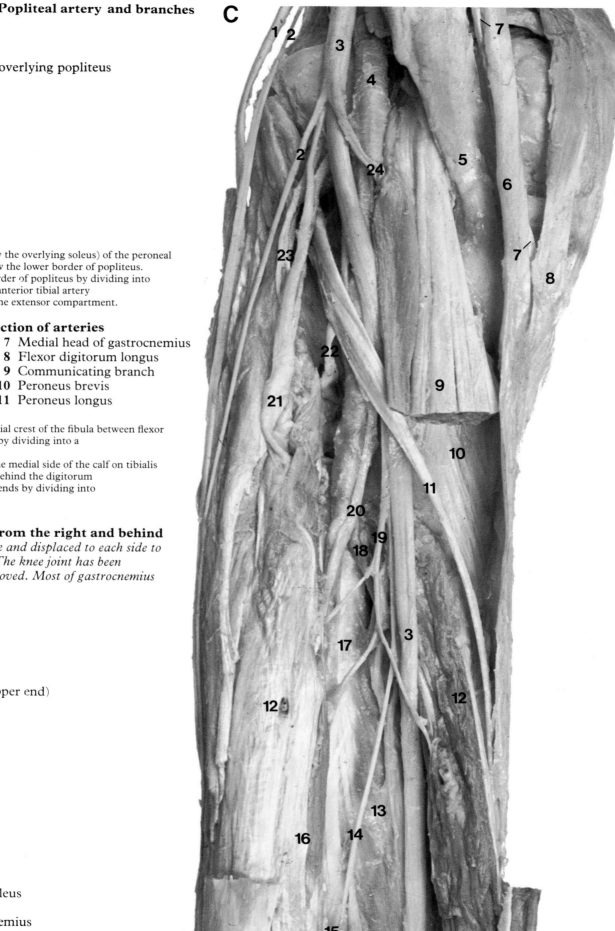

317

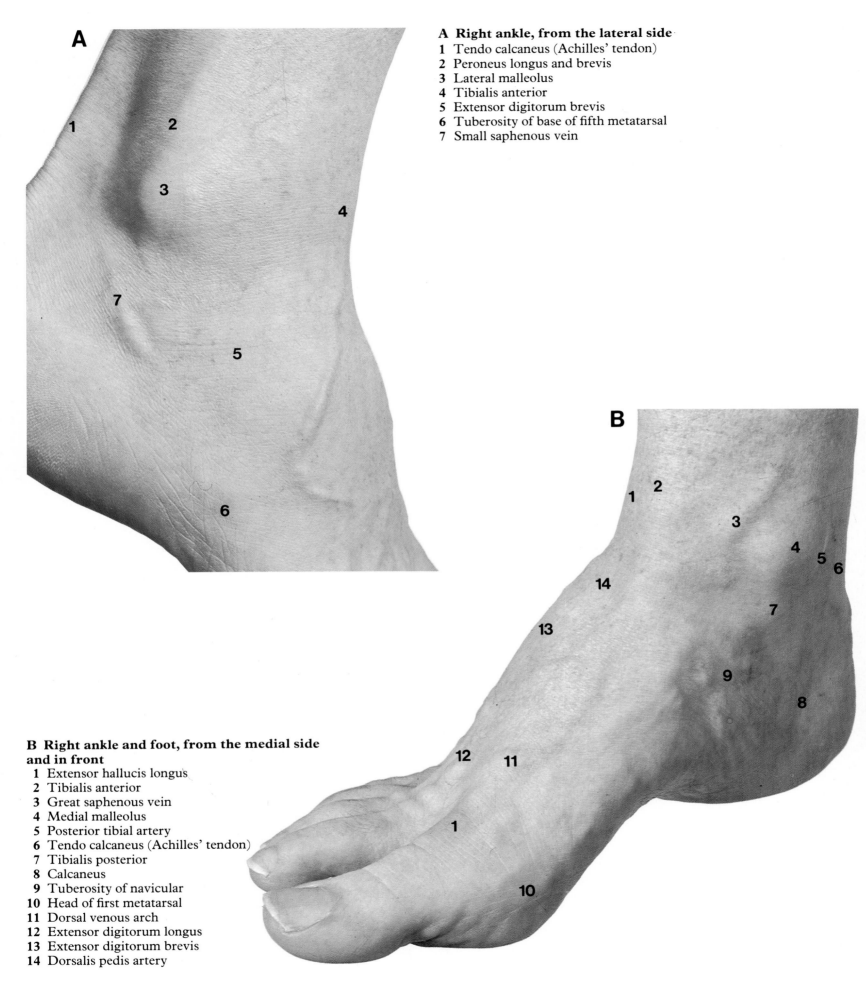

A Right ankle, from the lateral side
1 Tendo calcaneus (Achilles' tendon)
2 Peroneus longus and brevis
3 Lateral malleolus
4 Tibialis anterior
5 Extensor digitorum brevis
6 Tuberosity of base of fifth metatarsal
7 Small saphenous vein

B Right ankle and foot, from the medial side and in front
1 Extensor hallucis longus
2 Tibialis anterior
3 Great saphenous vein
4 Medial malleolus
5 Posterior tibial artery
6 Tendo calcaneus (Achilles' tendon)
7 Tibialis posterior
8 Calcaneus
9 Tuberosity of navicular
10 Head of first metatarsal
11 Dorsal venous arch
12 Extensor digitorum longus
13 Extensor digitorum brevis
14 Dorsalis pedis artery

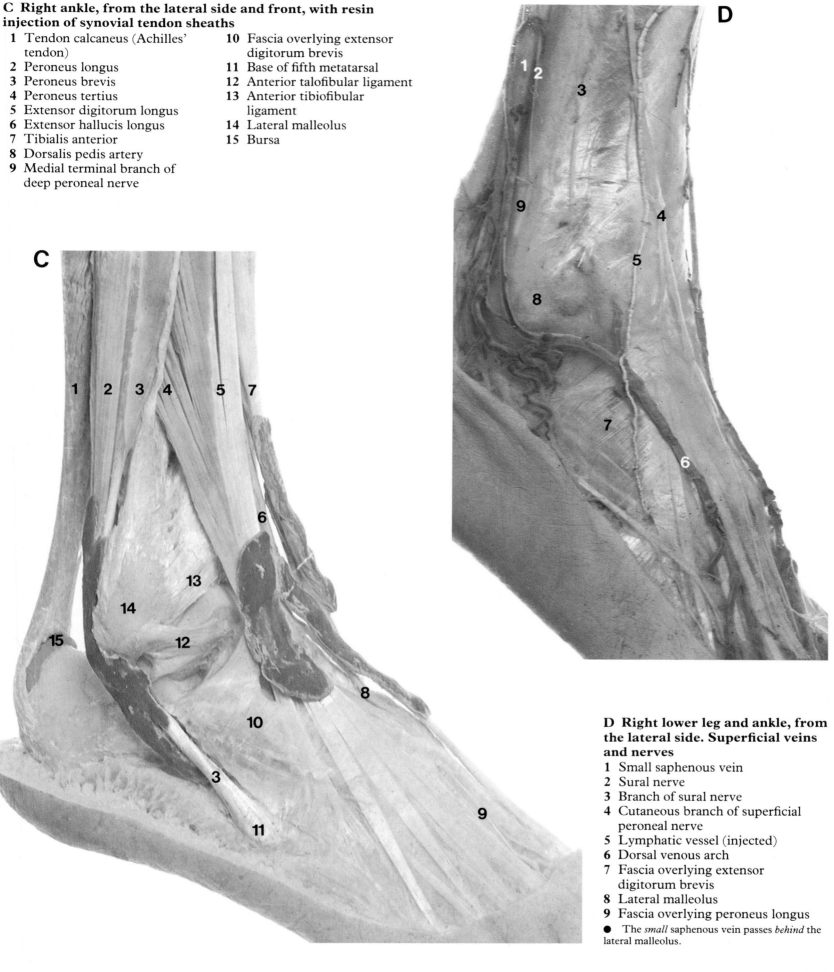

C Right ankle, from the lateral side and front, with resin injection of synovial tendon sheaths

1 Tendon calcaneus (Achilles' tendon)
2 Peroneus longus
3 Peroneus brevis
4 Peroneus tertius
5 Extensor digitorum longus
6 Extensor hallucis longus
7 Tibialis anterior
8 Dorsalis pedis artery
9 Medial terminal branch of deep peroneal nerve
10 Fascia overlying extensor digitorum brevis
11 Base of fifth metatarsal
12 Anterior talofibular ligament
13 Anterior tibiofibular ligament
14 Lateral malleolus
15 Bursa

D Right lower leg and ankle, from the lateral side. Superficial veins and nerves

1 Small saphenous vein
2 Sural nerve
3 Branch of sural nerve
4 Cutaneous branch of superficial peroneal nerve
5 Lymphatic vessel (injected)
6 Dorsal venous arch
7 Fascia overlying extensor digitorum brevis
8 Lateral malleolus
9 Fascia overlying peroneus longus

● The *small* saphenous vein passes *behind* the lateral malleolus.

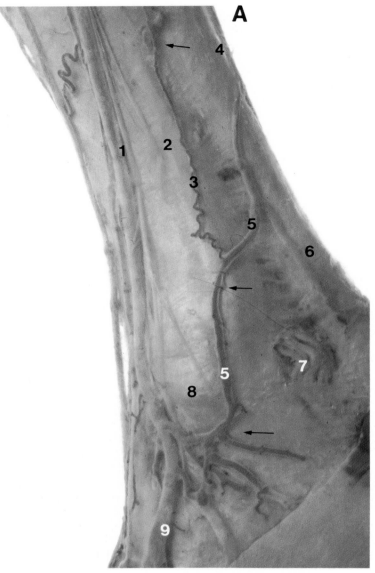

A Right lower leg and ankle from the medial side. Superficial veins and nerves

1 Great saphenous vein and saphenous nerve
2 Tibialis posterior and flexor digitorum longus underlying deep fascia
3 Posterior arch vein
4 Small saphenous vein
5 Communication between great and small saphenous veins
6 Tendo calcaneus (Achilles' tendon)
7 Posterior tibial vessels and tibial nerve
8 Medial malleolus
9 Dorsal venous arch

● The arrows indicate common levels for perforating veins (communications between superficial and deep veins).
● The *great* saphenous vein passes *in front of* the medial malleolus. The *small* saphenous vein passes *behind* the lateral malleolus (see page 318).

B Right ankle and sole, in plantar flexion, from the medial side and below

1 Tibialis posterior
2 Flexor digitorum longus
3 Posterior tibial artery and tibial nerve
4 Flexor hallucis longus
5 Plantaris
6 Tendo calcaneus (Achilles' tendon)
7 Medial calcanean branches
8 Lateral plantar artery and nerve
9 Abductor digiti minimi
10 Flexor accessorius
11 Medial plantar artery and nerve
12 Tuberosity of navicular

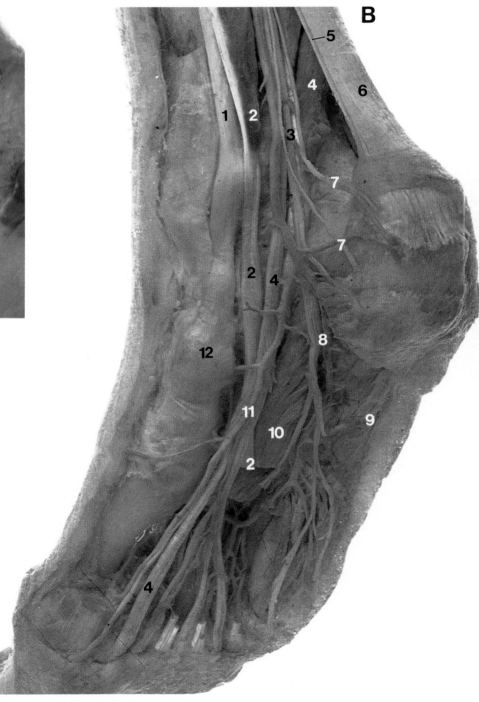

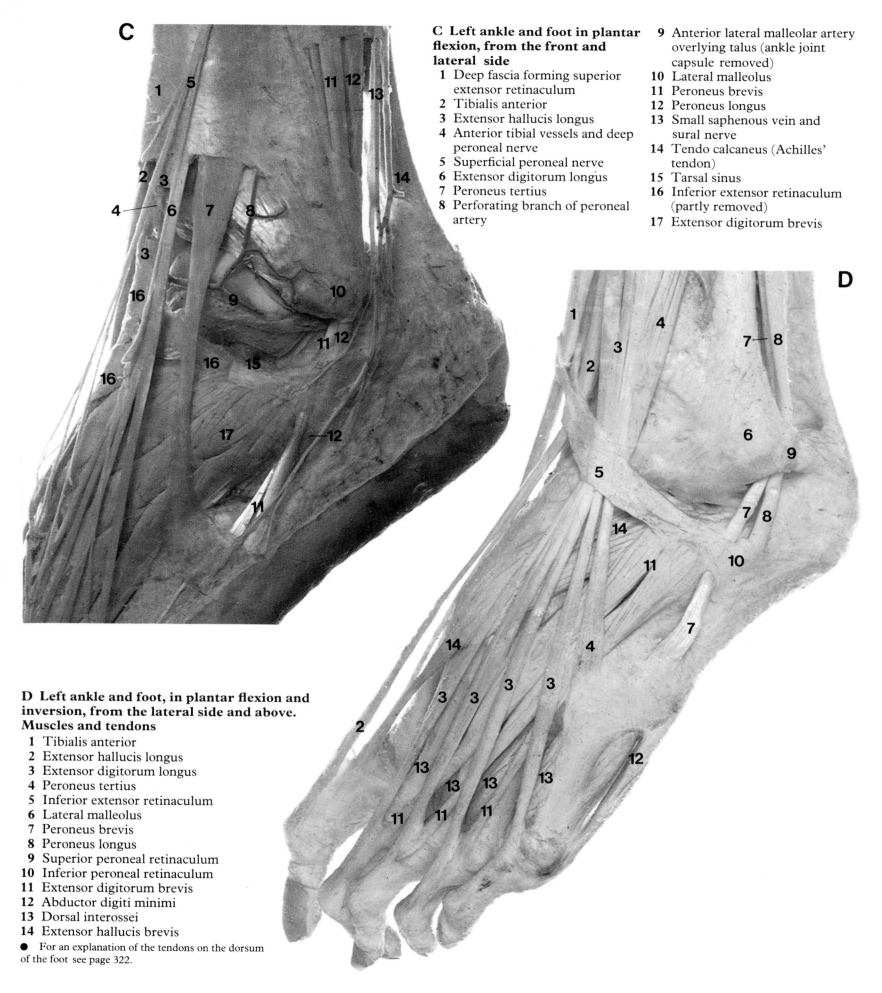

C Left ankle and foot in plantar flexion, from the front and lateral side

1 Deep fascia forming superior extensor retinaculum
2 Tibialis anterior
3 Extensor hallucis longus
4 Anterior tibial vessels and deep peroneal nerve
5 Superficial peroneal nerve
6 Extensor digitorum longus
7 Peroneus tertius
8 Perforating branch of peroneal artery
9 Anterior lateral malleolar artery overlying talus (ankle joint capsule removed)
10 Lateral malleolus
11 Peroneus brevis
12 Peroneus longus
13 Small saphenous vein and sural nerve
14 Tendo calcaneus (Achilles' tendon)
15 Tarsal sinus
16 Inferior extensor retinaculum (partly removed)
17 Extensor digitorum brevis

D Left ankle and foot, in plantar flexion and inversion, from the lateral side and above. Muscles and tendons

1 Tibialis anterior
2 Extensor hallucis longus
3 Extensor digitorum longus
4 Peroneus tertius
5 Inferior extensor retinaculum
6 Lateral malleolus
7 Peroneus brevis
8 Peroneus longus
9 Superior peroneal retinaculum
10 Inferior peroneal retinaculum
11 Extensor digitorum brevis
12 Abductor digiti minimi
13 Dorsal interossei
14 Extensor hallucis brevis

● For an explanation of the tendons on the dorsum of the foot see page 322.

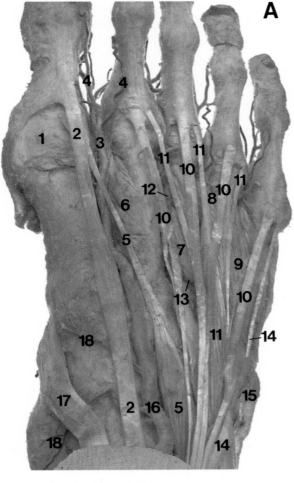

A Dorsum of the right foot. Muscles, tendons and arteries

1 First metatarsophalangeal joint
2 Extensor hallucis longus
3 First dorsal metatarsal artery
4 Digital arteries
5 Extensor hallucis brevis
6 First ⎫
7 Second ⎬ dorsal interosseous
8 Third ⎪
9 Fourth ⎭
10 Extensor digitorum longus
11 Extensor digitorum brevis
12 Second dorsal metatarsal artery
13 Arcuate artery
14 Peroneus tertius
15 Tuberosity of base of fifth metatarsal and peroneus brevis
16 Dorsalis pedis artery
17 Tibialis anterior
18 Tarsal arteries

● Extensor digitorum longus sends its tendons to the four lateral toes, while extensor digitorum brevis sends its tendons to the four medial toes. The part of extensor digitorum brevis that goes to the great toe is known as extensor hallucis brevis.
● The dorsalis pedis artery enters the sole by passing between the two heads of the first dorsal interosseous muscle.

B Right talocalcanean and talocalcaneonavicular joints, from above with the talus removed

1 Dorsal venous arch
2 Tibialis anterior
3 Extensor hallucis longus
4 Dorsalis pedis artery and vena comitans
5 Deep peroneal nerve
6 Extensor digitorum longus
7 Extensor digitorum brevis
8 Calcaneonavicular part of bifurcate ligament
9 Cervical ligament
10 Interosseous talocalcanean ligament
11 Inferior extensor retinaculum
12 Peroneus brevis
13 Peroneus longus
14 Small saphenous vein
15 Sural nerve
16 Tendo calcaneus (Achilles' tendon)
17 Abductor hallucis
18 Flexor hallucis longus
19 Posterior tibial vessels and medial and lateral plantar nerves
20 Flexor digitorum longus
21 Tibialis posterior
22 Deltoid ligament
23 Posterior ⎫
24 Middle ⎬ articular surface on calcaneus for talus
25 Anterior ⎭
26 Plantar calcaneonavicular ligament
27 Articular surface on navicular for talus

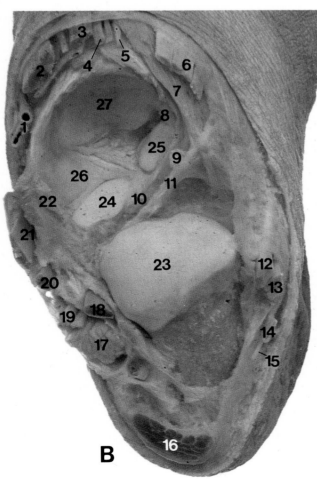

Left ankle and foot. Ligaments, C from the medial side, D from the lateral side, E from behind

1 Groove on talus for flexor hallucis longus between lateral and medial tubercles
2 Medial malleolus
3 Deltoid ligament (marker between superficial and deep parts)
4 Groove on sustentaculum tali for flexor hallucis longus
5 Plantar calcaneonavicular ligament (above marker)
6 Tuberosity of navicular
7 Short plantar ligament (below marker)
8 Long plantar ligament
9 Neck of talus
10 Cervical ligament
11 Tarsal sinus
12 Anterior talofibular ligament
13 Lateral malleolus
14 Calcaneofibular ligament
15 Calcaneocuboid ⎫ parts of bifur-
16 Calcaneonavicular ⎬ cate ligament
17 Groove on lateral malleolus for peroneus brevis
18 Posterior tibiofibular ligament
19 Inferior transverse ligament
20 Groove on tibia for flexor hallucis longus
21 Tibial slip of posterior talofibular ligament
22 Groove on medial malleolus for tibialis posterior
23 Posterior talofibular ligament
24 Posterior tibiotalar ⎫ parts of del-
25 Tibiocalcanean ⎬ toid ligament
26 Tendo calcaneus (Achilles' tendon)

● The deltoid ligament is the medial ligament of the ankle joint. On the lateral side of the ankle there are three separate ligaments – anterior and posterior talofibular and calcaneofibular.

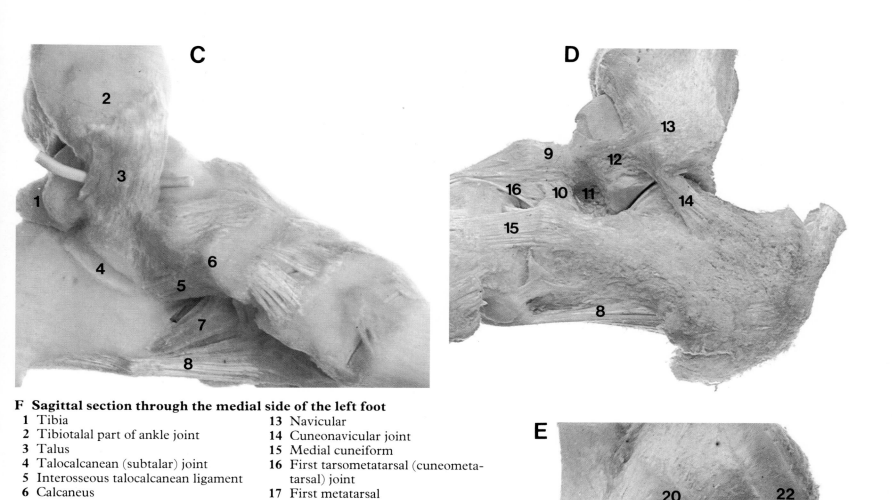

F Sagittal section through the medial side of the left foot

1 Tibia
2 Tibiotalal part of ankle joint
3 Talus
4 Talocalcanean (subtalar) joint
5 Interosseous talocalcanean ligament
6 Calcaneus
7 Tendo calcaneus (Achilles' tendon)
8 Flexor accessorius
9 Flexor digitorum brevis
10 Plantar aponeurosis
11 Plantar calcaneonavicular ligament
12 Talonavicular part of talocalcaneonavicular joint

13 Navicular
14 Cuneonavicular joint
15 Medial cuneiform
16 First tarsometatarsal (cuneometa-
tarsal) joint
17 First metatarsal
18 Sesamoid bone
19 Metatarsophalangeal joint of great
toe
20 Proximal phalanx
21 Interphalangeal joint
22 Distal phalanx

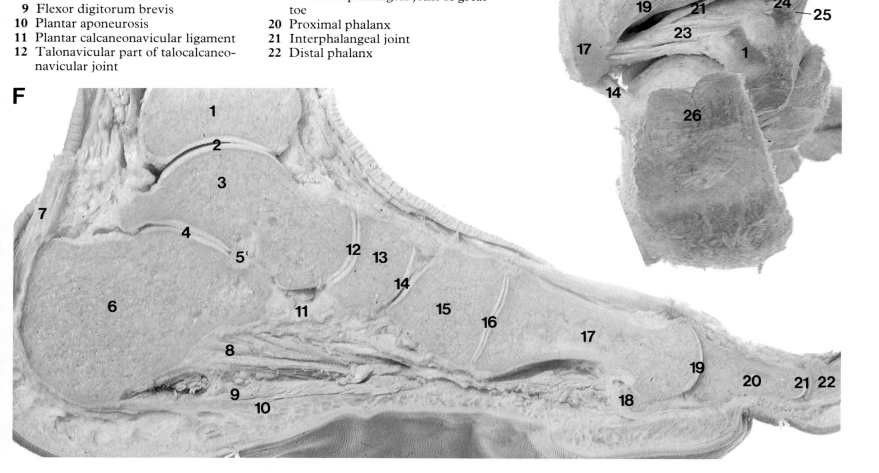

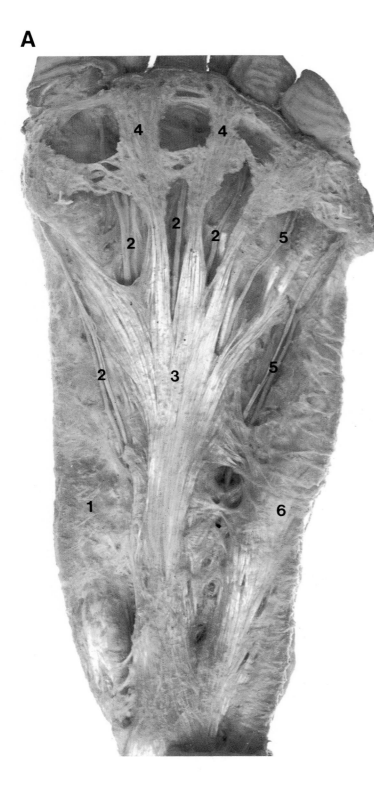

A

A Sole of the left foot. Plantar aponeurosis
1 Medial part of aponeurosis overlying abductor hallucis
2 Digital branches of medial plantar nerve and artery
3 Central part of aponeurosis overlying flexor digitorum brevis
4 Superficial stratum of digital slip of aponeurosis
5 Digital branches of lateral plantar nerve and artery
6 Lateral part of aponeurosis overlying abductor digiti minimi

B Sole of the right foot. Plantar nerves with flexor digitorum brevis removed
1 Fourth tendon of flexor digitorum longus (fourth lumbrical absent)
2 Common plantar digital branch of lateral plantar nerve
3 Transverse head of adductor hallucis
4 Third tendon of flexor digitorum brevis
5 Second lumbrical and common plantar digital branch of medial plantar nerve
6 Oblique head of adductor hallucis
7 Flexor hallucis brevis
8 Flexor hallucis longus
9 Abductor hallucis
10 Medial plantar nerve
11 Flexor accessorius
12 Lateral plantar nerve
13 Long plantar ligament
14 Abductor digiti minimi
15 Deep branch of lateral plantar nerve
16 Second plantar interosseous
17 Fourth dorsal interosseous
18 Third plantar interosseous
19 Flexor digiti minimi brevis

● The flexor digitorum brevis corresponds to the flexor digitorum superficialis of the upper limb: the tendons split to allow the longus tendons to pass through, and the phalangeal attachments of the tendons are similar.
● The medial plantar nerve normally supplies abductor hallucis, flexor digitorum brevis, flexor hallucis brevis and the first lumbrical. All the other muscles of the sole are supplied by the lateral plantar nerve.
● In the foot there are four dorsal and three plantar interossei (in the hand there are four dorsal and four palmar).

C Sole of the left foot. Plantar nerves and deep muscles
1 Flexor hallucis brevis
2 Flexor hallucis longus
3 Oblique head of adductor hallucis
4 First ⎤
5 Second ⎥ lumbrical
6 Third ⎥
7 Fourth ⎦
8 Flexor digitorum brevis
9 Flexor digitorum longus
10 First ⎤
11 Second ⎥
12 Third ⎥ dorsal interosseous
13 Fourth ⎦
14 First ⎤
15 Second ⎥ plantar interosseous
16 Third ⎦
17 Abductor digiti minimi
18 Flexor digiti minimi brevis
19 Peroneus longus
20 Flexor accessorius
21 Plantar aponeurosis
22 Lateral plantar artery
23 Lateral plantar nerve
24 Medial plantar nerve
25 Abductor hallucis
26 Deep branch of lateral plantar nerve
27 Plantar digital nerve of great toe

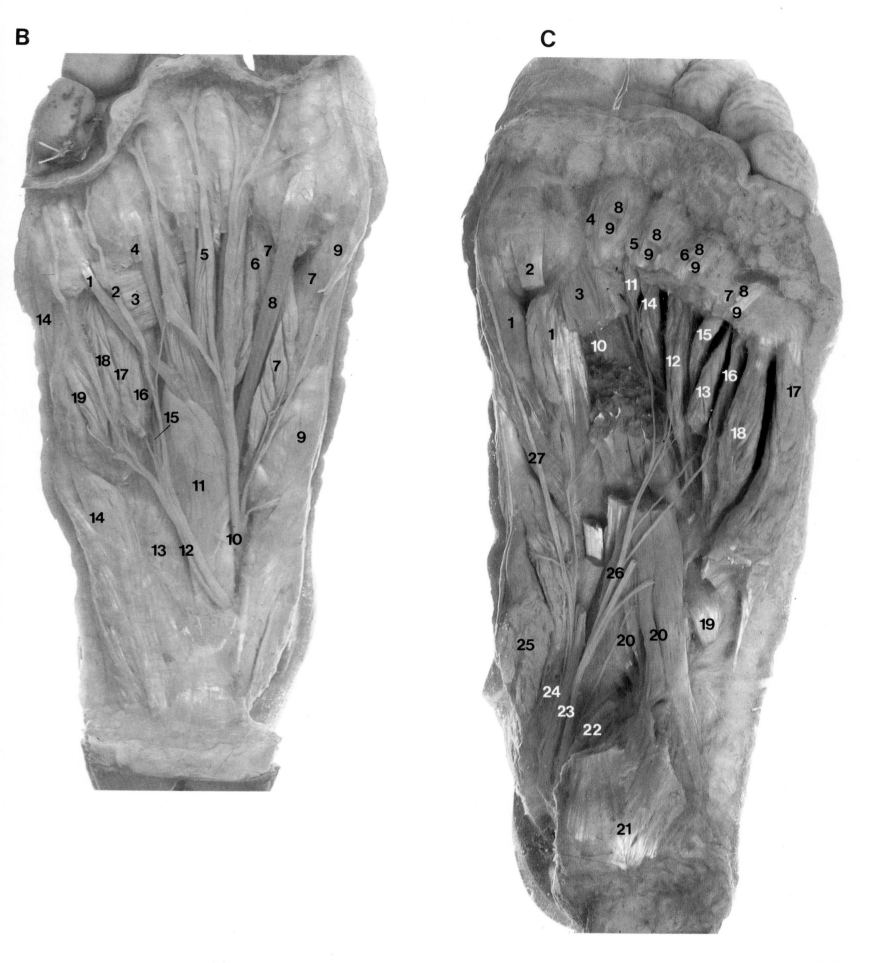

B

C

● Unlike the palm of the hand which has superficial and deep arterial arches, the sole of the foot has one plantar arch, formed by the lateral plantar artery anastomosing with the dorsalis pedis artery which enters the sole by passing between the two heads of the first dorsal interosseous muscle. The arch gives off plantar metatarsal arteries, and these divide to form the plantar digital vessels.

B Sole of the left foot. Deep muscles
 1 Abductor hallucis
 2 Flexor hallucis brevis
 3 Flexor hallucis longus
 4 Oblique ⎫ head of adductor hallucis
 5 Transverse ⎭
 6 Interossei
 7 Flexor digiti minimi brevis
 8 Abductor digiti minimi
 9 Flexor digitorum brevis
10 Deep branch of lateral plantar nerve
11 Medial plantar nerve
12 Flexor digitorum longus
13 Tibial nerve
14 Tibialis posterior

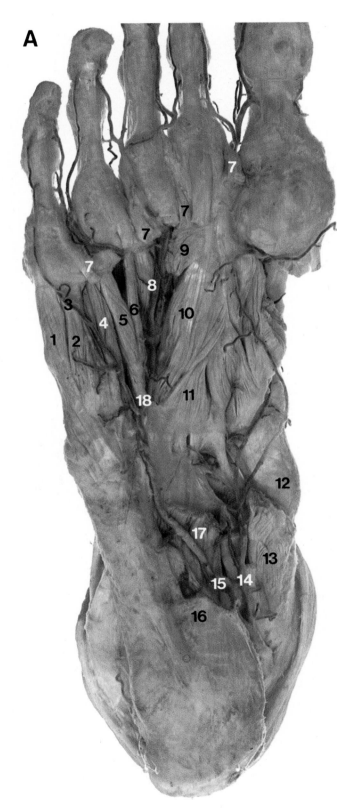

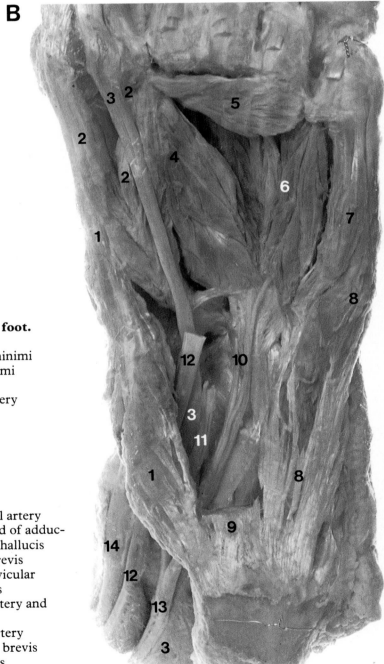

A Sole of the right foot. Arteries
 1 Abductor digiti minimi
 2 Flexor digiti minimi brevis
 3 Plantar digital artery
 4 Third plantar interosseous
 5 Fourth dorsal interosseous
 6 Second plantar interosseous
 7 Lumbrical
 8 Plantar metatarsal artery
 9 Transverse ⎫ head of adduc-
10 Oblique ⎭ tor hallucis
11 Flexor hallucis brevis
12 Tuberosity of navicular
13 Abductor hallucis
14 Medial plantar artery and nerve
15 Lateral plantar artery
16 Flexor digitorum brevis
17 Flexor accessorius
18 Plantar arch

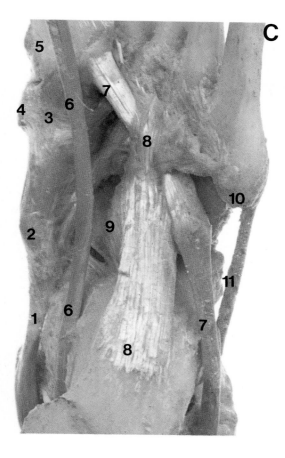

C Sole of the left foot. Long plantar ligament and peroneus longus

1 Tibialis posterior
2 Tuberosity of navicular
3 Medial cuneiform
4 Tibialis anterior
5 Base of first metatarsal
6 Flexor hallucis longus
7 Peroneus longus
8 Long plantar ligament
9 Short plantar ligament
10 Tuberosity of base of fifth metatarsal
11 Peroneus brevis

● Tibialis anterior is attached to the medial sides of the medial cuneiform and base of the first metatarsal; peroneus longus is attached to the lateral sides of the same bones.
● The short plantar ligament is largely under cover of the long plantar ligament.
● The long plantar ligament converts the groove on the cuboid into a tunnel for the peroneus longus tendon.

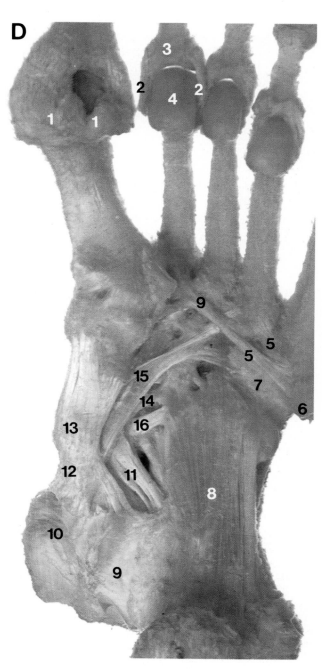

D Sole of the left foot. Ligaments with superficial fibres of the long plantar ligament removed

1 Sesamoid bone
2 Collateral ligament of metatarsophalangeal joint
3 Base of proximal phalanx
4 Head of second metatarsal
5 Plantar metatarsal ligament
6 Tuberosity of base of fifth metatarsal
7 Groove on cuboid for peroneus longus
8 Deep fibres of long plantar ligament
9 Groove on sustentaculum tali for flexor hallucis longus
10 Deltoid ligament
11 Plantar calcaneonavicular ligament
12 Tibialis posterior
13 Tuberosity of navicular
14 Plantar cuneonavicular ligament
15 Fibrous slip from tibialis posterior
16 Plantar cuboideonavicular ligament

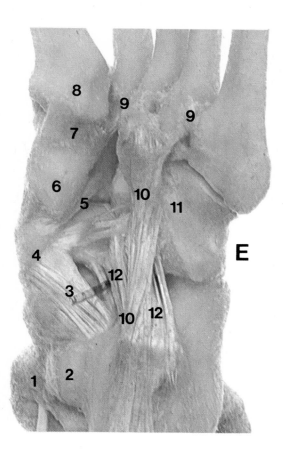

E Sole of the left foot. Plantar ligaments

1 Deltoid ligament
2 Groove on sustentaculum tali for flexor hallucis longus
3 Plantar calcaneonavicular ligament
4 Tuberosity of navicular
5 Plantar cuneonavicular ligament
6 Medial cuneiform
7 Plantar tarsometatarsal ligament
8 Base of first metatarsal
9 Plantar metatarsal ligaments
10 Long plantar ligament
11 Groove on cuboid for peroneus longus
12 Short plantar ligament (glass marker at medial margin)

● The blue marker passes between the superficial and deep parts of the deltoid ligament.
● The plantar calcaneonavicular ligament is commonly called the spring ligament. Its upper surface supports part of the head of the talus (see page 322).

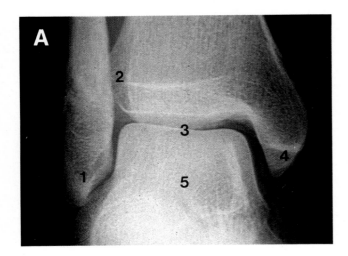

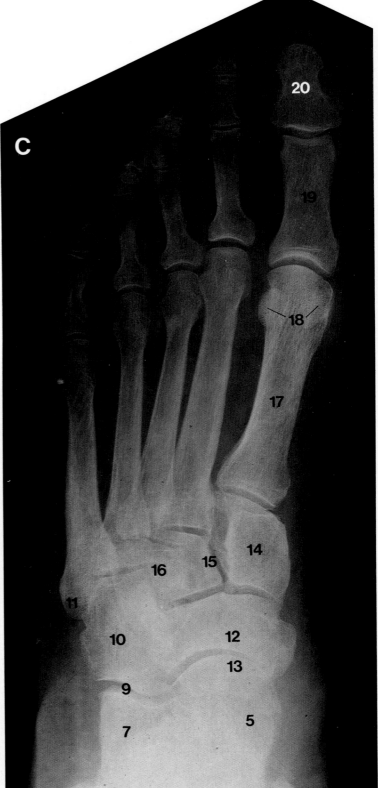

Radiographs of the ankle and foot, A from behind, B from the lateral side, C from below

1 Lateral malleolus
2 Inferior tibiofibular syndesmosis
3 Ankle joint
4 Medial malleolus
5 Talus
6 Talocalcanean (subtalar) joint
7 Calcaneus
8 Tarsal sinus
9 Calcaneocuboid joint
10 Cuboid
11 Tuberosity of base of fifth metatarsal
12 Navicular
13 Talonavicular part of talocalcaneonavicular joint
14 Medial ⎫
15 Intermediate ⎬ cuneiform
16 Lateral ⎭
17 First metatarsal
18 Sesamoid bones in flexor hallucis brevis
19 Proximal ⎫ phalanx of
20 Distal ⎬ great toe

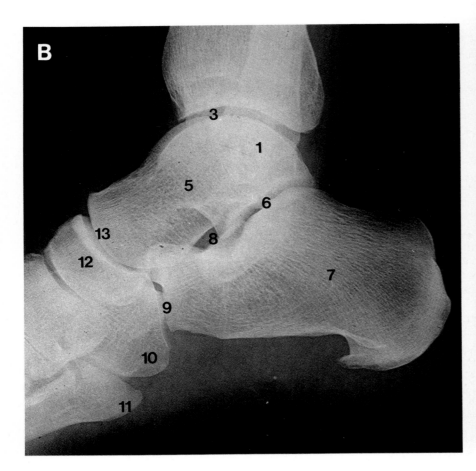

Appendix

The reference lists of vessels and nerves have been arranged for quick identification of parent trunks and branches. Thus, the left common carotid artery is one of the three branches of the arch of the aorta, while the right common carotid is one of the branches of the brachiocephalic trunk.

The arrows indicate a continuity (instead of branching) with a change of name.

The generally accepted standard pattern has been given. For common variations, which are particularly frequent among veins, reference should be made to standard texts. (The articular and vascular branches of nerves have been omitted.)

The inclusion of items in these lists does not necessarily imply that they are illustrated in the atlas; many of the smaller vessels and nerves are not shown but have been included in the lists for reference purposes.

Arteries

AORTA AND BRANCHES

Ascending aorta → arch of aorta → thoracic aorta → abdominal aorta

Ascending aorta
Right coronary
  Marginal
  Posterior interventricular
Left coronary
  Circumflex
  Anterior interventricular

Arch of aorta
Brachiocephalic trunk
  Right common carotid
    Right internal carotid
    Right external carotid
  Right subclavian → axillary → brachial
  Thyroidea ima (occasional)
Left common carotid
  Left internal carotid
  Left external carotid
Left subclavian → axillary → brachial

Thoracic aorta
Pericardial
Right bronchial
Oesophageal
Mediastinal
Phrenic
Posterior intercostal (3–11)
  Left bronchial (from third)
Subcostal

Abdominal aorta
Coeliac trunk
Superior mesenteric
Inferior mesenteric
Middle suprarenal
Renal
  Inferior suprarenal
Testicular (ovarian)
Inferior phrenic
  Superior suprarenal
Lumbar
Median sacral
Common iliac
  Internal iliac
  External iliac → femoral

CAROTID ARTERIES AND BRANCHES

Internal carotid
Caroticotympanic
Pterygoid
Cavernous
Hypophysial
Meningeal
Ophthalmic
  Central of retina
  Lacrimal
    Lateral palpebral
    Zygomatic
    Recurrent meningeal
  Muscular
    Anterior ciliary
  Long posterior ciliary
  Short posterior ciliary
  Supra-orbital
  Posterior ethmoidal
  Anterior ethmoidal
  Anterior meningeal
  Medial palpebral
  Supratrochlear
  Dorsal nasal
Anterior cerebral
Middle cerebral
Posterior communicating
Anterior choroidal

External carotid
Ascending pharyngeal
Superior thyroid
  Infrahyoid
  Sternocleidomastoid
  Superior laryngeal
  Cricothyroid
Lingual
Facial
  Ascending palatine
  Tonsillar
  Glandular
  Submental
  Inferior labial
  Superior labial
    Septal
  Lateral nasal
Occipital
Posterior auricular
Superficial temporal
  Transverse facial
Maxillary → sphenopalatine
  Deep auricular
  Anterior tympanic
  Middle meningeal
  Accessory meningeal
  Inferior alveolar
    Dental
    Mylohyoid
    Mental
  Deep temporal
  Pterygoid
  Masseteric
  Buccal
  Infra-orbital
    Anterior superior alveolar
    Dental
  Posterior superior alveolar
    Dental
  Greater palatine
    Lesser palatine
  Pharyngeal
  Artery of pterygoid canal

Arteries

SUBCLAVIAN ARTERY AND BRANCHES

Subclavian ➤ axillary ➤ brachial
Vertebral
  Spinal
  Meningeal
  Anterior spinal
  Posterior spinal
  Posterior inferior cerebellar
Internal thoracic
  Pericardiacophrenic
  Mediastinal
  Thymic
  Sternal
  Perforating
    Mammary
  Anterior intercostal
  Musculophrenic
  Superior epigastric
Thyrocervical trunk
  Inferior thyroid
    Ascending cervical
    Inferior laryngeal
    Glandular
    Pharyngeal
    Oesophageal
    Tracheal
  Suprascapular
  Superficial cervical
Costocervical trunk
  Superior intercostal
  Deep cervical
Dorsal scapular

Basilar (union of vertebrals)
Pontine
Labyrinthine
Anterior inferior cerebellar
Superior cerebellar
Posterior cerebral

AXILLARY ARTERY AND BRANCHES

Axillary ➤ brachial
Superior thoracic
Thoraco-acromial
  Acromial
  Clavicular
  Deltoid
  Pectoral
Lateral thoracic
  Lateral mammary
Subscapular
  Circumflex scapular
  Thoracodorsal
Anterior circumflex humeral
Posterior circumflex humeral

Brachial
Profunda brachii
  Posterior descending
  Radial collateral
Nutrient
Superior ulnar collateral
Inferior ulnar collateral
Radial
  Radial recurrent
  Palmar carpal
  Superficial palmar
  Dorsal carpal
  Dorsal metacarpal
    Dorsal digital
  First dorsal metacarpal
  Princeps pollicis
  Radialis indicis
  Deep palmar arch
    Palmar metacarpal
    Perforating
Ulnar
  Anterior ulnar recurrent
  Posterior ulnar recurrent
  Common interosseous
    Anterior interosseous
      Median
    Posterior interosseous
      Interosseous recurrent
  Palmar carpal
  Dorsal carpal
  Deep carpal
  Superficial palmar arch
    Common palmar digital
    Palmar digital

SOME BRANCHES OF THE ABDOMINAL AORTA

Coeliac trunk
Left gastric
  Oesophageal
Common hepatic
  Hepatic
    Cystic
  Gastroduodenal
    Right gastro-epiploic
    Superior pancreaticoduodenal
    Supraduodenal
  Right gastric
Splenic
  Pancreatic
  Short gastric
  Left gastro-epiploic

Superior mesenteric
Inferior pancreaticoduodenal
Jejunal and ileal
Ileocolic
  Ascending
  Anterior caecal
  Posterior caecal
  Appendicular
  Ileal
Right colic
Middle colic

Inferior mesenteric
Left colic
Sigmoid
Superior rectal

Internal iliac
Anterior trunk
  Superior vesical
  Inferior vesical
  Middle rectal
  Uterine
  Vaginal
  Obturator
  Internal pudendal
    Inferior rectal
    Perineal
    Artery of the bulb
    Urethral
    Deep artery of penis (clitoris)
    Dorsal artery of penis (clitoris)
  Inferior gluteal
Posterior trunk
  Iliolumbar
  Lateral sacral
  Superior gluteal

External iliac ➤ femoral
Inferior epigastric
  Cremasteric
  Pubic (abnormal obturator)
Deep circumflex iliac

Arteries

FEMORAL ARTERY AND BRANCHES
Femoral → popliteal
  Superficial epigastric
  Superficial circumflex iliac
  Superficial external pudendal
  Deep external pudendal
  Profunda femoris
    Lateral circumflex femoral
    Medial circumflex femoral
    Perforating
  Descending genicular

Popliteal
  Sural
  Superior genicular
  Middle genicular
  Inferior genicular
  Anterior tibial → dorsalis pedis
    Posterior tibial recurrent
    Anterior tibial recurrent
    Anterior medial malleolar
    Anterior lateral malleolar
    Dorsalis pedis → plantar arch
      Tarsal
      First dorsal metatarsal
        Dorsal digital
      Arcuate
        Dorsal metatarsal (2–4)
          Dorsal digital
  Posterior tibial
    Circumflex fibular
    Peroneal
      Nutrient
      Perforating
      Communicating
      Lateral malleolar
      Calcanean
    Nutrient
    Communicating
    Medial malleolar
    Calcanean
    Medial plantar
      Superficial digital
    Lateral plantar → plantar arch
      Superficial
      Plantar metatarsal
        Common plantar digital
          Plantar digital
      Perforating

Veins

TRIBUTARIES OF MAJOR VEINS
SUPERIOR VENA CAVA
Superior vena cava
  Left brachiocephalic
    Left internal jugular
    Left subclavian
    Left vertebral
    Left supreme (first posterior) intercostal
    Left superior intercostal (2–4)
    Inferior thyroid
    Thymic
    Pericardial
  Right brachiocephalic
    Right internal jugular
    Right subclavian
    Right vertebral
    Right supreme (first posterior) intercostal
  Azygos
    Right superior intercostal (2–4)
    Right posterior intercostal (5–11)
    Right subcostal
    Right ascending lumbar and/or lumbar
      azygos
    Right bronchial
    Oesophageal
    Pericardial
    Mediastinal
    Vertebral venous plexuses
    Hemiazygos
      Left ascending lumbar and/or lumbar
        azygos
      Left subcostal
      Left posterior intercostal (9–11)
      Oesophageal
      Pericardial
      Mediastinal
      Vertebral venous plexuses
    Accessory hemiazygos
      Left posterior intercostal (5–8)
      Left bronchial
      Oesophageal
      Pericardial
      Mediastinal
      Vertebral venous plexuses

INFERIOR VENA CAVA
Inferior vena cava
  Common iliac (right and left)
  Fourth lumbar (right and left)
  Third lumbar (right and left)
  Testicular (ovarian) (right)
  Renal (right and left)
  Suprarenal (right)
  Inferior phrenic (right and left)
  Hepatic (right, middle and left)
  (Upper lumbar veins join ascending lumbar.
    Left testicular or ovarian and suprarenal
    veins join left renal)

INTERNAL JUGULAR VEIN
Internal jugular
  Inferior petrosal sinus
  Pharyngeal
  Lingual
  Facial
  Superior thyroid
  Middle thyroid

EXTERNAL JUGULAR VEIN
External jugular
  Posterior auricular
  Posterior branch of retromandibular
  Occipital
  Posterior external jugular
  Suprascapular
  Transverse of neck
  Anterior jugular

RETROMANDIBULAR VEIN
Retromandibular
  Superficial temporal
  Maxillary
  Transverse facial
  Pterygoid plexus
    Middle meningeal
    Greater palatine
    Sphenopalatine
    Buccal
    Dental
    Deep facial
    Inferior ophthalmic
  Anterior branch to join facial
  Posterior branch to external jugular

FACIAL VEIN
Facial
  Supratrochlear
  Supra-orbital
  Superior ophthalmic
  Palpebral
  External nasal
  Labial
  Deep facial
  Submental
  Submandibular
  Tonsillar
  External palatine (paratonsillar)

GREAT SAPHENOUS VEIN
Great saphenous
  Dorsal venous arch
  Perforating
  Accessory saphenous
  Anterior femoral cutaneous
  Superficial epigastric
  Superficial circumflex iliac
  Superficial external pudendal
  Deep external pudendal
  (Small saphenous vein communicates with great
    saphenous but usually drains to popliteal
    vein)

Veins

CARDIAC VEINS
Coronary sinus
Great cardiac
Middle cardiac
Small cardiac
Posterior of left ventricle
Oblique of left atrium
Anterior cardiac
Venae cordis minimae

DURAL VENOUS SINUSES
Posterosuperior group
Superior sagittal
Inferior sagittal
Straight
Transverse
Sigmoid
Petrosquamous
Occipital

Antero-inferior group
Cavernous
Intercavernous
Inferior petrosal
Superior petrosal
Sphenoparietal
Basilar
Middle meningeal veins

HEPATIC PORTAL SYSTEM
Portal vein
Superior mesenteric
Jejunal and ileal
Right gastro-epiploic
Pancreatic
Pancreaticoduodenal
Ileocolic
Appendicular
Right colic
Middle colic
Splenic
Pancreatic
Short gastric
Left gastro-epiploic
Inferior mesenteric
Left colic
Sigmoid
Superior rectal
Left gastric
Right gastric
Prepyloric
Paraumbilical (to left branch)
Cystic (to right branch)

PORTAL-SYSTEMIC ANASTOMOSES
Oesophageal branches of the left gastric vein with the hemiazygos vein
Superior rectal branch of the inferior mesenteric vein with the middle and inferior rectal veins (internal iliac)
Paraumbilical veins of the falciform ligament with anterior abdominal wall veins
Retroperitoneal colonic veins with posterior abdominal wall veins
Bare area of the liver with diaphragmatic veins

Lymphatic System

THORACIC DUCT AND CISTERNA CHYLI TRIBUTARIES
Thoracic duct
Left jugular trunk
Left subclavian trunk
Left bronchomediastinal trunk

Right lymphatic duct
Right jugular trunk
Right subclavian trunk
Right bronchomediastinal trunk

Cisterna chyli
Left lumbar trunk
Right lumbar trunk
Intestinal trunks

LYMPH NODES OF THE HEAD AND NECK
Deep cervical
Superior (including jugulodigastric)
Inferior (including jugulo-omohyoid)

Draining superficial tissues in the head
Occipital
Retro-auricular (mastoid)
Parotid
Buccal (facial)

Draining superficial tissues in the neck
Submandibular
Submental
Anterior cervical
Superficial cervical

Draining deep tissues in the neck
Retropharyngeal
Paratracheal
Lingual
Infrahyoid
Prelaryngeal
Pretracheal

LYMPH NODES OF THE UPPER LIMB AND MAMMARY GLAND
Draining the upper limb
Axillary
Apical
Central
Lateral
Pectoral (anterior)
Subscapular (posterior)
Infraclavicular
Supratrochlear
Cubital

Draining the mammary gland
Pectoral
Subscapular
Apical
Parasternal
Intercostal

LYMPH NODES OF THE THORAX
Draining thoracic walls
Superficial
Pectoral
Subscapular
Parasternal
Inferior deep cervical
Deep
Parasternal
Intercostal
Phrenic
Diaphragmatic

Draining thoracic contents
Brachiocephalic
Posterior mediastinal
Tracheobronchial
Paratracheal
Superior tracheobronchial
Inferior tracheobronchial
Bronchopulmonary
Pulmonary

LYMPH NODES OF THE ABDOMEN AND PELVIS
Lumbar
Pre-aortic
Coeliac
Gastric
Left gastric
Right gastro-epiploic
Pyloric
Hepatic
Pancreaticosplenic
Superior mesenteric
Inferior mesenteric
Lateral aortic
Common iliac
External iliac
Internal iliac
Inferior epigastric
Circumflex iliac
Sacral
Retro-aortic

LYMPH NODES OF THE LOWER LIMB
Superficial inguinal
Upper
Lower
Deep inguinal
Popliteal

Nerves

CRANIAL NERVES AND BRANCHES

I Olfactory (from olfactory mucous membrane)

II Optic (from retina)

III Oculomotor
Superior ramus (to superior rectus and levator palpebrae superioris)
Inferior ramus (to medial rectus, inferior rectus, inferior oblique and ciliary ganglion)

IV Trochlear (to superior oblique)

V Trigeminal
Ophthalmic
Lacrimal
Frontal
Supratrochlear
Supra-orbital
Nasociliary ➞ anterior ethmoidal ➞ external nasal
Internal nasal (from anterior ethmoidal)
Ciliary ganglion
Long ciliary
Infratrochlear
Posterior ethmoidal
Maxillary ➞ infra-orbital
Meningeal
Pterygopalatine
Orbital
Palatine
Nasal
Pharyngeal
Zygomatic
Posterior superior alveolar
Middle superior alveolar
Anterior superior alveolar
Palpebral
Nasal } (from infra-orbital)
Superior labial
Mandibular
Meningeal
Nerve to medial pterygoid (and tensor veli palatini and tensor tympani)
Anterior trunk
Buccal
Masseteric
Deep temporal
Nerve to lateral pterygoid
Posterior trunk
Auriculotemporal
Lingual
Inferior alveolar
Mental

VI Abducent (to lateral rectus)

VII Facial
Greater petrosal
Nerve to stapedius
Chorda tympani
Posterior auricular (to occipitalis and auricular muscles)
Nerve to posterior belly of digastric
Nerve to stylohyoid
Temporal
Zygomatic
Buccal } to frontalis and muscles of facial expression
Marginal mandibular
Cervical

VIII Vestibulocochlear
Cochlear (from coils of cochlea)
Vestibular (from utricle, saccule and ampullae of semicircular ducts)

IX Glossopharyngeal
Tympanic
Lesser petrosal
Carotid
Pharyngeal
Muscular (to stylopharyngeus)
Tonsillar
Lingual

X Vagus
Meningeal
Auricular
Pharyngeal (to muscles of pharynx and soft palate except stylopharyngeus and tensor veli palatini)
Carotid body
Superior laryngeal
Internal laryngeal
External laryngeal (to cricothyroid)
Right recurrent laryngeal (to muscles of larynx except cricothyroid)
Cardiac (cervical)
Cardiac (thoracic)
Left recurrent laryngeal (to muscles of larynx except cricothyroid)
Pulmonary
Oesophageal
Anterior trunk
Gastric
Hepatic
Posterior trunk
Coeliac
Gastric

XI Accessory
Cranial root (to muscles of palate and possibly larynx via vagus)
Spinal root (to sternocleidomastoid and trapezius)

XII Hypoglossal
Meningeal
Descending (upper root of ansa cervicalis, from first cervical nerve joining lower root from second and third cervical nerves, to form ansa and supply sternohyoid, sternothyroid and superior and inferior bellies of omohyoid)
Nerve to thyrohyoid (from first cervical nerve)
Muscular (to geniohyoid and muscles of tongue except palatoglossus)

SOME HEAD AND NECK NERVE SUPPLIES

All the muscles of	Supplied by	Except	Supplied by
Pharynx	Pharyngeal plexus	Stylo-pharyngeus	Glosso-pharyngeal nerve
Palate	Pharyngeal plexus	Tensor veli palatini	Nerve to medial pterygoid
Larynx	Recurrent laryngeal nerve	Crico-thyroid	External laryngeal nerve
Tongue	Hypoglossal nerve	Palato-glossus	Pharyngeal plexus
Facial expression (including buccinator)	Facial nerve		
Mastication	Mandibular nerve		

CERVICAL PLEXUS AND BRANCHES

Lesser occipital C2
Great auricular C2, 3
Transverse cutaneous of neck C2, 3
Supraclavicular C3, 4
Phrenic (to diaphragm) C3, 4, 5
Communicating (with vagus and hypoglossal nerves and superior cervical sympathetic ganglion)
Muscular (to rectus capitis lateralis, rectus capitis anterior, longus capitis and longus colli, and by lower root of ansa cervicalis (descending cervical) to sternohyoid, sternothyroid and inferior belly of omohyoid) C1, 2, 3

TYPICAL THORACIC NERVE BRANCHES

Thoracic spinal nerve
Dorsal ramus
Medial
Lateral
Ventral ramus ➞ anterior cutaneous
Recurrent
Collateral
Lateral cutaneous
Posterior
Anterior

Nerves

BRACHIAL PLEXUS AND BRANCHES

Supraclavicular branches
From the roots
    To scalenes and longus colli C5, 6, 7, 8
    To join phrenic nerve C5
    Dorsal scapular (to rhomboids) C5
    Long thoracic (to serratus anterior) C5, 6, 7

From the upper trunk
    Nerve to subclavius C5, 6
    Suprascapular (to supraspinatus and
      infraspinatus) C5, 6

Infraclavicular branches
From the lateral cord
    Lateral pectoral (to pectoralis major and
      minor) C5, 6, 7
    Musculocutaneous C5, 6, 7
    Lateral root of the median C(5), 6, 7

From the medial cord
    Medial pectoral (to pectoralis major and
      minor) C8, T1
    Medial root of the median C8, T1
    Medial cutaneous of arm C8, T1
    Medial cutaneous of forearm C8, T1
    Ulnar C(7), 8, T1

From the posterior cord
    Upper subscapular (to subscapularis) C5, 6
    Thoracodorsal (to latissimus dorsi) C6, 7, 8
    Lower subscapular (to subscapularis and
      teres major) C5, 6
    Axillary C5, 6
    Radial C5, 6, 7, 8, T1

Musculocutaneous C5, 6, 7
Muscular (to coracobrachialis, biceps and
    brachialis)
Lateral cutaneous of forearm

Median C(5), 6, 7, 8, T1
In the arm
    To pronator teres (occasional)
In the forearm
    Muscular (to pronator teres, flexor carpi
      radialis, palmaris longus and flexor
      digitorum superficialis)
    Anterior interosseous (to flexor pollicis
      longus, flexor digitorum profundus and
      pronator quadratus)
    Palmar cutaneous
    Communicating (with ulnar nerve)
In the hand
    Muscular (to abductor pollicis brevis, flexor
      pollicis brevis, opponens pollicis and the
      two lateral lumbricals)
    Common palmar digital
      Palmar digital

Ulnar C(7), 8, T1
Muscular (to flexor carpi ulnaris and flexor
    digitorum profundus)
Palmar cutaneous
Dorsal
    Dorsal digital
Superficial terminal
    Nerve to palmaris brevis
    Common palmar digital
      Palmar digital
Deep terminal (to abductor digiti minimi,
    opponens digiti minimi, flexor digiti
    minimi brevis, adductor pollicis, all the
    interossei and the two medial lumbricals)

Axillary C5, 6
Muscular (to deltoid and teres minor)
Upper lateral cutaneous of arm

Radial C5, 6, 7, 8, T1
Muscular (to triceps, anconeus,
    brachioradialis, extensor carpi radialis longus
    and brachialis)
Posterior cutaneous of arm
Lower lateral cutaneous of arm
Posterior cutaneous of forearm
Superficial terminal
    Dorsal digital
Deep terminal (posterior interosseous) (to
    extensor carpi radialis brevis, supinator,
    extensor digitorum, extensor digiti minimi,
    extensor carpi ulnaris, extensor pollicis
    longus, extensor indicis, abductor pollicis
    longus and extensor pollicis brevis)

LUMBAR PLEXUS AND BRANCHES
Muscular (to psoas major and minor, quadratus
    lumborum and iliacus) T12, L1, 2, 3, 4
Iliohypogastric (to part of internal oblique and
    transversus abdominis) L1
Ilio-inguinal (to part of internal oblique and
    transversus abdominis) L1
Genitofemoral L1, 2
    Genital branch (to cremaster)
    Femoral branch
Lateral cutaneous of thigh L2, 3
Femoral L2, 3, 4
    Nerve to pectineus
    Anterior division
      Intermediate cutaneous of thigh
      Medial cutaneous of thigh
      Nerve to sartorius
    Posterior division
      Saphenous
      Nerves to quadriceps femoris
Obturator L2, 3, 4
    Anterior branch
      Muscular (to adductor longus, adductor
        brevis and gracilis)
    Posterior branch
      Muscular (to obturator externus and
        adductor magnus)
Accessory obturator (occasional) (to pectineus)
    L3, 4

SACRAL PLEXUS AND BRANCHES
Nerve to quadratus femoris and inferior gemellus
    L4, 5, S1
Nerve to obturator internus and superior gemellus
    L5, S1, 2
Nerve to piriformis S(1), 2
Superior gluteal (to gluteus medius and minimus
    and tensor fasciae latae) L4, 5, S1
Inferior gluteal (to gluteus maximus) L5, S1, 2
Posterior cutaneous of thigh S2, 3
Sciatic L4, 5, S1, 2, 3
    Muscular (to biceps, semitendinosus,
      semimembranosus and adductor magnus)
    Tibial L4, 5, S1, 2, 3
      Muscular (to gastrocnemius, plantaris,
        soleus, popliteus, tibialis posterior, flexor
        digitorum longus and flexor hallucis
        longus)
      Sural
      Medial calcanean
      Medial plantar
        Common plantar digital
          Plantar digital
        Muscular (to abductor hallucis, flexor
          digitorum brevis, flexor hallucis brevis
          and first lumbrical)
      Lateral plantar
        Muscular (to flexor accessorius and
          abductor digiti minimi)
        Superficial
          Muscular (to flexor digiti minimi brevis,
            and fourth dorsal and third plantar
            interossei)
          Common plantar digital
            Plantar digital
        Deep (to adductor hallucis, first to third
          dorsal and first and second plantar
          interossei, and second to fourth
          lumbricals)
    Common peroneal L4, 5, S1, 2
      Recurrent
      Lateral cutaneous of calf
      Peroneal communicating
      Superficial peroneal
        Muscular (to peroneus longus and
          peroneus brevis)
        Medial dorsal cutaneous
        Intermediate dorsal cutaneous
          Dorsal digital
      Deep peroneal
        Muscular (to tibialis anterior, extensor
          hallucis longus, extensor digitorum
          longus, peroneus tertius and extensor
          digitorum brevis)
        Dorsal digital
Perforating cutaneous S2, 3
Pudendal S2, 3, 4
    Inferior rectal
    Perineal
      Posterior scrotal (labial)
      Muscular (to perineal muscles and levator
        ani)
    Dorsal nerve of penis (clitoris)
Nerve to levator ani, coccygeus and external anal
    sphincter S4
Pelvic splanchnics (nervi erigentes) S2, 3, (4)

Muscles

MUSCLES OF THE HEAD
Muscles of the scalp
Epicranius
  Occipitofrontalis
  Temporoparietalis

Muscles of the nose
Procerus
Nasalis

Muscles of the eyelids
Orbicularis oculi
Corrugator supercilii

Muscles of mastication
Masseter
Temporalis
Lateral pterygoid
Medial pterygoid

Muscles of the mouth
Levator labii superioris alaeque nasi
Levator labii superioris
Zygomaticus minor
Zygomaticus major
Levator anguli oris
Mentalis
Depressor labii inferioris
Depressor anguli oris
Buccinator
Orbicularis oris
Risorius

MUSCLES OF THE NECK
Superficial and lateral muscles
Platysma
Splenius cervicis
Sternocleidomastoid

Anterior vertebral muscles
Longus colli
Longus capitis
Rectus capitis anterior
Rectus capitis lateralis

Lateral vertebral muscles
Scalenus anterior
Scalenus medius
Scalenus posterior

Suprahyoid muscles
Digastric
Stylohyoid
Mylohyoid
Geniohyoid

Infrahyoid muscles
Sternohyoid
Sternothyroid
Thyrohyoid
Omohyoid

MUSCLE GROUPS IN HEAD AND NECK
Muscles of the pharynx
Superior constrictor
Middle constrictor
Inferior constrictor
Stylopharyngeus
Palatopharyngeus
Salpingopharyngeus

Muscles of the palate
Palatoglossus
Palatopharyngeus
Tensor veli palatini
Levator veli palatini
Musculus uvulae

Muscles of the larynx
Cricothyroid
Posterior crico-arytenoid
Lateral crico-arytenoid
Transverse arytenoid
Oblique arytenoid
Aryepiglottic
Thyro-arytenoid and vocalis
Thyro-epiglottic

Muscles of the tongue
Extrinsic
  Genioglossus
  Hyoglossus and chondroglossus
  Styloglossus
  Palatoglossus
Intrinsic
  Superior longitudinal
  Inferior longitudinal
  Transverse
  Vertical

Muscles of the orbit
Levator palpebrae superioris
Orbitalis
Muscles of the eyeball
  Superior rectus
  Inferior rectus
  Medial rectus
  Lateral rectus
  Superior oblique
  Inferior oblique

MUSCLES OF THE TRUNK
Suboccipital muscles
Rectus capitis posterior major
Rectus capitis posterior minor
Obliquus capitis inferior
Obliquus capitis superior

Deep muscles of the back
Splenius capitis
Splenius cervicis
Erector spinae
  Iliocostalis
  Longissimus
  Spinalis
  Transversospinalis
    Semispinalis
    Multifidus
    Rotator
  Interspinal
  Intertransverse

Muscles of the thorax
External intercostal
Internal intercostal
Innermost intercostal
Subcostal
Transverse thoracic
Levatores costarum
Serratus posterior superior
Serratus posterior inferior
Diaphragm

Muscles of the abdomen
Anterolateral muscles
  External oblique
  Internal oblique
  Cremaster
  Transversus abdominis
  Rectus abdominis
  Pyramidalis
Posterior muscles
  Psoas major
  Psoas minor
  Iliacus
  Quadratus lumborum

Muscles of the pelvis
Piriformis
Obturator internus
Levator ani
Coccygeus

Muscles of the perineum
Anal muscle
  External anal sphincter
Urogenital muscles
  Superficial transverse perinei
  Bulbospongiosus
  Ischiocavernosus
  Deep transverse perinei
  Sphincter urethrae

MUSCLES OF THE UPPER LIMB
Connecting limb and vertebral column
Trapezius
Latissimus dorsi
Levator scapulae
Rhomboid major
Rhomboid minor

Connecting limb and thoracic wall
Pectoralis major
Pectoralis minor
Subclavius
Serratus anterior

Scapular muscles
Deltoid
Subscapularis
Supraspinatus
Infraspinatus
Teres minor
Teres major

Muscles

Muscles of upper arm
Biceps brachii
Coracobrachialis
Brachialis
Triceps

Muscles of the forearm
Anterior forearm muscles
Superficial flexor group
Pronator teres
Flexor carpi radialis
Palmaris longus
Flexor carpi ulnaris
Flexor digitorum superficialis
Deep flexor group
Flexor digitorum profundus
Flexor pollicis longus
Pronator quadratus
Posterior forearm muscles
Superficial extensor group
Brachioradialis
Extensor carpi radialis longus
Extensor carpi radialis brevis
Extensor digitorum
Extensor digiti minimi
Extensor carpi ulnaris
Anconeus
Deep extensor group
Supinator
Abductor pollicis longus
Extensor pollicis brevis
Extensor pollicis longus
Extensor indicis

Muscles of the hand
Thenar group
Abductor pollicis brevis
Flexor pollicis brevis
Opponens pollicis
Adductor pollicis
Lumbricals (four)
Dorsal interossei (four)
Palmar interossei (four)
Hypothenar group
Palmaris brevis
Abductor digiti minimi
Flexor digiti minimi brevis
Opponens digiti minimi

MUSCLES OF THE LOWER LIMB
Muscles of the iliac region
Psoas major
Psoas minor
Iliacus

Muscles of the gluteal region
Gluteus maximus
Gluteus medius
Gluteus minimus
Piriformis
Obturator internus
Superior gemellus
Inferior gemellus
Quadratus femoris
Obturator externus

Muscles of the thigh
Anterior femoral group
Tensor fasciae latae
Sartorius
Quadriceps femoris
Rectus femoris
Vastus lateralis
Vastus medialis
Vastus intermedius
Articularis genu
Medial femoral group
Gracilis
Pectineus
Adductor longus
Adductor brevis
Adductor magnus
Posterior femoral group
Biceps femoris
Semitendinosus
Semimembranosus

Muscles of the leg
Anterior muscles
Tibialis anterior
Extensor hallucis longus
Extensor digitorum longus
Peroneus tertius
Lateral muscles
Peroneus longus
Peroneus brevis
Posterior muscles
Superficial group
Gastrocnemius
Soleus
Plantaris
Deep group
Popliteus
Flexor hallucis longus
Flexor digitorum longus
Tibialis posterior

Muscles of the foot
Dorsal muscle – extensor digitorum brevis
Plantar muscles
First layer
Abductor hallucis
Flexor digitorum brevis
Abductor digiti minimi
Second layer
Flexor accessorius
Lumbricals (four)
Third layer
Flexor hallucis brevis
Adductor hallucis
Flexor digiti minimi brevis
Fourth layer
Dorsal interossei (four)
Plantar interossei (three)

Index

350